Sensory-Enhanced Yoga® for Children and Adolescents

by the same author

Sensory-Enhanced Yoga® for Self-regulation and Trauma Healing
Lynn Stoller
ISBN 978 1 91208 513 2
eISBN 978 1 91208 514 9

of related interest

Yoga Therapy for Children and Teens with Complex Needs
A Somatosensory Approach to Mental, Emotional and Physical Wellbeing
Shawnee Thornton Hardy
Foreword by Amy Wheeler
ISBN 978 1 78775 225 2
eISBN 978 1 78775 226 9

Yoga Therapy for Fear
Treating Anxiety, Depression and Rage with the Vagus Nerve and Other Techniques
Beth Spindler
ISBN 978 1 84819 374 1
eISBN 978 0 85701 331 6

Trauma-informed Yoga for Pain Management
A Practical Manual for Simple Stretching, Gentle Strengthening, and Mindful Breathing
Yael Calhoun with Mona Bingham
ISBN 978 1 83997 800 5
eISBN 978 1 83997 801 2

The Chakras in Grief and Trauma
A Tantric Guide to Energetic Wholeness
Karla Helbert
Illustrations by Rachel Rosenkoetter
ISBN 978 1 84819 365 9
eISBN 978 0 85701 324 8

SENSORY-ENHANCED YOGA®

FOR CHILDREN AND ADOLESCENTS

HEALING CHILDHOOD TRAUMA, ANXIETY, AND STRESS THROUGH THE KOSHAS

LYNN STOLLER AND
MEG HENNESSEY SCHOFIELD

SINGING DRAGON
LONDON AND PHILADELPHIA

First published in Great Britain in 2024 by Singing Dragon,
an imprint of Jessica Kingsley Publishers
Part of John Murray Press

1

A CIP catalogue record for this title is available from the
British Library and the Library of Congress

ISBN 978 1 80501 105 7
eISBN 978 1 80501 106 4

Printed and bound in the United States by Integrated Books International

Jessica Kingsley Publishers' policy is to use papers that are natural, renewable and recyclable products and made from wood grown in sustainable forests. The logging and manufacturing processes are expected to conform to the environmental regulations of the country of origin.

Singing Dragon
Carmelite House
50 Victoria Embankment
London EC4Y 0DZ

www.singingdragon.com

John Murray Press
Part of Hodder & Stoughton Limited
An Hachette UK Company

Contents

Part 3: The Practice

Acknowledgments

We would like to deeply thank our family and friends for their endless support during this book writing process. Whether it was taking over home responsibilities when we were on writing weekends away, making meals when we couldn't leave the computer, giving opinions on images or cover ideas, or offering to read over sections to help with the editing process, each gesture of support helped us immensely.

We are also very grateful to the JKP publishing team for their invaluable support and guidance during our writing journey. We really appreciated their patience, understanding, and gentle nudging that kept us on track when life got in the way.

In addition, a debt of gratitude is owed to Dr. Erin O'Neill, who contributed her valuable expertise during the initial incubation of the ideas, structure for the book, and writing process. Dr. O'Neill also developed and authored the initial fidelity measure for the SMYLE™ program, for which we are deeply appreciative.

We would also like to extend a special thank you to the models of our book, Matias and Nicholas Avila, Allie and Charlotte Grove, and Jason and Melissa Stoller, who helped bring our SMYLE™ practices to life in a way that others could learn from.

Finally, we would like to thank each other for our mutual commitment to the project, which involved uncountable face-to-face and virtual meetings where we built off each other's strengths and taught each other so much! Congratulations! We did it!

List of Acronyms

5-HT	5-hydroxytryptamine (serotonin)
ACE	Adverse Childhood Experiences (Study)
ACTH	adrenocorticotropic hormone
ADHD	attention deficit hyperactivity disorder
ANS	autonomic nervous system
CDC	Centers for Disease Control and Prevention
CEN	central executive network
CRH	corticotropin-releasing hormone
dACC	dorsal anterior cingulate cortex
DCML	dorsal column–medial lemniscal
dlPFC	dorsolateral PFC
DMN	default mode network
dmPFC	dorsomedial PFC
EEG	electroencephalography
GABA	gamma-aminobutyric acid
HPA	hypothalamic–pituitary–adrenal (axis)
MBCT	mindfulness-based cognitive therapy
MBSR	mindfulness-based stress reduction
MDD	major depressive disorder
mPFC	medial prefrontal cortex

MRI magnetic resonance imaging

PBIS Positive Behavioral Interventions and Supports

PCC posterior cingulate cortex

PFC prefrontal cortex

PNS parasympathetic nervous system (branch of the ANS)

PPC posterior parietal cortex

PTSD post-traumatic stress disorder

SEL social-emotional learning

SMYLE™ Sensory and Mindfulness-based Yoga for Learning Environments™

SN salience network

SNS sympathetic nervous system (branch of the ANS)

vlPFC ventrolateral prefrontal cortex

vmPFC ventromedial PFC

PART 1

The Science

CHAPTER 1

Introduction

The brain is a truly magnificent organ in the human body. It is referred to as "plastic" in the field of neuroscience, meaning that over time, the brain can change. These changes can be positive, as with learning new skills, or they can be negative, causing disruption to cognitive and motor functioning. Some individuals are born with differences within the structures of the brain that impact how they are able to complete daily tasks, routines, and responsibilities. For others, the brain may change, for better or worse, due to events that occur during their life.

The incidence of deleterious brain changes caused by trauma or other forms of toxic stress is unfortunately fairly high among children and adolescents across societies. For example, more than two-thirds of children in the USA have reported at least one traumatic event (SAMHSA 2023), and 5 percent of adolescents have met the criteria for post-traumatic stress disorder (PTSD) in their short lifetime (Kessler *et al.* 2012). In the UK, 31 percent of 18-year-olds reported experiencing a serious traumatic event during their childhood, and 7.7 percent reported having had PTSD (Lewis *et al.* 2019). On top of that, stress levels in children have become significantly exacerbated by the COVID-19 pandemic (Triggle 2021). Those who experienced toxic stress or trauma but did not go on to develop PTSD often have residual responses in the autonomic nervous system (ANS), which can lead to serious physical and mental health ailments as adults (Burke Harris 2018). We sometimes know when children and adolescents are suffering from an unresolved stress response, but oftentimes we don't, and we are not trained to look for the signs.

Fortunately, mindfulness-based treatments can be enormously helpful in healing PTSD, anxiety, toxic stress, and related mental health conditions (Khalsa *et al.* 2016), including in children (Miller *et al.* 2020). Yoga and mindfulness practices have been found to change the brain in a positive direction, taking advantage of the already naturally occurring neuroplasticity. As can be seen in Figure 1.1, yoga practices including postures, breathwork, relaxation, and meditation influence physical, cognitive, and emotional aspects of the body, which can ultimately affect behaviors and quality of life (Butzer *et al.* 2016).

Many studies have found benefits of yoga and mindfulness practices with children. Unsurprisingly, many of these studies have been conducted in school settings, where children spend a major portion of their lives. Benefits have been found in children as young as preschool through adolescence. Yoga has been shown to positively influence motor performance including balance, strength, and flexibility (Folleto, Pereira, and Valentini 2016) as well as reaction time, planning, execution time, and motor speed (Galantino, Galbavy, and Quinn 2008).

In the study by Folleto *et al.* (2016) of first grade students, positive changes were also found in ratings of social behavior and generalization of learned skills from the yoga classes, such as independence in dealing with challenging emotions and the use of breathing techniques. Razza, Bergen-Cico, and Raymond (2013) found positive changes in attention, gratification, and impulse control in preschool children following a mindful yoga intervention. As little as 10 minutes per day has been found to reduce anxiety in elementary-age children (Rosenberg 2018). Additionally, Nilsoge *et al.* (2016) found improvements in memory and attention following a yearlong yoga intervention.

This is just the tip of the iceberg. A literature review of studies published since 2010 conducted by Butzer *et al.* (2016) found school-based yoga improved many parameters of psychosocial well-being, including, but not limited to, the following:

- Ability to function under pressure
- Aggression
- Anger control
- Anxiety
- Attention
- Classroom behavior
- Concentration
- Coping frequency
- Depression
- Emotional arousal
- Fatigue
- General distress
- Hostility
- Hyperactivity
- Internalizing
- Intrusive thoughts
- Mood
- Mood disturbance
- Mood state
- Negative affect
- Physical arousal
- Resilience
- Rumination
- Self-awareness
- Self-control
- Self-esteem
- Self-regulation.

To explain their findings, they developed a theoretical model to suggest how a school-based yoga program may effectively help school children to develop self-regulation, mind–body awareness, and physical fitness skills, which, in turn, would facilitate improved behaviors, mental state, health, and performance (see

Figure I.I). While these investigations mostly involved small pilot studies with no control group, thus resulting in tentative conclusions, the evidence presented by the growing list of studies shows the potential of yoga to positively influence self-regulation, learning, and occupational performance in children. But how, exactly, is yoga producing these positive effects? And which yoga and mindfulness practices work best to help children heal from trauma, manage toxic stress, self-regulate, maximize their learning potential, and live an empowered and fully engaged life?

To answer these questions, we have integrated evidence from the fields of yoga, occupational therapy, neuroscience, and trauma psychology to produce a process-oriented theoretical model that addresses all facets of a child's being to help them feel ***safe, calm, clear, uplifted, and empowered***. We have found the model and associated guidelines for practice to be highly applicable across various contexts—school, home, healthcare, and community settings. We are excited to offer you this book to present the model and its science base, as well as the practices and techniques we use to implement the program.

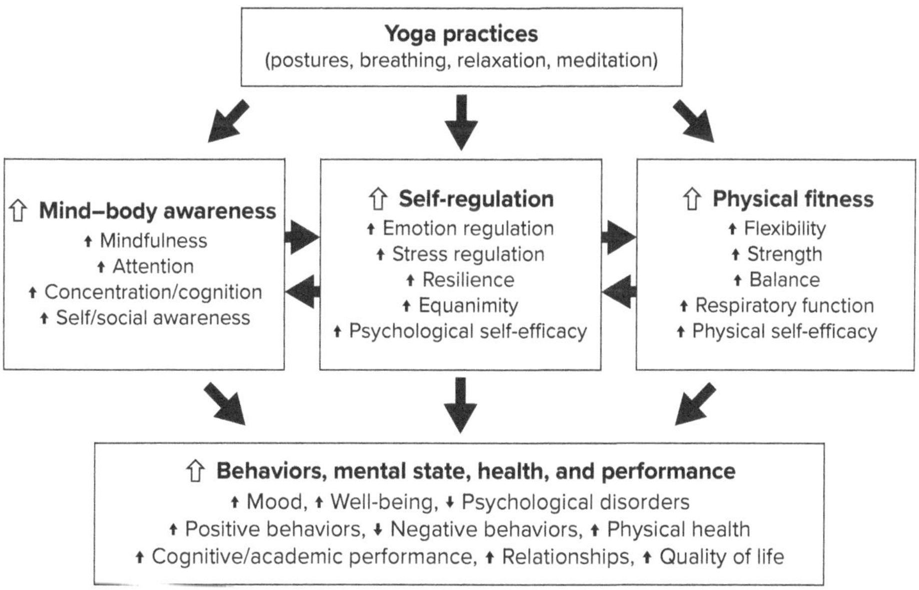

FIGURE I.I: HYPOTHESIZED ASSOCIATIONS BETWEEN YOGA PRACTICE, MIND–BODY AWARENESS, SELF-REGULATION, PHYSICAL FITNESS, AND BEHAVIORS, MENTAL STATE, HEALTH, AND PERFORMANCE[1]

Reproduced from Butzer et al. (2016)

1 Reprinted with permission of Emerald Publishing Limited, UK.

THE SMYLE™ PROGRAM

The Sensory-Enhanced Yoga® program was initially developed to address combat stress and other related mental health conditions. Our child- and adolescent-focused version of the program, called ***SMYLE™ (Sensory and Mindfulness-based Yoga for Learning Environments™)***, presents as a unique, neuroscience-based intervention for use with children of all ages and abilities. SMYLE™ addresses all five layers of a child's being (as described by the ancient yogic kosha model) to promote health, well-being, and sense of empowerment—all of which have a profound effect on learning and overall occupational performance. These five aspects include the ***physical layer*** (the solid part of ourselves); the ***energy layer*** (the "life energy" that fills the physical body, which is strongly influenced by the ANS); the ***mental/emotional layer*** (the emotions, reflexive mental chatter, and sensorimotor-related "thoughts" that fill our waking life); the ***wisdom layer*** (the higher mind, e.g., conscience, morality, and judgment, which mature over the course of our development); and the ***bliss layer***, or, as we like to call it, the ***layer of integration***, which is the product of the optimal functioning of the previous four layers where we achieve an optimal sense of "well-being" and "well-doing."

SMYLE™ uses carefully crafted and selected yoga forms and movements, breathing techniques, and mindfulness practices to address these layers to allow a child to function within their optimal state of being. Many children today function in dysregulated states marked by hyper and/or hypoarousal due to innate characteristics, trauma, or toxic stress. Dysregulated states of arousal in turn affect attention, and emotional and behavioral regulation. SMYLE™ follows principles that harness the power of neuroplasticity and neurochemical reactions to bring children from states of dysregulation to calmer states of being where they may be able to learn, develop friendships, and reach their full potential.

The SMYLE™ program was especially created to help school children:

- Effectively manage stress before it leads to emotional dysregulation and/or inappropriate behaviors.
- Develop emotional resiliency, i.e., the ability to rise to meet a challenge or threat as well as easily calm once it has passed.
- Decrease hypervigilance and overreaction to sensory input (e.g., visual, crowds, touch, noise, movement).
- Improve quality of sleep and energy levels to support wellness and enhance daily productivity.
- Decrease intrusive thoughts by learning to become present through breath and body awareness.
- Enhance sense of self-worth and personal empowerment.

HOW THIS BOOK IS ORGANIZED

The book consists of three parts, the science, the theory, and the practice.

Part 1: The Science describes how toxic stress and/or trauma can often lead to neurological disruption in the excitation–inhibition balance within the brain, which can negatively impact optimal functioning and well-being. The neurophysiology of both the normal and unresolved stress response is discussed to explain how this imbalance occurs. PTSD is a common outcome of an unresolved stress response, and is explained from a sensory processing and developmental perspective. Part 1 concludes by discussing brain changes that frequently occur in PTSD and in mindfulness-based practices to describe the inverse relationship between the two. All these topics are discussed through a child-focused lens.

Part 2: The Theory introduces and weaves the ancient yogic kosha model into the Western science perspective that was presented in Part 1 to produce the ***Transdisciplinary Model for Post-Traumatic Growth in Children***. Those who are familiar with the adult-focused Sensory-Enhanced Yoga® program will recognize that the model used by SMYLE™ is almost identical, with just a slight word tweak here and there to reflect its focus on children. This is because the original model applies to people of all ages and conditions. The child version of the ***guiding principles of Sensory-Enhanced Yoga*** are closely based on the SMYLE™ model, and are presented with a detailed description of how to implement these principles within yoga in child-friendly ways.

Part 3: The Practice offers suggestions on how to set up and structure yoga and mindfulness practices across various contexts (i.e., school, community, and home) to help children and adolescents achieve and maintain a calm state of alertness that is conducive to learning and living an engaged life. We include yoga form descriptions, photographs, and visual supports that have been found to be effective in helping children to self-regulate and navigate through all of the stresses and challenges presented at school, home, and beyond. Yoga lessons of various lengths are described for certain time points and purposes during a day, such as morning routines, transitions between activities, after lunch, short calming and energizing routines, as well as "mindful moments." Longer lessons are also included that can be used for full-length yoga classes. Readers will learn how to tailor the practices to meet the individual needs of the child they are working with.

We have found that incorporating these practices within the school setting can be a highly effective way to help students self-regulate throughout the day, which is necessary to optimize their ability to access the school curriculum. These practices can also be effective in the home setting as part of the child's daily or weekly routines. More and more child yoga classes are being taught in community and health settings, both in person and online. The more opportunities we offer children to do yoga, the greater its potential to help children to resolve past traumas and manage current stressors in their lives. Yoga can enable children to see the beauty of the world with fresh eyes, as well as a whole big bright future ahead of them. We wish all this and more for them.

Finally, we acknowledge that there are significantly more gaps in the knowledge base for children and adolescents than there are for adults, both in the study of PTSD/toxic stress and in the study of yoga and other mindfulness-based practices, and at times we have extrapolated from these adult studies to make some of our key points. We look forward to refining our theory and information as new research becomes available, and invite you to contact us through the Sensory-Enhanced Yoga® Institute[2] if you have any questions on the presented material or to provide suggestions or other feedback. We wish you an enjoyable learning journey!

2 www.sensoryenhancedyoga.org

CHAPTER 2

Stress in Children

Stress. We know this word down to our very bones, as it affects every organ in the human body. Many people experience an immediate bodily reaction upon hearing the word. Yet the American Institute of Stress (2020) has suggested that this word is so subjective as to defy definition. Hans Selye, a pioneering endocrinologist, coined the term "stress" in 1936 to mean "the non-specific response of the body to any demand." Selye created this term based on his experiments with small laboratory animals, which he exposed to extreme and prolonged sensory and emotional stimuli, such as bright lights, loud sounds, extreme cold, and frustrating situations. No matter the stressor, the effects were the same: gastric ulcers, shrinkage of lymphoid tissue, and adrenal enlargement (Tan and Yip 2018), which became known as the "universal triad" of stress (Rogers 2016). Selye later discovered that persistent stress over extended lengths of time caused these animals to develop various diseases similar to those seen in humans, such as heart attacks, stroke, and kidney disease. The idea that many different types of stressors could cause the same disease turned the current thinking of the day on its head, as it was then believed that most conditions were caused by disease-specific pathogens (Rogers 2016).

Over the years, researchers and doctors have adapted Selye's definition to better encompass the experiences and responses of individuals in today's society. According to the National Center for Complementary and Integrative Health, stress is "a physical and emotional reaction that people experience as they encounter demands or changes in life" (NIH 2020). These demands can be anything from exercise, school, work, social experiences, major life transitions, or traumatic events. What makes stress such a subjective phenomenon is that even though all individuals have had stress in some form throughout their lives, how they experience, process, and cope with stress can be drastically different. For instance, some children are undisturbed by serious threats while others may experience minor threats as traumatic (American Academy of Pediatrics 2016). There are many factors that influence someone's reaction to stress, including age, attachment history with caregivers, cognitive and sensory processing abilities, personal experiences, genetics, environmental factors, and more.

The quality of attachment to a child's caregivers is among the most influential factors affecting their response to stress (Donadon, Martin-Santos, and Osório 2018). In fact, it has been shown that insecure attachment puts a child at risk for PTSD (Ogle, Rubin, and Siegler 2015). It is well known that the quality of the mother–infant bond is strongly influenced by hormones, particularly oxytocin. This hormone is released by the pituitary gland in mothers during breastfeeding, and also plays a huge role in the formation of all loving bonds, including romantic relationships (Algoe, Kurtz, and Grewen 2017). Oxytocin has a powerful regulating effect on the hypothalamic–pituitary–adrenal (HPA) axis, which is the hormonal response to stress (Donadon *et al.* 2018). Children are highly dependent on their caregivers to help them stay regulated through activation of this biobehavioral system. Caregivers not only include parents, but also school teachers, healthcare workers, club leaders, and babysitters, among others. These co-regulatory relationships significantly shape the developing brain, setting the foundation for the child's mental health later in life (Phillips *et al.* 2022).

If children do not have the means to process and properly manage the stress in their lives, whether through co-regulation and/or self-regulation strategies, it will compound over time. Just as Selye discovered in his research, compounded persistent stress over extended lengths of time can lead to lifelong negative health consequences (Middlebrooks and Audage 2008). Furthermore, stress levels—which were already "off the charts" across all ages, demographics, and societies of the world—became significantly exacerbated by the COVID-19 pandemic (APA 2020; BBC News 2019). Children who relied heavily on positive relationships with school caregivers to help compensate for insecure or disorganized attachments in their home setting became even more vulnerable to the stressful and isolating impacts of the pandemic (Rajkumar 2020). It is thus vital for people to become aware of and monitor the stress in their lives and to learn how to effectively manage it (NIH n.d.). Without such awareness, individuals, especially children, will not have the means to process what is happening in their bodies and minds, or learn how to cope with it. This stress education process needs to start as soon as a child is developmentally ready for it.

In this chapter, you will learn more about stress and its effects on child development, how the body responds to stress, and how an overwhelming event or even chronic toxic stress can completely disrupt the body's ability to resolve the stress reaction and return to homeostasis (physiological balance). Later chapters will cover best practices for managing both current and chronic stress.

THE THREE TYPES OF STRESS

An extensive body of research has revealed that excessive or prolonged stress response activation in the body and brain of a child can completely disrupt that child's development (Center on the Developing Child n.d.-a, n.d.-b). It is not difficult to see why it could have such a devastating effect, since the stress response "includes biochemical changes to the neurologic, endocrine, and immune systems" (Franke 2014, p.391)—systems that are vitally important for normal human growth and development. When these systems become dysregulated, it can have profound consequences.

However, not all stress produces negative effects. The National Scientific Council on the Developing Child (2005) described three distinguishable kinds of responses to stress, which are especially well summarized by Franke (2014, pp.391–392; emphasis added):

> A ***positive stress response*** is a normal stress response and is essential for the growth and development of a child. Positive stress responses are infrequent, short-lived, and mild. The child is supported through this stressful event with strong social and emotional buffers such as reassurance and parental protection. The child gains motivation and resilience from every positive stress response, and the biochemical reactions that occur with such a stressful event return to baseline. Examples include meeting new people or learning a new task.
>
> ***Tolerable stress*** responses are more severe, frequent or sustained. The body responds to a greater degree, and these biochemical responses have the potential to negatively affect brain architecture. Examples include divorce or the death of a loved one. In tolerable stress responses, once the adversity is removed, the brain and organs recover fully given the condition that the child is protected with responsive relationships and strong social and emotional support.
>
> ***Toxic stress*** results in prolonged activation of the stress response, with a failure of the body to recover fully. It differs from a normal stress response in that there is a lack of caregiver support, reassurance, or emotional attachments. The insufficient caretaker support prevents the buffering of the stress response or the return of the body to baseline function. Examples of toxic stress include abuse, neglect, extreme poverty, violence, household dysfunction, and food scarcity. Caretakers with substance abuse or mental health conditions also predispose a child to a toxic stress response.

Franke (2014) points out that exposure to less severe but chronic ongoing daily stressors can also fall under the category of toxic stress. Occurring early in life, toxic stress is a risk factor for an unhealthy lifestyle, socioeconomic inequity, and poor health down the road. In contrast, the increased heart rate and adrenaline produced by positive stress enables a child to effectively meet a "just right challenge." Healthy development of the stress response system requires that a child experiences both positive and tolerable stress. This allows the key hormonal and neural mechanisms that make up the stress response to react normally in the face of stressors. But for every adverse childhood experience a child has, the risk of tolerable stress tipping over into toxic stress increases, as the system responds more frequently and intensely to multiple stressors (Burke Harris 2019).

It is the balance of positive and negative experiences ***weighed against each other and in relation to the child's biopsychosocial makeup*** that determines the outcome for the child. To explain this concept, the Center on the Developing Child at Harvard University (2015) likens child development to a balance scale or seesaw, with positive and negative experiences on opposing sides and a fulcrum representing the child's intrinsic personal factors. These factors affect the position of the fulcrum and thus how easily the scale tips toward negative or positive outcomes. Our modified version of this scale is presented as Figure 2.1.

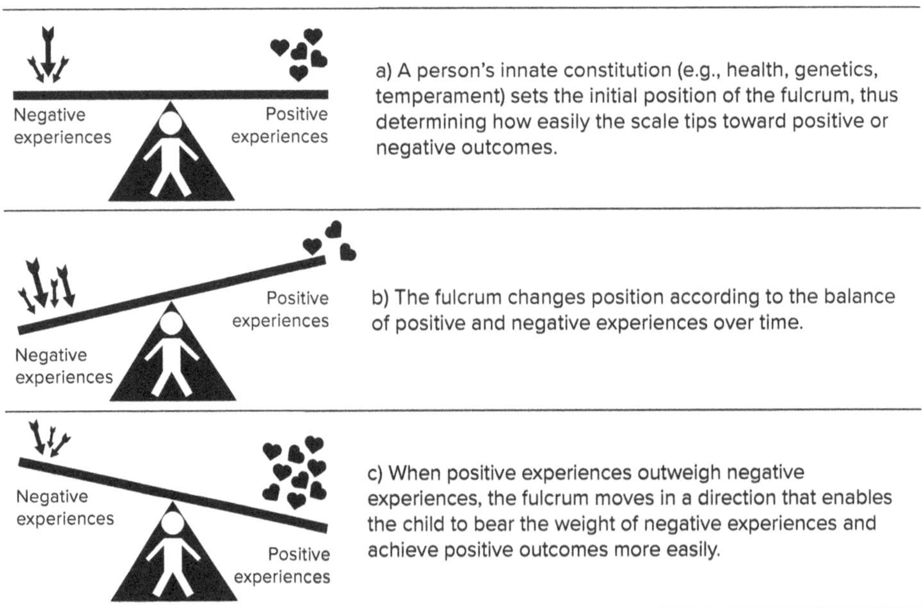

FIGURE 2.1: INFLUENCE OF POSITIVE AND NEGATIVE LIFE EXPERIENCES ON THE BODYMIND

Inspired by an image titled "Tipping the scale toward positive outcomes" from the National Scientific Council on the Developing Child (2015)

Initially, these intrinsic factors consist of an individual's innate temperament and abilities (including genetic differences). Over time, the cumulative effects of life experiences influence a child's biopsychosocial constitution, and can thus shift the fulcrum's location. The Center on the Developing Child (2015) explains that building the skills needed to manage stress moves the fulcrum to a position that makes the scale better able to bear the weight of negative experiences. They list these skills as the ability to focus attention, solve problems, plan, adapt to novel situations, self-regulate, and control impulses. Most of these skills fall within the umbrella of executive functioning skills, which are controlled by the prefrontal cortex (PFC). Toxic stress impacts the functioning of the PFC, and thus the acquisition of these skills (Arnsten *et al.* 2015).

FORMS OF CHILDHOOD STRESS

No person is too young to experience stress. As Dr. Bruce McEwen (2008) pointed out, we are aging from the moment of conception, and our early life experiences strongly affect the quality and length of our lives. For example, prenatal stress is believed to be a factor in causing preterm birth, as well as full term birth with low birth weight (Barker 1995; Wadhwa, Sandman, and Garite 2001). Due to the high neuroplasticity of their brains, children are particularly sensitive to stress, especially when it is repetitive or prolonged.

Childhood stress comes in many forms and degrees of severity. It can range from mild daily stressors such as running late for the school bus to extreme stressors such as abuse, neglect, and family dysfunction. All of these factors can have a profound impact on the trajectory of an individual's life. The Adverse Childhood Experiences (ACE) Study is a landmark investigation that demonstrated a strong correlation between the latter types of stress and the development of risky behaviors and health problems in adulthood (Middlebrooks and Audage 2008).

The ACE Study was conducted by the Centers for Disease Control and Prevention (CDC) and Kaiser Permanente's Health Appraisal Center in San Diego with over 17,000 adult participants. It is one of the largest studies ever conducted on this topic. This was a retroactive study that relied on the participants' memories regarding the events of their childhood. Specifically, it studied the participants' exposure to ***abuse*** (emotional, physical, sexual), ***neglect*** (emotional, physical), and ***household dysfunction*** (mother being treated violently, household substance abuse, household mental illness, parental separation or divorce, incarcerated household member). It found that almost two-thirds of participants reported at least one ACE, and more than one in five reported three or more ACEs. The number of health conditions the participants had was strongly correlated to the number of ACEs they had experienced. Specifically, they found that a greater number of ACEs put a person at greater risk in adulthood for experiencing one or more of the conditions listed on the following page (Middlebrooks and Audage 2008).

- Alcoholism
- Chronic obstructive pulmonary disease
- Depression
- Fetal death
- Illicit drug use
- Ischemic heart disease
- Liver disease
- Multiple sexual partners
- Risk for intimate partner violence
- Sexually transmitted diseases
- Smoking
- Suicide attempts
- Unintended pregnancies.

ACEs were also found to be associated with risky health behaviors in childhood and adolescence, including pregnancies, suicide attempts, early smoking, sexual activity, and illicit drug use (Middlebrooks and Audage 2008). Also, as pointed out by Dr. Nadine Burke Harris in her 2014 TED Talk, "In high doses, [childhood trauma] affects brain development, the immune system, hormonal systems, and even the way our DNA is read and transcribed. Folks who are exposed in very high doses have triple the lifetime risk of heart disease and lung cancer and a ***20-year difference in life expectancy***" (emphasis added).

Children are also exposed to other more common forms of stress on a daily basis, such as hearing an argument between their parents, being disciplined by a teacher, forgetting their lunchbox, saying something awkward to their crush, being snubbed by a peer, not understanding a class assignment, getting a low score on a test, being last to be picked for a team in gym class, or being left out of a play date between friends. These experiences, too, impact the ANS and potentially a child's mental health depending on cumulative load and where the child's "fulcrum" is positioned with regard to the balance of positive and negative life experiences, using our seesaw analogy. Many children with special challenges know no other way but to "sweat the small stuff" due to the innate wiring of their nervous systems and added stress that comes with having the disability in the first place.

We also need to consider ***sensory input*** as a potential stressor in a child's daily life. Throughout the hours of the day, our minds have an infinite amount of information to process—ambulance sirens blasting in the distance, dogs barking next door, people conversing around us, bright rays from new UV lights in schools, teachers lecturing in front of the classroom, and the list goes on. The mind needs to filter through all of this information and sort out what is most necessary to attend to, what can be ignored, and, most importantly, what can cause the person harm. Toxic stress significantly impairs these sensory filters, causing generalized hyperarousal, which further compounds a child's stress level.

THE NORMAL STRESS RESPONSE

To help understand how the stress response works, let's imagine a situation that would cause it to be activated. Picture yourself at home in bed sleeping when you hear someone breaking in through your front door. Immediately your brain transmits signals to prepare your body and mind to fight for your life. Your breath quickens, your heart starts pounding, your muscles tighten, and your pupils dilate. All of these physiological changes work together to prepare you for a situation your brain has interpreted as dangerous. Your brain subconsciously activated certain safeguards that allow you to now be ready to fight the burglar or flee as fast as you can. This phenomenon is more commonly referred to as the ***fight–flight*** response. Without thinking about it, our brain naturally sets this response into motion when it thinks we are under excessive pressure, and it is designed to protect us from any form of danger.

But what happens if the burglar starts to ascend the stairs and heads towards your bedroom? Your brain now interprets this new situation and believes there is no possible means of escape, so it employs its most primitive branch of the stress response, the freeze, or immobility, response. You immediately hide under your bed, slow down your breathing, and do all that you can to not move a muscle. You close your eyes and hope that the burglar searches your room without knowing you are there and will then quickly move on to the next room. And just so you can relax now, we will pretend he did in fact move on and quickly left the house and was promptly caught, arrested, and jailed!

We will now describe what happened in the body during the "fight–flight" and freeze responses that were elicited during the home invasion. Let's rewind the tape and take the story from the point at which the burglar enters the home. In such situations, the body will quickly detect the threat and respond in two ways:

- *Through the nervous system*, which controls the sympathetic branch of the ***ANS***; and
- *Through the endocrine (hormonal) system*, by initiating a series of hormonal responses of the ***HPA axis***.

Figure 2.2 depicts the series of events that occurs in the stress response, which will be discussed in more detail in the following pages.

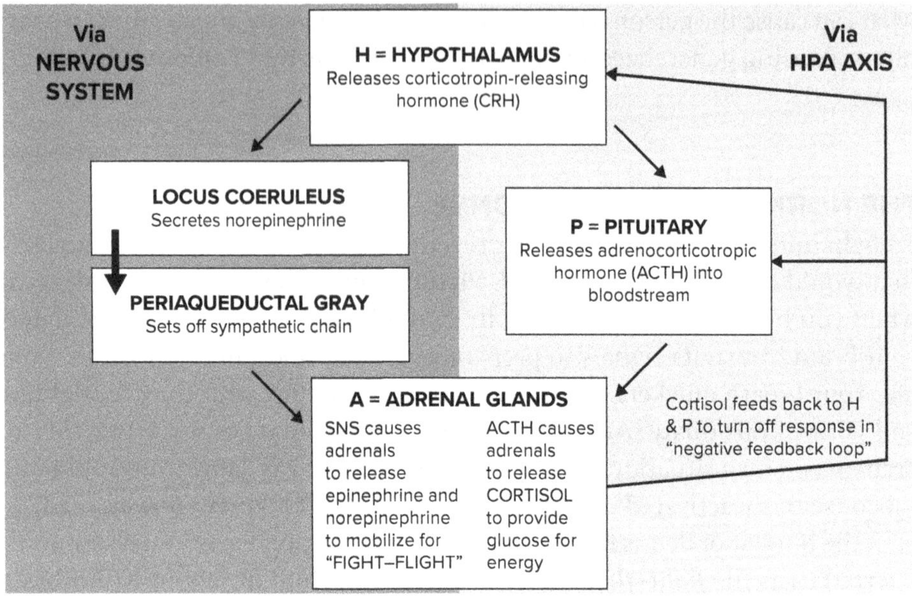

FIGURE 2.2: THE NORMAL STRESS RESPONSE

Processing stress through the nervous system

The ***ANS*** is the branch of the peripheral nervous system that sends signals from the central nervous system to all of the tissues and organs of the body except for the skeletal muscles. It is referred to as the "involuntary nervous system" as humans typically have little control over it. The ANS makes significant contributions to the homeostasis, or balance, of the body, including regulation of blood pressure, digestion, urinary bladder contractions, eye dilation, and body temperature (McCorry 2007).

Historically, the ANS has been depicted as having two opposing branches, the ***sympathetic nervous system (SNS)***, aka the "fight–flight" system, and the ***parasympathetic nervous system (PNS)***, aka the "rest and digest" system. Figure 2.3 shows a breakdown of the physiological effects that the SNS and PNS branches have on the body. Usually, both of these systems actively work together at the same time to varying degrees, using many different pathways to target particular organs and tissues (Jänig 2006). Yet in the face of a serious threat, there is typically a "full force" effort on the part of the SNS to deal with it, with an associated decrease in activation of the PNS.

The two-branched ANS model is still helpful for understanding the basics of how the peripheral body responds to stress; however, we need to add an additional layer of complexity to it. According to Dr. Stephen Porges' polyvagal theory (2011), there are actually ***three*** divisions to the ANS: one sympathetic and ***two*** parasympathetic (see Figure 2.4). The parasympathetic system is divided into a primitive ***dorsal vagal*** branch and a newer ***ventral vagal*** branch.

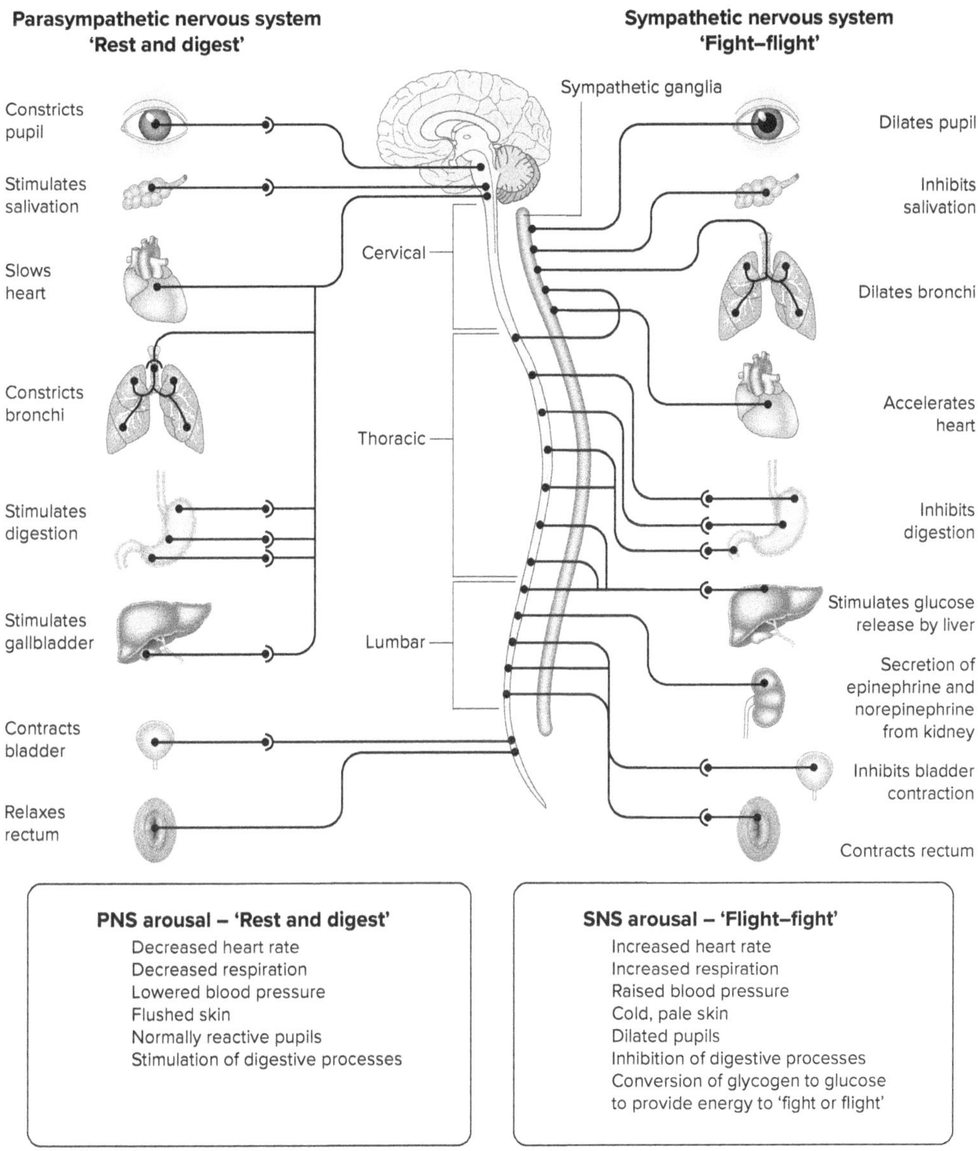

FIGURE 2.3: THE AUTONOMIC NERVOUS SYSTEM

Reproduced from Stoller (2019)

According to Dr. Porges' polyvagal theory, humans have a hierarchical response system to stress that is based on our evolutionary history. If we sense safety in the environment, we employ our most highly developed system of engagement, which is the **ventral vagal branch of the PNS**, otherwise known as the **social engagement system**, which keeps us in a state of optimal arousal. This system can modulate the fight–flight system and its associated symptoms of hyperarousal. If we sense danger, the **SNS** kicks in, which is responsible for the ***fight–flight response***. However, if we are in a situation of threat to life with no perceivable means of escape, we employ the most primitive branch of the PNS, which is the **dorsal vagal** system, responsible for the ***freeze***, or immobility, response, and characterized by extreme hypoarousal.

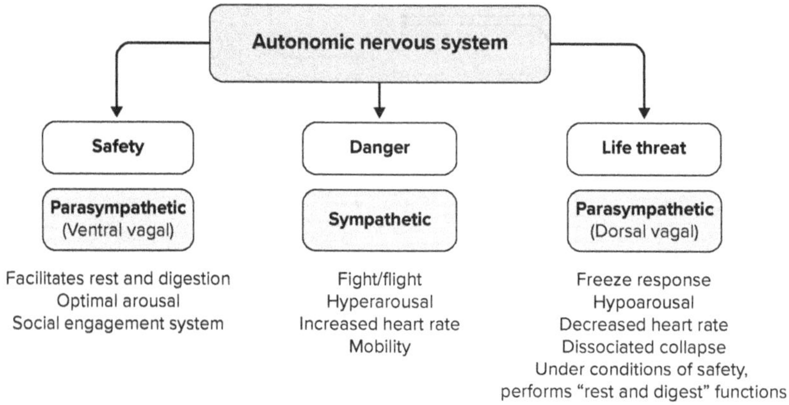

FIGURE 2.4: PORGES' THREE DIVISIONS OF THE AUTONOMIC NERVOUS SYSTEM
Reproduced from Stoller (2019)

Now, let's take a deeper look at the nervous system response to stress from a sensory perspective (please refer to Figure 2.5 to follow along). First, sensory information arrives to the brain from the senses, and is filtered through the **brainstem** until it reaches the **thalamus**, which is a major sensory processing center of the brain. The thalamus further filters that information and packages it into a form that the cortex can understand. But it also sends information to the amygdala, a small almond-shaped structure deep in the limbic system (i.e., the "emotional brain") that is responsible for our raw emotions, especially anxiety. The amygdala is said to be the "trigger of triggers."

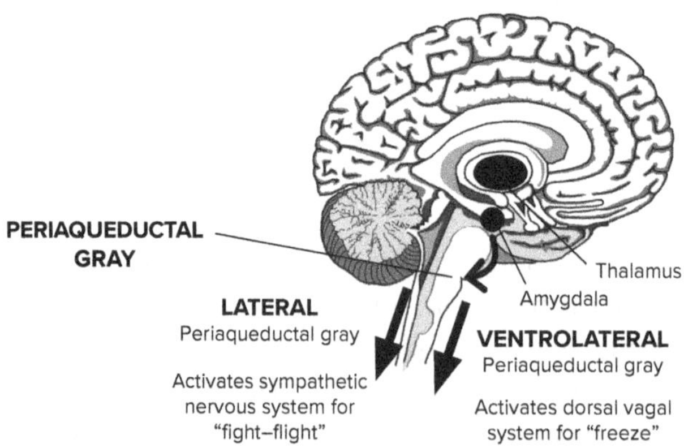

FIGURE 2.5: KEY STRUCTURES IN THE NERVOUS SYSTEM RESPONSE TO STRESS
Base image from Nickbyrd, Wikimedia Commons

The **amygdala** gets information about the potential threat before the cortex has even processed it. That is why, if we see a long-coiled object on the path as we are walking through the woods, we will jump away from it, thinking it might be a snake, but then the cortex fills in the details to let us know that it is just a discarded piece of garden hose.

Conversely, we may notice a threat and our first instinct is to go into fight–flight mode, but then our cortex, especially the medial prefrontal cortex (mPFC), fills in the information for us and tells us ***"Nope, this isn't going to work! This is a life threat! You have to freeze!"*** All that information goes to the **periaqueductal gray** in the midbrain, located at the top of the brainstem.

If it is determined that a **fight–flight response** is appropriate, the **lateral** and **dorsolateral periaqueductal gray** will activate the SNS. They do this by signaling the **locus coeruleus** (also in the brainstem) to release norepinephrine (aka noradrenaline) and by stimulating the sympathetic **chain of nerves** along the spinal column. These actions produce the changes in the body depicted in the SNS column of Figure 2.3, including the release of adrenaline and noradrenaline from the adrenal glands that sit on top of the kidneys. The release of these chemicals (as well as cortisol by the hormonal response to stress) works to increase blood glucose levels to provide the boost of energy needed to face the challenge. The heart races and the breath quickens, speeding the delivery of that glucose-rich blood to the muscles to aid in fighting or fleeing. Once the threat has passed, cortisol normally resolves the fight–flight response through a negative feedback loop to the brain, and then life resumes as usual, with no lasting effects.

However, if a **freeze response** is appropriate, it will activate the ***ventro*lateral periaqueductal gray**, which, in turn, activates the dorsal vagal branch of the PNS. The freeze response is accompanied by an "opioid-mediated analgesia" (Porges 2011), presumed to spare animals from agonizing pain when being devoured by a predator (Levine 1997). According to Dr. Peter Levine, it is the residue of undischarged energy from the "freeze" response, that is, the ***dorsal vagal response***, that is said to be responsible for the symptom of **dissociation**, in which the mind has lost its connection to the body and to the "here and now" of the present moment. In his highly recommended book *Waking the Tiger*, Dr. Levine writes:

> Traumatic symptoms are not caused by the "triggering" event itself. They stem from the frozen residue of energy that has not been resolved and discharged; this residue remains trapped in the nervous system where it can wreak havoc on our bodies and spirits. The long-term, alarming, debilitating, and often bizarre symptoms of PTSD develop when we cannot complete the process of moving in, through, and out of the "immobility" or "freezing" state. (Levine 1997, p.19)

The HPA axis: the brain's hormonal response to stress

To explain how and why the undischarged energy from an unresolved fight-flight response wreaks havoc in the bodymind, we need to dive deeper into the brain's hormonal response to stress, called the ***hypothalamic-pituitary-adrenal axis***, aka the ***HPA axis***. During the "fight-flight" response, the hypothalamus not only activates the sympathetic "fight-flight" branch of the nervous system; it also activates a chain of hormonal responses. As with the SNS, the HPA axis is always operating to maintain homeostasis with regard to many bodily functions, and particularly with regard to an organism's energy needs. During our everyday lives, the HPA axis is kept in balance by the inhibitory influences of other brain structures (Hopper *et al.* 2007; Lanius *et al.* 2010; Sherin and Nemeroff 2011). In turn, the ***thalamus***—when working well—helps to keep those structures humming sweetly along so they can perform their roles effectively.

The neurotransmitter serotonin (5-hydroxytryptamine [5-HT]) also helps to regulate the HPA axis. Serotonin modulates stress and emotional responses, and is implicated in mood and anxiety disorders. Neurons that secrete serotonin originate in the brainstem and project to many areas of the brain, and interact with other neurotransmitters to help keep the nervous and hormonal systems regulated (Sherin and Nemeroff 2011). So for people who are not under chronic stress, experiencing other mental health issues, or dealing with prior trauma, this is the situation on the ground before the "tiger" shows up, as the person goes through the normal ups and downs of nervous system arousal but generally stays self-regulated.

However, in response to a highly stressful or traumatic situation (the "tiger," or home invader, as it may be), the normal HPA drive is greatly boosted to meet the challenge (Herman *et al.* 2016). This HPA chain reaction is described in Figure 2.6 (see also Figure 2.2). The hypothalamus significantly increases its release of the corticotropin-releasing hormone (CRH), which, within minutes, stimulates the anterior pituitary to release an extra pulse of ACTH. The ACTH travels through the bloodstream to the adrenal glands, causing the adrenals to pump out a rush of cortisol.

Cortisol produces various effects to promote short-term survival, one of which is to raise the "blood sugar" to provide energy to respond to the threat. Normally, once the threat has passed and the cortisol reaches a certain threshold in the brain, it **turns off** the "fight-flight" response via a negative feedback loop, similar to how a thermostat works in a home. When the temperature in a home is lower than the temperature the thermostat was set at, the thermostat signals the furnace to turn on. Then, when the home reaches the set temperature, it turns the heat off. This is called a "negative feedback loop."

The negative feedback loop of the HPA axis works as follows: cortisol feeding back to the brain from the bloodstream shuts off the stress response ("thermostat") by (a) binding to receptors in the hypothalamus, thus shutting off the release of CRH, and (b) binding to receptors in the pituitary, thus shutting off the release of ACTH (Cooper *et al.* 2017).

STRESS RESPONSE GONE WRONG

In PTSD, this negative feedback loop fails. One prominent theory is that the pituitary becomes hypersensitive to the cortisol feeding back to it, thus causing it to release an insufficient amount of ACTH (Cooper *et al.* 2017; Sherin and Nemeroff 2011). This, in turn, causes the adrenal glands to release less cortisol into the bloodstream (Yehuda *et al.* 2015), which is insufficient to turn off the stress response at the level of the hypothalamus. So CRH (a form of cortisol) continues to be released by the hypothalamus, upsetting the chemistry balance in the brain. Higher levels of norepinephrine and epinephrine also continue to circulate in the bloodstream, contributing to the hyperarousal and hypervigilance seen in PTSD (Cooper *et al.* 2017). Over time, the brain chemistry changes alter brain networks and structures (discussed in the coming chapters) (Herman 2013).

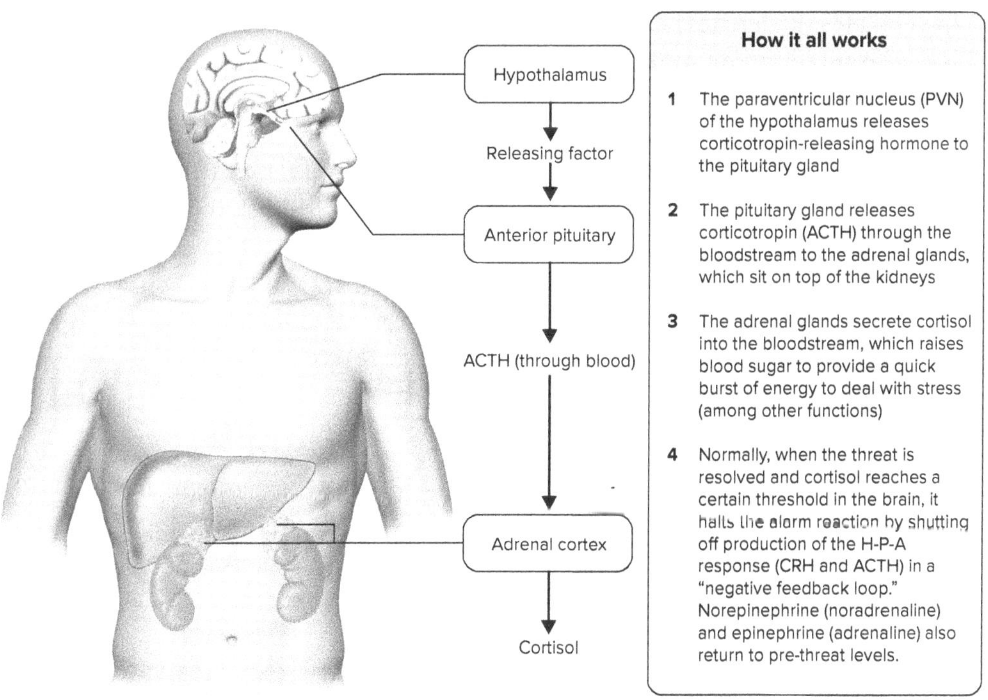

FIGURE 2.6: THE HPA AXIS
Reproduced from Stoller (2019)

The process described here not only occurs as a result of an acute traumatic event, but also in response to chronic stress due to a prolonged HPA axis response (Cooper *et al.* 2017). Furthermore, there is evidence to suggest that an individual's genetic makeup may influence how they respond to traumatic events (Yehuda *et al.* 2015). Children are at especially high risk for negative outcomes, as their brains are not yet fully developed. Their teachers and therapists may not even be aware that they are experiencing toxic stress in their lives, which makes it even more important to establish programs in school, community, and healthcare settings that address emotional self-regulation in ***all*** children.

WINDOW OF TOLERANCE

When working with children, where do you begin to help them avoid the deleterious effects of stress? Of paramount importance is finding ways to help children stay within their ***window of tolerance***, a concept often discussed in clinical treatment in reference to self-regulation (Siegel 1999; Wilbarger and Wilbarger 1990, 1997). Dr. Porges' polyvagal view of the ANS closely parallels this concept. Normally, in everyday life, people fluctuate between higher and lower states of alertness, but they usually stay within the normal range, which is represented by the middle bar in Figure 2.7. However, when experiencing an extremely stressful or traumatic event, it is common for people to veer far outside the window of tolerance into hyperarousal, controlled by the SNS, or into hypoarousal, controlled by the dorsal vagal branch of the PNS. There is evidence that different emotions are associated with different patterns of sympathetic activation accompanied by different degrees of parasympathetic deactivation (Rainville *et al.* 2006). The "window" is the range of arousal states where emotions are tolerable and experiences can be integrated (Siegel 1999).

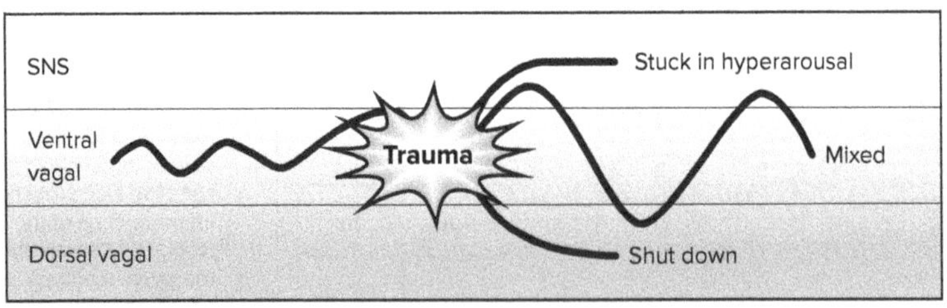

FIGURE 2.7: WINDOW OF TOLERANCE

Siegel (1999); Wilbarger and Wilbarger (1990, 1997), reproduced from Stoller (2019). Based on neuroimaging studies, Bremner (1999) and Lanius et al. (2006) proposed two general patterns of PTSD: a flashback/re-living/hyperarousal PTSD group and a dissociated PTSD group

The Beacon House Therapeutic Services and Trauma Team[1] described the concept of the window of tolerance with regard to children:

> Every individual has a unique window of tolerance. When they are within their window of tolerance they feel regulated, calm and able to learn, love and play to the best of their ability. When something triggers them, making them feel worried or scared, they are pushed outside of their window of tolerance. A child can be pushed just outside of their window, or way outside of their window, leading to either mild or extreme distress. A child who has experienced trauma and loss has a narrower window of tolerance compared with children who have had a secure, stable and safe early childhood. In other words, small "everyday" triggers can be intolerable and unbearable for traumatized children.

When a child is within their window of tolerance, sensory information, language, and thoughts can be processed and integrated, but when they veer outside their window of tolerance, limbic processing takes precedence, which causes the thinking and speech centers of the brain to go offline (van der Kolk 2014). When that occurs, they are unable to articulate their "story" or engage in executive thinking processes including planning, organizing, sequencing, and flexible thinking. Thus, we cannot expect that verbal negotiation will work to pull them back within their window (van der Kolk 2014).

Children who are operating outside their window of tolerance need to develop their ***emotional regulation*** skills (a subset of executive functioning skills) to help them manage their attention, emotions, and arousal levels (Nappa 2016). A crucial developmental pathway to emotional regulation is ***co-regulation***, through which a caretaker shows that they are listening and validating the child's feelings, and teaches them that their emotions can be tolerated. Validating responses have been shown to reduce the effects of a stressor, and are thus thought to be more conducive to emotional regulation even during a stressful condition (Shenk and Fruzzetti 2011). As children are ready, and in stages, we teach them how to regulate their own arousal, emotional, and behavioral states (discussed in more detail in the next chapter).

THE EFFECT OF YOGA ON THE ANS AND HPA AXIS

From the foregoing discussion, it is clear that we need effective ways to help individuals better manage their response to stressors so they do not lead to such destructive brain changes and symptoms. Among the current treatments for PTSD, yoga is arguably among the best for this purpose, and there is evidence

1 https://beaconhouse.org.uk/resources, paras 1, 2, 3.

to back up this assertion. For example, a systemic review and meta-analysis was conducted of 42 randomized controlled trials that each included yoga (with or without mindfulness-based stress reduction), an active control group, and physiological measures of comparison. The researchers found that "practices that include yoga asanas [forms] appear to be associated with improved regulation of the sympathetic nervous system and hypothalamic–pituitary–adrenal system in various populations" (Pascoe, Thompson, and Ski 2017, abstract). When compared to active control, yoga asana interventions (which varied between studies) were associated with reduced evening cortisol, waking cortisol, ambulatory systolic blood pressure, resting heart rate, high frequency heart rate variability, fasting blood glucose, cholesterol, and low-density lipoprotein. All without any pharmaceutical intervention!

While most of these studies were conducted with adults, children's studies are quickly catching up. In a recent review of 27 yoga studies investigating the effects of yoga on anxiety and/or depression in children with various health conditions, 70 percent of the studies overall showed improvements (James-Palmer *et al.* 2020). Of the studies that investigated both anxiety and depression, 58 percent showed reductions in both symptoms, while 25 percent only demonstrated reductions in anxiety. Seventy percent of the studies that investigated anxiety alone showed improvements, while 40 percent of studies that only investigated depression showed improvements. The yoga interventions varied widely, but were included if they incorporated the use of yoga postures. They may have included breathing, meditation, and/or relaxation elements as well.

Although the studies were generally of reduced quality, the totality of findings show that the practice of yoga postures typically leads to some reduction in anxiety and depression, regardless of the style of yoga intervention and health status of the children. Later in this book we discuss various ways to help students move back within their window of tolerance, using the yoga tools of asana, breathwork, and meditation, provided within the context of a safe and nurturing environment.

CHAPTER 3

PTSD and Sensory Processing

In the previous chapter, you learned how an unresolved "fight–flight" response due to trauma, acute or chronic stress, or even a genetic predisposition to anxiety can lead to long-term chemistry changes in the brain. In this chapter, we will focus on the observable symptoms that can result from these changes, and, more specifically, the diagnosis of PTSD and its relationship to sensory processing.

WHAT IS PTSD?

In order to receive an official diagnosis of PTSD, certain causal and symptom criteria must be met, which are listed in the American Psychiatric Association's *Diagnostic and Statistical Manual of Mental Disorders* (DSM-5) (APA 2013). The causal criteria include directly experiencing or witnessing actual or threatened death or serious injury (for children, especially when it happens to caregivers), learning that a close relative or friend was exposed to such trauma, or being repeatedly exposed to aversive details of the trauma. However, many trauma experts believe the causal criteria should not be defined (Dohrenwend 2010; Roberts *et al.* 2012) as there are many other causes of trauma, such as "early loss or lack of consistent caregivers; emotional, physical, or sexual abuse; various forms of neglect; surgical procedures; and life-saving measures in the neonatal intensive care unit" (Koomar 2009, p.1). People also exhibit different degrees of sensitivity and vulnerability to stressors, due to genetics and their environmental history (Brewin *et al.* 2009).

It is also not uncommon for the symptom criteria to fail to fully describe the consequences of a qualifying traumatic event for a particular person, which leads to additional diagnoses. In fact, many of the conditions listed in the DSM-5 are often caused by highly stressful or traumatic events, including those with a childhood onset. However, the criteria set forth in the DSM-5 provide a good starting basis for our discussion of PTSD. The DSM-5 organizes these symptoms under four symptom clusters, which include the following:

- **Persistent *re-experiencing* symptoms**, such as intrusive thoughts, memories, images, or perceptions. In children this may be expressed as play re-enactment or frightening dreams in which they re-experience the content or emotions of the traumatic event. They may also have flashbacks in which they respond as though the trauma is occurring in the present moment. Re-experiencing symptoms often causes emotional distress or physical reactions, which can be particularly harmful for children because they do not have the cognitive ability to process what is happening to them.
- **Persistent *avoidance of reminders of the trauma***, which could come in the form of any of the following:
  - Activities
  - Bodily sensations (e.g., pain)
  - Conversations
  - Feelings
  - Memories
  - Objects
  - People
  - Places
  - Stimuli from other senses (e.g., specific sights, sounds, smells, or tastes)
  - Thoughts.

  Adults can deliberately avoid situations in a subtle manner, by purposefully distracting themselves, or by generating reasonable excuses for missing social events or other opportunities. Children, on the other hand, don't yet have the cognitive ability to subtly avoid situations. Instead, when children are met with triggering stimuli, their distress is often visible to others via strong emotional expressions (e.g., meltdown, physical aggression, bullying) or extreme disengagement (e.g., shutdown, isolating behavior, becoming very quiet).
- **Persistent *numbing* of general responsiveness and *negative cognitions or mood*.** Numbing is a feeling of detachment from your own emotions, and is often associated with limited facial expressions or even flat affect. In children, this may manifest as increased expression of negative emotions (such as fear, sadness, guilt, or shame) and reduced expressions of positive emotions, social withdrawal, and restriction in play activities.
- **Persistent symptoms of *increased arousal* (not present before the trauma)** such as:
  - Hyperalertness
  - Hypervigilance
  - Sleep difficulties

- Rising quickly to anger (e.g., temper tantrums)
- Having difficulty concentrating
- Exaggerated startle response to unexpected stimuli (e.g., sound, touch, or a particular sight).

To qualify for the PTSD diagnosis, a certain number of symptoms need to be met in each of these categories, and be present for at least a month. However, when at least nine symptoms are present in *any* category, occurring from three days to one month following the traumatic event, the individual qualifies for a diagnosis of ***acute stress disorder*** according to the DSM-5.

DISSOCIATIVE SUBTYPE OF PTSD

The DSM-5 also identifies a ***dissociative subtype of PTSD*** (APA 2013). Dissociation is a state in which the person loses awareness of the immediate surroundings, and includes even mild forms such as daydreaming or getting lost in a book or a movie. However, during trauma, stronger forms of dissociation may be used as a defense to enable the mind to escape the overwhelming situation, since the body can't. As the trauma is occurring, the mind blocks off the thoughts, perceptions, feelings, and memories, which makes it difficult to remember the details of the trauma later on. Following the trauma, dissociative symptoms in children may appear as overwhelm or shutdown, or the child may appear to be completely disengaged from their surroundings (Koomar 2009). Although some forms of dissociation are embedded into the core criteria of PTSD, the DSM-5 recognizes that a subgroup of those who have PTSD experience additional dissociative symptoms, which include the following:

- ***Depersonalization***, a perception of *your sense of self* as being unreal. The person feels as if they are disconnected from the self, watching the self act while having no control over those actions, and feeling like the world has become less real and more dream-like. Depersonalization is often accompanied by emotional numbing.
- ***Derealization***, a perception of the *external world* as being unreal or strange. Familiar places may seem alien or surreal. Derealization often co-occurs with depersonalization.

Alan Schore defines dissociation as ***"a disruption of primary consciousness"*** (2012, p.291; emphasis added). He explains primary consciousness as a right-brained process in which information coming in through the senses from the outside world creates bodily sensations and emotions, enabling us to feel present inside our skin and in our surroundings. When disrupted, the "here and now" of the present moment loses meaning and can seem distant and beyond reach. An intact mind-body connection—often referred to as a sense of ***embodiment***—is essential for finding meaning in life, and when you lose that connection, you lose hope. It is thus not surprising that dissociation is associated with an increased risk of suicidality (Calati, Bensassi, and Courtet 2017).

HYPERAROUSAL = CORE SYMPTOM OF PTSD

Of the four symptom clusters discussed above, hyperarousal is considered to be the core symptom of PTSD and the key to understanding the phenomenon of the condition, as it underlies the development of the other symptom clusters (Costanzo *et al.* 2016). As renowned trauma expert and social worker Babette Rothschild explained:

> People who suffer from PTSD are plagued with frightening body symptoms which are characteristic of hyperarousal: accelerated heartbeat, cold sweating, rapid breathing, heart palpitations, hypervigilance, and hyper startle response (jumpiness). These symptoms lead to sleep disturbances, loss of appetite, sexual dysfunction and difficulties in concentrating, which are further hallmarks of PTSD. Hyperarousal both instigates flashbacks and is also increased by them, and hyperarousal is the underlying cause of the symptom of avoidance, as traumatic reminders increase ANS arousal. Through understanding hyperarousal, the phenomenon of PTSD becomes comprehendible. (1997, para. 6)

In her paper on the physiological correlates of child abuse, Kendall-Tackett (2000, abstract) found that chronic hyperarousal underlies the symptoms of PTSD, depression, and irritable bowel syndrome, which frequently co-occur in this population. She further noted, "Persons who have experienced traumatic events are often 'primed' to overreact to subsequent stressors, making them more vulnerable to these events." This points to an alteration in how the nervous system processes sensory input following a traumatic event.

In fact, disturbances in sensory processing are believed to play a prominent role in the hyperarousal symptoms of PTSD (Newport and Nemoroff 2000)—and vice versa. According to Dr. Bessel van der Kolk (1997, 2014), the extreme hyperarousal that is often experienced during a traumatic event can disrupt how the event is processed in the brain, resulting in memories that present as highly fragmented sensory impressions that are often as vivid as the moment the actual event occurred. Dr. van der Kolk further explains that these sensory elements often fail to integrate together into a cohesive, narrative story that can be verbally expressed, which explains why talk therapies have had only limited success.

Robinson and Brown also described how hyperarousal can alter sensory processing, and how the resulting memory fragmentation may present in the bodymind:

> Heightened sensory awareness can mean that environmental features, which might otherwise have gone unnoticed, can become powerfully imprinted as associations with traumatic events. For some, this response is encoded as explicit memories where the person can make sense of their responses and understand it through narrative (Briere, 2002; Rothschild, 2000), whereas for others, the traumatic memories can become fragmented into visual, sensory and emotional pieces causing implicit memories and drives. Such fragmentation can mean that memories appear as disjointed images, physical sensations and intense emotional reactions (van der Kolk, 2014). (Robinson and Brown 2016, para. 2)

The resulting fragmentation of memory is a direct result of the chemical changes that occur during the stress response. You will recall from the last chapter that adrenaline (epinephrine) is released from the adrenal glands to provide energy to meet the threat. This same adrenaline also enhances the coding of ***implicit memories***, that is, our unconscious sensory, perceptual, and emotional memories, all of which are stored in the regions of the brain where they were originally processed. At the same time, the strong boost of CRH in the brain deactivates the hippocampus, which plays a key role in consolidating these various bits of sensory information into a narrative storyline (***explicit memories***). Therefore, the hippocampus is unable to pull the memory fragments together from various parts of the brain to create the story (see Figure 3.1).

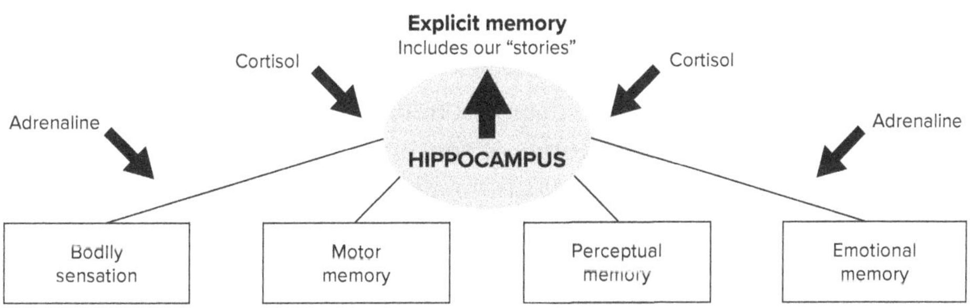

1. Adrenaline increases the coding of implicit memory.
2. At the same time, cortisol has neurotoxic effects on the hippocampus, reducing its activity level and volume.
3. The result is that the trauma is stored as a dis-integrated array of sensations, emotions, and perceptions, further fueling the hyperarousal.

FIGURE 3.1: HOW TRAUMA AFFECTS MEMORY ENCODING
Inspired by Siegel (Siegel and Buczynski, n.d.)

Following the trauma, those who go on to develop PTSD often show difficulties with sensory filtering, that is, the ability of the brain to sort relevant from irrelevant information, which reinforces hyperarousal (Stewart and White 2008). While anxiety, stress, and sensory-filtering issues have long been known to associate together, a study by Stewart and White (2008) has shown that re-experiencing and numbing symptoms are also associated with disruption in sensory filtering.

THE SENSORY ELEMENTS OF HYPERAROUSAL

Sensory symptoms were barely understood in traumatized children until the 1990s, when researchers began to examine sensory processing in children who lived in Romanian orphanages. Although Dr. Jean Ayres' sensory integration theory was developed in the 1960s and 1970s, her professional focus was on treating children with learning disorders, not children with trauma histories (Ayres 1972). However, some of the occupational therapists she mentored did conduct research. Taken together, their findings show that children who have been institutionalized are at significantly higher risk for sensory integration dysfunction, often expressed as impaired attention, motor planning, and modulation of sensory input from the environment, especially visual, auditory, tactile, and movement input (Cermak and Daunhauer 1997; Haradon *et al.* 1994; Lin *et al.* 2005; Wilbarger *et al.* 2010).

Dr. Jane Koomar, one of Dr. Ayres' mentees and an internationally renowned occupational therapist and sensory integration expert in her own right, explained that many children who have experienced trauma demonstrate dysregulated arousal states in tandem with sensory sensitivities that are often expressed by fight, flight, or freeze responses (Koomar 2009; also citing van der Kolk 2004). She cautioned that it is important to investigate sensory issues carefully to determine whether the child is triggered by specific sensory input (e.g., certain sounds or smells) associated with their past trauma and/or whether they become hyperaroused by broader categories of sensory input, as that information is important to inform the treatment intervention. In the latter situation, the child may be determined to have a ***sensory modulation disorder***.

The term ***sensory modulation*** is used in sensory integration theory to describe (a) the ability to regulate and organize reactions to sensory input in a graded and adaptive manner; and (b) the balancing of excitatory and inhibitory inputs and adapting to environmental changes (Bundy, Lane, and Murray 2002). To better understand these concepts, it is necessary to explain what sensory processing is in general.

WHAT IS "SENSORY PROCESSING?"

Sensory processing refers to how the neurons communicate together to process all of the incoming information from our senses in order to plan our movements, generate ideas, and produce other thoughts and behaviors (see Figure 3.2). Single neurons cannot "think," but when groups of neurons all interact together in a focused way for a particular purpose, the result is organized action or thought. The brain sorts through the sensory information, filtering out what is irrelevant and organizing and integrating the rest, in order to understand the situation and plan an appropriate response. In PTSD, the timing, filtering, and processing of sensory information is often impaired (Newport and Nemeroff 2000).

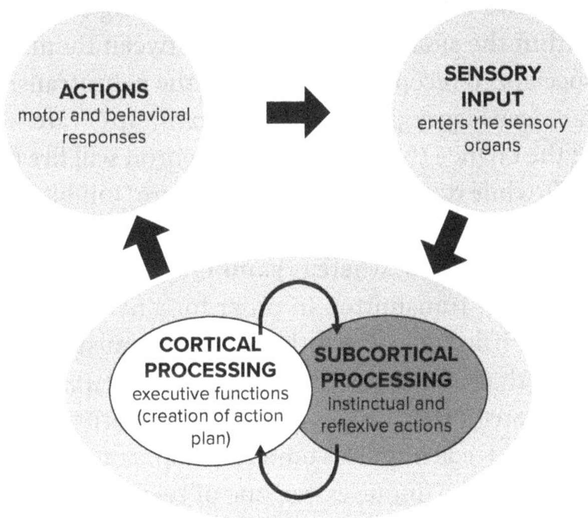

FIGURE 3.2: SENSORY PROCESSING

As a quick review, the major parts of a neuron are as follows:

- **Cell body:** the main part of the neuron that contains the nucleus and controls all functions of the cell.
- **Dendrite:** fibrous roots that extend out from the cell body in order to take in and process information from the axons of nearby neurons.
- **Axon:** nerve fiber that carries impulses away from the nerve cell body to transmit information to different neurons, muscles, and glands.
- **Neurotransmitters:** chemical messengers that are released at the end of an axon into the synaptic gap between neurons either near the dendrite or the cell body. A neurotransmitter influences a neuron in one of three ways: excites (boosts), inhibits (blocks), or modulates (balances).

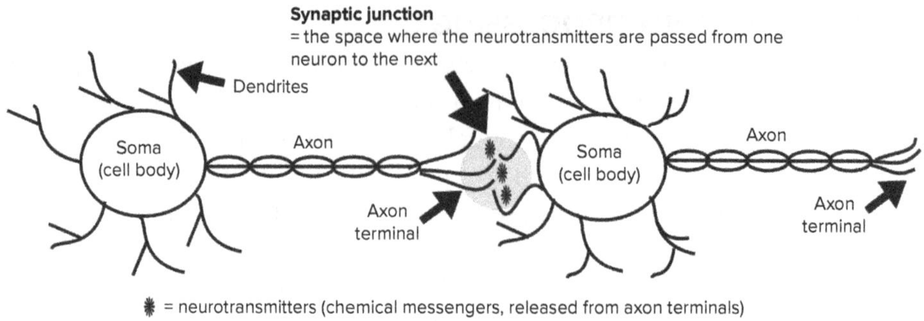

FIGURE 3.3: TRANSMISSION OF NEURAL IMPULSES

Neurons communicate with other neurons by releasing chemicals (i.e., neurotransmitters) within the small gap that exists between them. The "receiving" neurons have specialized receptor sites to allow the neurotransmitters to enter the cell membrane (see Figure 3.3). Some neurotransmitters are "excitatory," that is, they increase the chance that the receiving neuron will fire (i.e., produce an "action potential"), while other neurotransmitters are "inhibitory," and decrease the chance that the receiving neuron will fire. **Glutamate** is the principal excitatory transmitter in the brain, whereas **gamma-aminobutyric acid (GABA)** is the principal inhibitory transmitter. In order for a neuron to fire, the sum of excitatory and inhibitory post-synaptic potentials must be greater than the firing threshold for that particular neuron (see Figure 3.4).

The excitatory transmitters usually synapse on dendrites, whereas the transmitters that block electrical impulses tend to synapse on the cell bodies so they are in position to block the impulses. So, one of two things can happen: either the excitatory transmitters can overtake the inhibitory transmitters to ***open the gate*** and cause an electric impulse, or the inhibitory transmitters, commonly GABA, can ***close the gate*** and block an impulse. Without inhibition, the brain would not be able to filter out irrelevant sensory information. When we use sensory- and mindfulness-based treatments to affect brain function, we are purposely opening or closing the gates at the neuronal level.

Inhibitory neural processes have a huge influence on a person's subjective emotional experience. According to Thayer and Lane's (2000, 2009) ***neurovisceral integration model***, to experience emotion consciously, subcortical emotion-laden information must reach the cerebral cortex, and as this information makes its journey upward, higher-level cortical structures exert their top-down inhibitory influence on this information (such as through the powers of reasoning and memory recall) to shape the nature of the emotional experience. As they explain, "This is consistent with the more general principle that inhibition serves to 'sculpt' excitatory neural action at all levels of the neuraxis to produce context appropriate responses to environmental demands" (Thayer and Lane 2009, p.83).

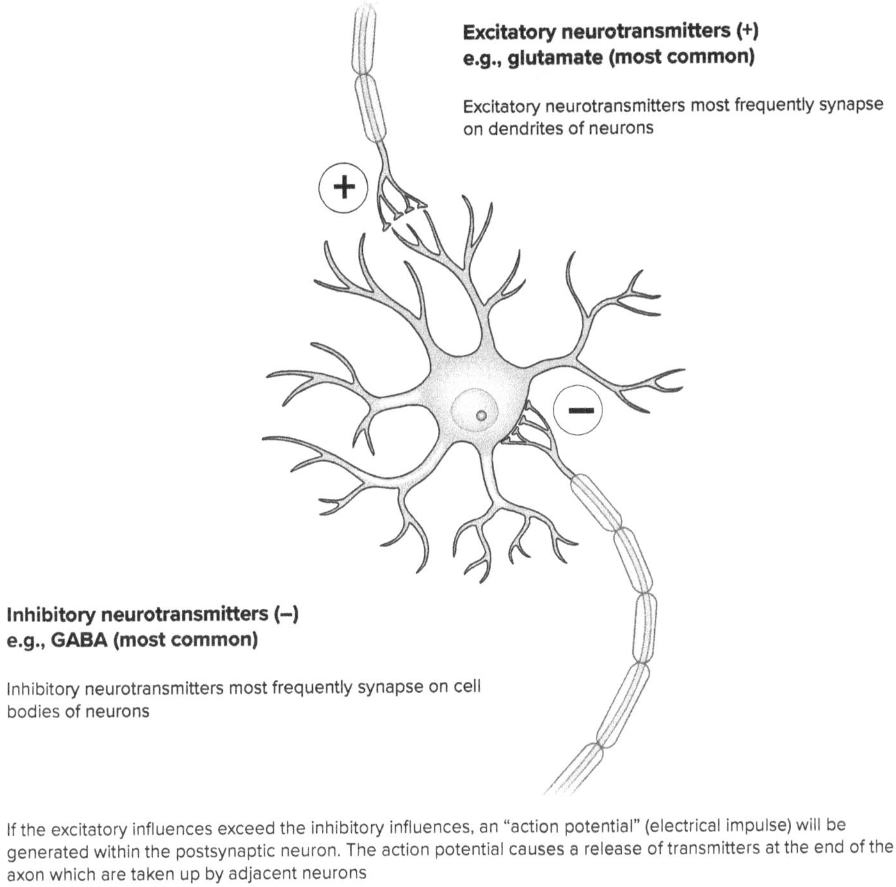

FIGURE 3.4: EXCITATORY AND INHIBITORY NEUROTRANSMITTERS
Reproduced from Stoller (2019)

How attachment sculpts brain processes

For children, nurturing caretakers play a very important role in helping to sculpt inhibitory processes. In Chapter 2, you learned how good quality caretaking dampens the hyper-responsivity of the HPA axis in early childhood due to the inhibitory effects of oxytocin, aka the "bonding hormone" (Agorastos *et al.* 2019). Oxytocin stimulates the release of GABA, which, among many other roles, surrounds the HPA axis to keep it in check (Herman, Mueller, and Figueiredo 2004).

Bonding occurs as the caregiver helps the infant or young child to modulate sensory input in a manner that soothes their nervous system, such as by cuddling (tactile), rocking (vestibular), singing and speaking softly (auditory), feeding (gustatory), or simply by their very presence (visual; olfactory). Caretakers are also the young child's "stand-in" for their immature reasoning skills; they start out reasoning for them, and over time help children learn to reason for themselves. This process builds their mPFC, which plays a huge role in inhibiting the stress response. As you can see, attachment bonds play a huge role in helping young children develop their ability to self-regulate their nervous systems; thus, we should not be surprised that orphaned children and those who have suffered parental abuse or neglect are much more likely to have dysregulated nervous systems and difficulty modulating sensory input.

In fact, Lanius *et al.* (2010) hypothesized two pathways of emotional dysregulation and brain dysfunction in PTSD, one due to fear conditioning or stress sensitization following a traumatic event and the other due to the neurodevelopmental impacts of adverse childhood events, the latter of which increase vulnerability to PTSD later in life. The same group of researchers also presented evidence of genetic risk factors for PTSD (Yehuda *et al.* 2015). Whatever the cause, the failure of the HPA axis to resolve itself leads to actual changes in brain structure and function, including aberrations in sensory processing, which are key to understanding the phenomenon of PTSD (and toxic stress) as well as how it may be effectively resolved. We will delve deeper into these brain changes in the next chapter.

CHAPTER 4

Effects of Early Life Stress on Brain Function

In the previous chapters, you learned how an unresolved "fight–flight" response leads to long-term chemistry changes in the brain that become expressed as chronic stress reactions or PTSD. Over time, these chemistry changes alter the integrity of brain structures and networks, and in the case of children, the very course of brain development. This explains why early life stress and trauma can have an especially devastating effect on a child's health, development, and well-being. All of these brain changes begin at the neuronal level, so we will start our discussion with a glossary of some basic neuronal processes (from Bilimoria and Bonni 2013; Menon 2013; Toga, Thompson, and Sowell 2006; see Figure 4.1).

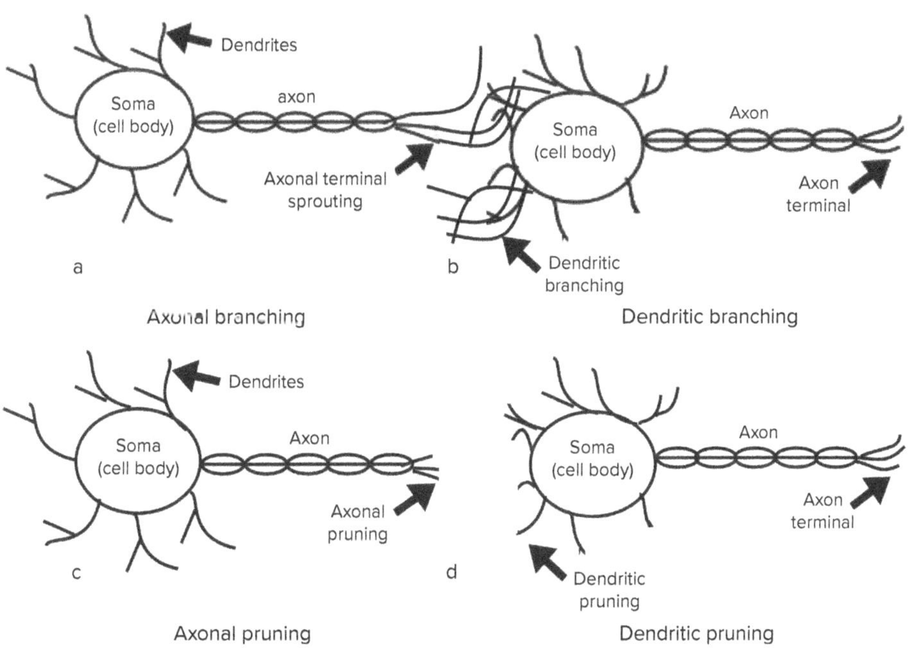

FIGURE 4.1: NEURONAL PROCESSES UNDERLYING BRAIN MATURATION

- ***Dendritic branching:*** Humans are born with approximately 100 billion neurons. With experience and sensory stimulation, the branching of neuronal dendrites increases, resulting in an increase in synaptic connections (Figure 4.1b).
- ***Myelination:*** As the dendrites are branching, the axons of neurons are undergoing the process of myelination. Myelination is the process of forming a myelin sheath (fatty lipid layer) around the axons of neurons, which serves to increase the speed of information transmission from one neuron to another.
- ***Axonal branching:*** The ends of an axon also undergo branching during development, called "arborization" (think of the crown of a tree), which enables the neuron to establish unique patterns of connectivity with other neurons (Figure 4.1a).
- ***Dendritic pruning:*** Dendritic pruning is a process that eliminates some dendrites and synapses that are no longer useful to create more efficient neuronal pathways to adapt to life's circumstances. Dendritic pruning occurs throughout life (Figure 4.1d).
- ***Axonal pruning:*** Axonal pruning also occurs during development and throughout life to help sculpt brain circuitry, in much the same manner as dendritic pruning (Figure 4.1c).
- ***Synaptic pruning:*** Synaptic pruning is the result of dendritic and/or axonal pruning; it just means that the neurons can no longer connect and synapse together, so there are fewer synapses.
- ***Brain networking:*** These processes enable the brain, over the first two decades of life, to develop a system of discrete neural networks that serve specific functions.

Each area of the brain develops at different developmental time points. This growth is characterized by rapid dendritic and axonal branching on a large scale to connect various regions within and between brain structures. This period of expansive growth is followed by dendritic and axonal pruning, which is necessary to create efficient and strong networks, much like how an arborist shapes a tree. Removing the weaker branches shifts resources to the ones that remain, helping them to build stronger and more stable networks (Sakai 2020).

Although there are certain time points during which accelerated branching and pruning normally occur in particular parts of the brain, these processes continue to occur throughout life. When these processes are impaired, it can lead to certain developmental neurological disorders (Riccomagno and Kolodkin 2015). For example, there is evidence to show that schizophrenia is characterized by excessive synaptic pruning, while autism is characterized by decreased synaptic pruning (Sakai 2020).

SEQUENCE OF BRAIN DEVELOPMENT

A child's brain reaches 90 percent of its adult size by the age of six; however, it undergoes massive changes in development in both the gray matter and white matter through adolescence (Riccomagno and Kolodkin 2015). Areas involved with basic sensory information, movement, and other elementary functions mature first, followed by areas in the ***parietal lobes*** involved with spatial orientation and language, which mature around 11–13 years of age, that is, the years of puberty (Agorastos *et al.* 2019; Marsh, Gerber, and Peterson 2008; see Figure 4.2). Areas involved in higher cortical processes including reasoning and other executive functions (e.g., ***PFC***; see Figure 4.3) mature through later adolescence (Marsh *et al.* 2008).

The ***temporal lobes***, ***amygdala*** and ***hippocampus***, which play key roles in language, emotion, and memory processing respectively, grow and change considerably between the ages of 4 and 18, which is consistent with critical periods of language acquisition, emotional growth, and memory skills (Lenroot and Giedd 2006; see Figure 4.3). In contrast, the ***basal ganglia***, a group of subcortical structures responsible for movement coordination, lose volume by puberty (Thompson *et al.* 2000; see Figure 4.4). The size of these structures may also depend on brain functions that are required at a given age, the developmental period, and environmental factors. Interestingly, the hippocampus continues to create new neurons into adulthood (Kuhn, Toda, and Gage 2018).

As a child matures, there is also a ***front-to-back wave of growth through the corpus callosum*** (Thompson *et al.* 2000; see Figure 4.5). This structure is a crucial fiber pathway that transmits information between the brain hemispheres. The fiber tracts of the corpus callosum (see Figure 4.6) that connect with the language and associative thinking areas of the brain grow more rapidly before and during puberty and then show significantly reduced growth after puberty; this pattern of growth coincides with the critical period for learning language (Thompson *et al.* 2000).

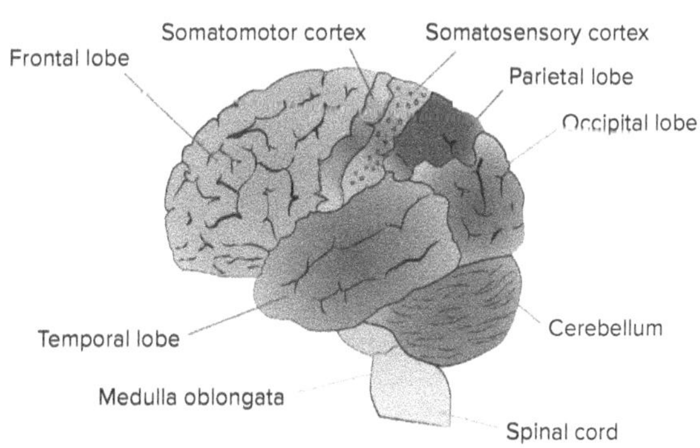

FIGURE 4.2: LOBES OF THE BRAIN
Vectorized by Jkwchui, Wikimedia Commons

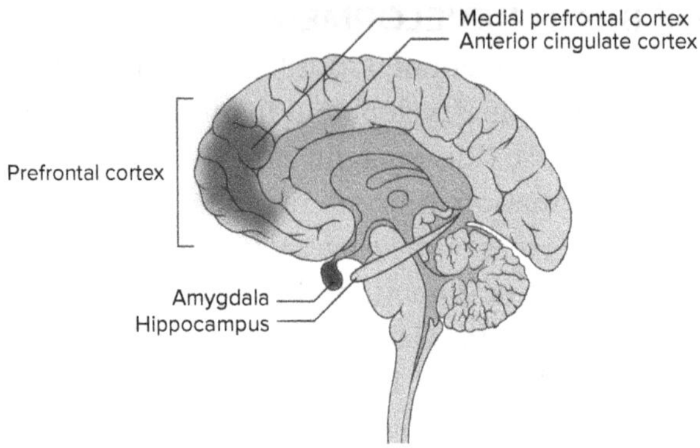

FIGURE 4.3: KEY STRUCTURES OF THE BRAIN
Patrick J. Lynch, medical illustrator, and C. Carl Jaffe, MD, cardiologist, Fvasconcellos, Whidou, Wikimedia Commons

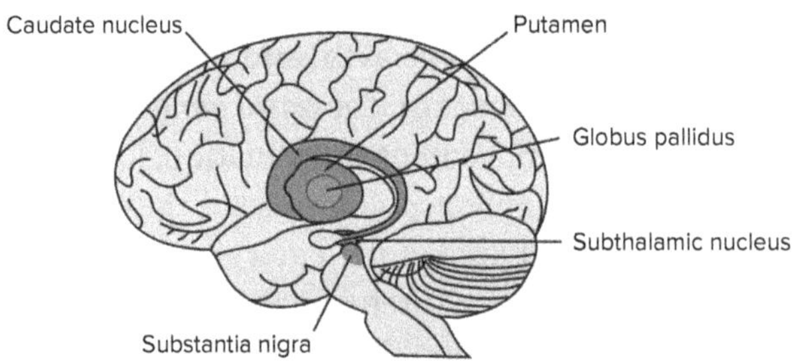

FIGURE 4.4: BASAL GANGLIA
Badseed utilizing the work of Leevanjackson and John Henkel, Wikimedia Commons

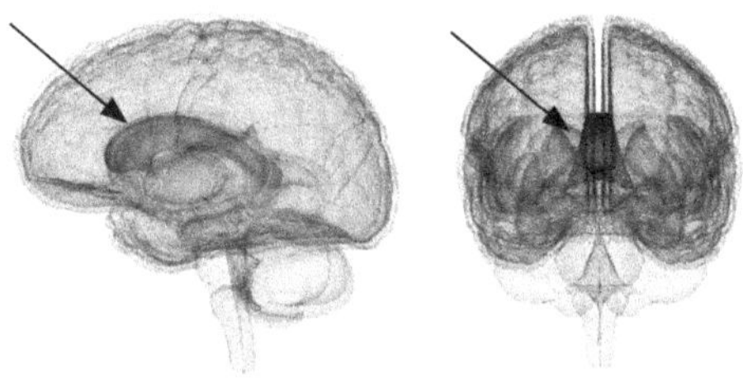

FIGURE 4.5: THE CORPUS CALLOSUM
Images generated by Life Science Databases (LSDB), Wikimedia Commons

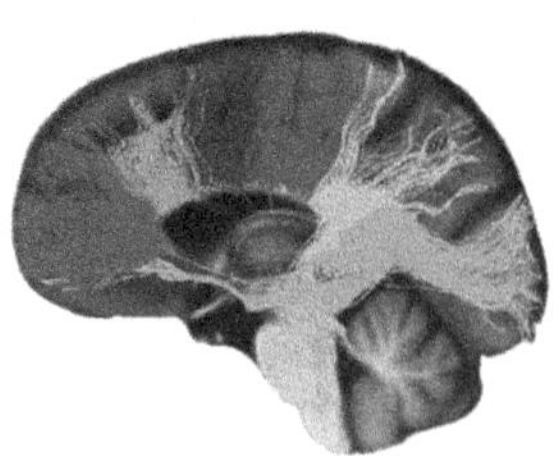

FIGURE 4.6: FIBER TRACTS OF THE CORPUS CALLOSUM
Margaret J. Rosenbloom and Adolf Pfefferbaum, MD, Wikimedia Commons

Negative experiences during critical periods of brain development can impair major neuroregulatory systems of the brain with profound and often permanent consequences (Anda *et al.* 2006), and can even change genes and their expression (McEwen 2008). Shonkoff and Phillips (2000) declared the "nature vs. nurture" debate solved, as we now know that genetic and environmental influences work very closely and dynamically together, setting a strong or fragile foundation for a child's future life trajectory.

THE NEUROCIRCUITRY MODEL OF PTSD

So how are brain processes and overall brain development affected by the long-term chemistry changes produced by an unresolved fight–flight response? The answer to this question first came to light following the invention of functional neuroimaging techniques in the 1990s (Bremner 2007). While participants are in a scanner, they are often asked to look at images, listen to auditory stimuli, and/or perform specific cognitive tasks that could be emotionally loaded and/or neutral. With regard to PTSD, a brain pattern emerged early on from these experiments, referred to as the ***Neurocircuitry Model of PTSD***. This model is still considered to be a highly valid theory to this day concerning the hyperaroused/re-experiencing subtype of the condition.

The basic neurocircuitry model is characterized by the following (Rauch, Shin, and Phelps 2006; see Figure 4.7):

- **Increased activation of the *amygdala***, the brain's threat detector, which instigates "knee-jerk" emotional reactions in the face of danger or a significant challenge.
- **Decreased activation of structures within the *mPFC***, which are involved in conscious rational thought processes and allow us to "reason away" our fears.
- **Decreased activation of the *hippocampus***, which puts situations into context based on personal memories.

These structures—the ***amygdala***, ***mPFC***, and ***hippocampus***, along with the anterior cingulate cortex and insula—are known to play a large role in regulating emotion and maintaining homeostasis (Roxo *et al.* 2011; van der Kolk 2014). (See the text boxes for more information on these brain structures.)

According to the ***Neurocircuitry Model of PTSD***, the higher brain centers, particularly the mPFC and hippocampus, are unable to effectively control the lower brain centers—especially the amygdala—leading to the emotional dysregulation seen in this condition. Inadequate top-down control causes the amygdala to overreact in the face of threat (Rauch *et al.* 2006; Shin and Liberzon

2010; Shin, Rauch, and Pitman 2005). The neurocircuitry model is supported by strong empirical evidence, including a large meta-analysis (Hayes, Hayes, and Mikedis 2012) and cross-sectional studies of children with PTSD (Herringa 2017). Decreased connectivity between the PFC and the amygdala, as well as dysfunction of the hippocampus, has also been found in studies of children and adults who have generalized anxiety disorder (Madonna *et al.* 2019; Patriquin and Mathew 2017).

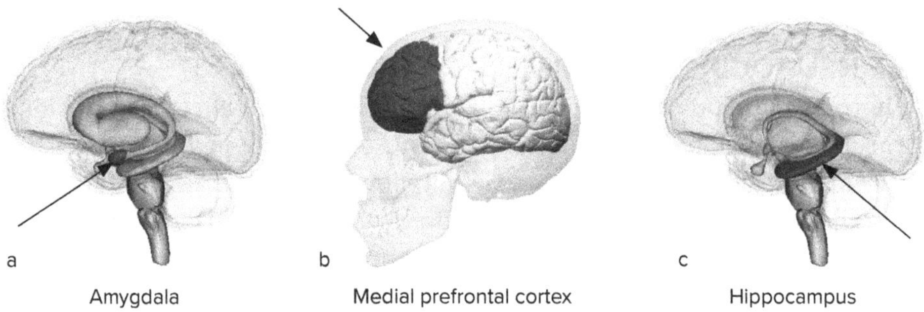

FIGURE 4.7: KEY BRAIN STRUCTURES IN THE NEUROCIRCUITRY MODEL OF PTSD
a: image was generated by Life Science Databases (LSDB), Wikimedia Commons; b: polygon data were generated by Database Center for Life Science (DBCLS), Wikimedia Commons; c: image was generated by Life Science Databases (LSDB), Wikimedia Commons

Amygdala

The amygdala is a small, almond-sized structure located deep in each temporal lobe. The amygdala constantly surveys the environment (as filtered through the thalamus and cerebral cortex) and assigns emotional significance to everything coming through the senses, whether positive or negative (Shin and Liberzon 2010). In particular, the amygdala plays a major role in the detection of threats and control of the body's response to threats (LeDoux 2015; Stephens and Wand 2012). It is the trigger that activates the HPA axis of the stress response (van der Werff *et al.* 2013). However, the amygdala only contributes to the feeling of fear indirectly, as this requires the engagement of conscious brain structures (LeDoux 2015).

Much like a pirate looking through a telescope from the watchtower, the amygdala constantly scans the environment to identify threats. If there are any, it triggers the hypothalamus to set off a fight–flight reaction, similar to signaling the other pirates on the ship to prepare for battle.

Hippocampus

The hippocampus is an essential brain structure for learning, memory, and cognition (Zeidman and Maguire 2016). It is involved in memory formation and storage, and in particular, assigns emotional meaning, time, and spatial context to our memories.

The anterior hippocampus is involved in episodic (autobiographical) memory, that is, it plays a key role in putting together the "story" of an event and placing it into context (Fanselow and Dong 2010; Zeidman and Maguire 2016). For example, it can remind us that most Labrador retrievers we've encountered in the past have been friendly dogs, so the one in front of us likely is, too, which keeps us calm. The anterior hippocampus also has neurons that code both space and time and can thus remind us where and when we saw that friendly dog (Jin and Maren 2015). However, if a dog bit us in the past, we might be very hesitant to approach one in the future. This is called contextual fear conditioning (Zeidman and Maguire 2016). Thus, the anterior hippocampus regulates the hormonal response to stress, that is, the HPA axis, in both directions—toward a sense of safety or threat—based on context and memory (Radley and Sawchenko 2011).

Think of the hippocampus as a GPS system: this device calculates time and place simultaneously and you can even drop a pin onto the GPS map and add detailed notes or pictures. Similarly, the hippocampus catalogs life events based on time and place. However, our memories are not stored in the hippocampus. Instead, different sensory and emotional elements are stored where they were originally processed (e.g., visual cortex, auditory cortex, limbic system). The hippocampus reconstructs the memory by pulling the pieces from these areas and organizes it by place and time so it is ready to be shown on the "big screen" in our brain.

Prefrontal cortex

The PFC is responsible for planning, reasoning, decision-making, and problem-solving (Funahashi 2017). It orchestrates our thoughts and can powerfully influence emotions through "top-down" inhibitory processes. The PFC has strong two-way connections with the thalamus and influences how it filters incoming sensory information (Wimmer *et al.* 2015). You might think of the PFC as the captain of the ship, as it plays such a key role in directing our thought processing. The captain takes in all of the important data—GPS coordinates, weather, other threats, integrity of the ship, etc.—and consults with past logs (relevant memories) and with the ship's officers (associated brain regions) to keep the ship on course and avoid obstacles, while filtering out the irrelevant happenings on the rest of the ship.

There are four parts of the PFC that are particularly relevant to our discussion:

- The medial PFC (mPFC) processes internal states relating to affect and motivation, and is involved in long-term memory processing. The mPFC helps to keep the HPA axis in check by providing top-down control over the emotional limbic system, including the amygdala (Shin, Rauch, and Pitman 2006). That is, it can help reason away our fears.
- The dorsolateral PFC (dlPFC) plays a large role in working memory tasks (Funahashi 2017) and is closely connected with the hippocampus (Goldman-Rakic, Selemon, and Schwartz 1984). It is active with cognitive tasks requiring focused attention, decision-making, and problem-solving (Funahashi 2017; Menon 2011).
- The ventromedial PFC (vmPFC) plays an important role in constructing emotional meaning (Roy, Shohamy, and Wager 2012) and regulating emotion (Andrewes and Jenkins 2019). It is concerned with embodied self-awareness, that is, our ability to be present in the moment to feel what is happening in our body and mind (i.e., sensations, emotions, movements), without judgment (Fogel 2009).
- The dorsomedial PFC (dmPFC) is concerned with conceptual self-awareness, that is, our self-judgment (Fogel 2009), appraisal, and evaluation (Hayes, Hayes and Mikedis 2012). It is continually active during waking states, and plays an important role in the stream of thought running through people's minds (Fogel 2009).

The role of the hippocampus in the neurocircuitry model has a special relevance in PTSD, as it is strongly implicated in the intrusiveness of traumatic memories. According to Dr. Jane Koomar, "In a child who is typically developing, the role of the hippocampus is to record and file event memories, putting them into chronological order and perspective before they become consolidated as narrative memories in the left frontal cortex" (2009, p.1). She explains that traumatic memories, by contrast, are not stored in the narrative memory centers, but are instead stored as somatic (body) sensations in limbic structures (serving emotional and survival processes) including the amygdala, where they may trigger physiological reactions in response to traumatic reminders (Koomar 2009).

A reduction in PFC volume is another frequent finding in the relatively few studies conducted with children with PTSD, most of whom were raised in institutions (Rinne-Albers *et al.* 2013). The PFC matures later in development, which explains why young children have decreased ability to inhibit their own impulses (Marsh *et al.* 2008). Given that trauma tends to deactivate the PFC, it stands to reason that children who have experienced trauma may show delayed and/or impaired development of inhibitory control over their emotions and behaviors. In fact, studies have shown a strong correlation between childhood trauma and self-injurious (Paivio and McCulloch 2004), self-destructive (van der Kolk, Perry, and Herman 1991), and impulsive behaviors (Roy 2005), the latter of which was also shown to be relevant to suicide behavior (Roy 2005).

THE NEUROCIRCUITRY MODEL OF PTSD AND DEPRESSION

The ***Neurocircuitry Model*** is not only applicable to PTSD and certain other anxiety disorders, but also depression. Depression is often stress-related, so it is no surprise that approximately half of trauma survivors who go on to develop PTSD also meet criteria for major depressive disorder (MDD) (Flory and Yehuda 2015). Flory and Yehuda (2015) have even raised the question of whether the co-occurrence of PTSD and depression represents a separate subtype of PTSD. Like PTSD, MDD is correlated with a decrease in neurons in the hippocampus and mPFC and an increase in neurons in the amygdala (Liu *et al.* 2017). In both conditions, elevated release levels of CRH (a form of cortisol) have been found, which raises the overall cortisol load in the brain (Flory and Yehuda 2015). There are particularly high concentrations of CRH in these three brain regions (Tyborowska *et al.* 2018), which explain the neuroimaging findings. These areas are especially sensitive to hormonal stress during the adolescent years (Tyborowska *et al.* 2018). This increase in cortisol upsets the balance of excitatory and inhibitory neurotransmitters, lowering GABA levels. Not surprisingly, lower levels of GABA are also a feature of major depression (Hare and Duman 2020) and PTSD (Averill *et al.* 2016).

THE IMPORTANT ROLE OF THE THALAMUS

The ***thalamus*** (see Figure 4.8) has also been implicated in PTSD, showing ***decreased activation*** in numerous studies (Bremner *et al.* 1999; Etkin and Wager 2007; Kim *et al.* 2007; Lanius *et al.* 2001, 2003) and more recently ***altered connectivity*** to various regions of the brain (Philip *et al.* 2016). For some unknown reason, the thalamus was not included in descriptions of the neurocircuitry model, despite the fact that it is a key subcortical structure supporting optimal functioning of the brain structures in the model (see the text box). Thus, the Sensory-Enhanced Yoga® program always included it in its own model since it pointed toward a bottom-up method for addressing the issue of PTSD (see Figure 4.9).

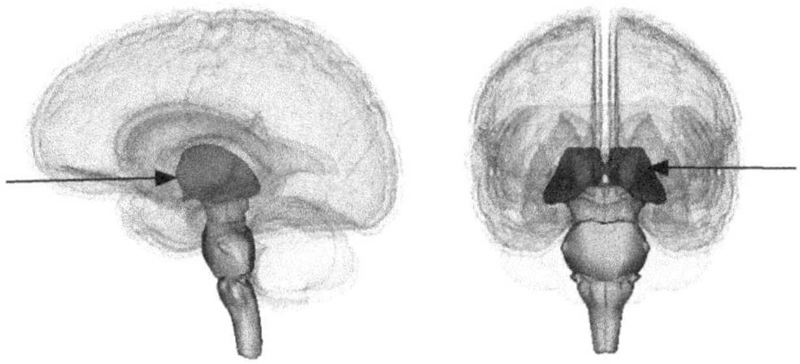

FIGURE 4.8: THALAMUS
Images generated by Life Science Databases (LSDB), Wikimedia Commons

Thalamus

The thalamus is the final relay station for sensory information before it is sent to the appropriate areas of the cerebral cortex for further processing (Courtiol and Wilson 2015; Hwang *et al.* 2017). It distills sensory information into a more interpretable form from which the cortex can then flesh out the details (Saalmann and Kastner 2015). It is theorized that a major role of the thalamus is to control functional connectivity within and across cortical regions (Nakajima and Halassa 2017, p.127; see also Hwang *et al.* 2017). It also helps to regulate sleep (Coulon, Budde, and Pape 2012). The integration of vestibular and somatosensory (body-based) input likely occurs in the thalamus (Wijesinghe, Protti, and Camp 2015).

It may be helpful to imagine the thalamus as an office receptionist who handles all communications, including throwing away the junk mail, answering the phones, sifting through emails, and forwarding the important stuff to the right departments. They have a very important role, because if they sleep on the job or get too stressed and overwhelmed, they will send "junk" to the other departments, disrupting the flow of information and decreasing efficiency in the office.

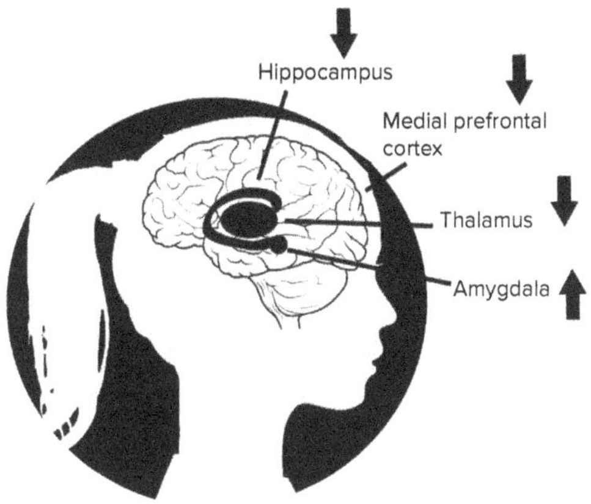

Arrows = the most common direction of activation in PTSD

FIGURE 4.9: SELECTED BRAIN CHANGES IN PTSD, THE EARLY FINDINGS

According to a research team at the Technical University of Munich (TUM), "All sensory perceptions converge [in the thalamus] first. As the main relay center, it therefore needs to reconcile the flood of incoming information and the brain's limited computing power" (2016, para. 2). So, if the thalamus is not working properly, it will affect the performance of all higher level brain structures, and thus our perceptions and understanding of the world around us. Bergmann (2008) asserted that altered thalamic functioning explains the cognitive and memory impairments, hemispheral imbalances, as well as the disturbed sensory integration often seen in PTSD. Examples of sensory disturbances include fragmented olfactory, auditory, taste, or visual memories or flashbacks, and/or kinesthetic/bodily sensations (Bergmann 2008).

Dr. Jean Ayres' (1972) sensory integration theory is based on the concept that carefully selected sensory input can influence the functioning of subcortical brain structures, including the thalamus, which, in turn, affect higher-level brain functioning. In the SMYLE™ program, we present carefully selected sensory input to help the thalamus function more optimally, in order to enhance higher level cortical processing. ***It is one of several key methods by which our program promotes self-regulation and healing from trauma, toxic stress, anxiety, and/or related mental health conditions.***

BRAIN DIFFERENCES IN THE DISSOCIATIVE SUBTYPE OF PTSD

More recent neuroimaging studies found additional brain structures impacted by PTSD, including the ***insula***; however, findings were mixed until Lanius and colleagues (2002, 2005, 2010; Harricharan *et al.* 2020; Hopper *et al.* 2007) discovered that different patterns of brain activation occur during the dissociative vs. hyperaroused/re-experiencing states of PTSD. Accordingly, they proposed a dissociative subtype, which ultimately became incorporated into the DSM-5.

The ***dissociative subtype*** is characterized by ***emotional overmodulation***, in which structures of the mPFC overinhibit the amygdala and insula, leading to detachment or numbing and other symptoms of dissociation (see Figure 4.10).

The insula plays a critical role in the ability to attend to interoceptive (body-based) sensation (Wang *et al.* 2019) and registers the bodily sensations as a "feeling state" (Harricharan *et al.* 2020), whereupon it communicates with higher cortical areas for emotion labeling and further processing (Torre and Lieberman 2018). However, in response to ***intolerable*** sensations and emotions, the mPFC exerts strong "top-down" inhibitory control over the amygdala and insula, in an effort to avoid emotional overwhelm (Menon and Uddin 2010; Yehuda *et al.* 2015).

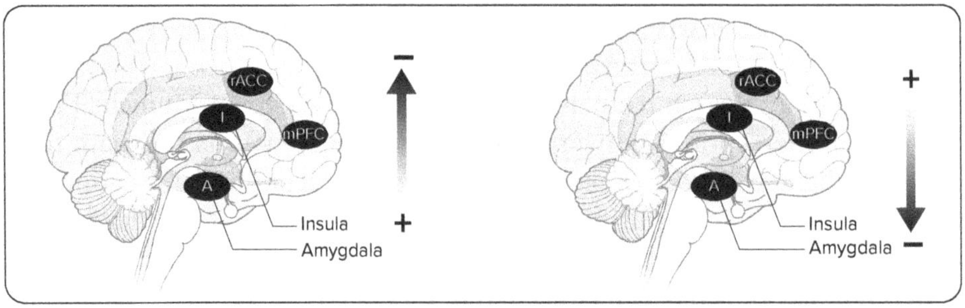

Hyperaroused/reexperiencing subtype

Decreased activation of structures within the medial prefrontal cortex, especially the ventral-medial PFC (vmPFC) and rostral anterior cingulate cortex (rACC), results in undermodulation (inadequate inhibitory control) of lower brain centers implicated in emotional arousal

Increased activation of neural substrates of emotion (amygdala and insula) overtake the regulatory influences of the mPFC

Either or both scenarios may result in symptoms of hyperarousal and reexperiencing

Dissociative subtype

Increased activation of structures within the medial prefrontal cortex, especially the ventral-medial PFC (vmPFC) and rostral anterior cingulate cortex (rACC), results in overmodulation (excessive inhibitory control) of lower brain centers implicated in emotional arousal

Decreased activation of neural substrates of emotion (amygdala and insula) are overpowered by the regulatory influences of the mPFC

Either or both scenarios may result in symptoms of dissociation, including emotional detachment and numbing

Traumatized individuals can also cycle between these two states or fall along a sliding scale from hyperarousal to hypoarousal
(Lanius *et al.* 2002, 2005, 2010; Hopper *et al.* 2007; Stark *et al.* 2015, p.217

FIGURE 4.10: THE TWO BASIC SUBTYPES OF PTSD
Reproduced from Stoller (2019)

In contrast, the more common ***hyperaroused/re-experiencing subtype*** is characterized by ***emotional undermodulation*** due to failure of the medial prefrontal structures to inhibit the limbic structures (Hopper *et al.* 2007; Lanius *et al.* 2010). Increased activation of the (right anterior) insula is associated with this subtype. It is also recognized that traumatized individuals can cycle between these two states (Lanius *et al.* 2010, 2015; Figure 4.10) or fall anywhere along a continuum from hypoarousal to hyperarousal (Stark *et al.* 2015, p.217).

THE TRIPLE NETWORK MODEL OF PTSD

As the neurocircuitry model was being refined, it became clear that there were many distinct networks in the brain. Soon, three core global brain networks emerged and were formulated by Menon (2011) into the ***triple network model***, which has piqued the interest of experts on trauma and other mental health conditions (see Figures 4.11 and 4.12). These networks are the ***central executive network (CEN)***, ***default mode network (DMN)***, and the ***salience network (SN)*** (Lanius *et al.* 2015; Menon 2011; Patel *et al.* 2012; Sridharan, Levitin, and Menon 2008;Yehuda *et al.* 2015). Menon characterized these core networks as consisting of a collection of brain regions, referred to as "nodes," and the connections that link them. He stated that a network may become altered by either faulty node functioning or faulty connections between them, which explains why some functional impairments may relate to a totally different part of the brain than the lesion location due to impaired connectivity with that lesion. According to Lanius and colleagues (2015), alterations in these networks affect the balance between excitatory and inhibitory neural processes, ***which highlights the relevance of these networks for treatment programs that utilize a sensory integrative approach, such as SMYLE™***. In fact, the careful selection and use of sensory and mindfulness-based techniques to influence brain networks could possibly impact the very nature of one's "self." As Menon (2019, p.2) asserts: "The harmonious functioning of the three core networks is responsible for the complex phenomenon that we understand as the 'mind' in the brain."

Let's now take a look at these three primary brain networks (see Figure 4.12):

- The ***CEN*** is responsible for helping us focus on a task at hand, and is primarily associated with the dlPFC and the posterior parietal cortex (PPC), along with other interconnected brain regions. This network helps with attention, working memory, decision-making, and other executive functions that allow us to control our thoughts, emotions, and behavior. When the CEN isn't working properly, it can lead to problems with cognitive function (Akiki, Averill, and Abdallah 2017; Lanius *et al.* 2015; Yehuda *et al.* 2015).
- The ***DMN*** is responsible for our self-reflective thinking, and is primarily associated with the posterior cingulate cortex (PCC)/precuneus and mPFC, as well as the lateral parietal lobes. This network is active when we're thinking about our own emotions, memories, or the future, and it's important for our sense of self over time (Bluhm *et al.* 2009; Lanius *et al.*

2015; van der Kolk 2014, p.90; Yehuda *et al.* 2015). When the DMN isn't working properly, it can lead to problems with self-referential processing, which may include dissociative symptoms such as depersonalization (Lanius *et al.* 2015; Yehuda *et al.* 2015).

- The ***SN*** is responsible for switching between the CEN and DMN based on what's most important at the moment. It's primarily associated with the insula and dorsal anterior cingulate cortex (dACC), and works with other brain regions to generate appropriate behavioral responses to salient information (Menon 2011; Patel *et al.* 2012). When the SN isn't working properly, it can lead to problems with arousal and interoception (Lanius *et al.* 2015; Seeley *et al.* 2007; Yehuda *et al.* 2015).

Overall, the CEN helps us focus on a task, the DMN helps us think about ourselves, and the SN helps us switch between the two.

The SN is controlled by two key brain structures:

- The ***dACC*** is ***externally focused***, and helps control our body's nervous system by assessing danger in our surroundings. It has a strong connection to the amygdala, which is known as the brain's "fear accelerator," and can be overactive in PTSD (VanElzakker *et al.* 2014).
- The ***insula***, on the other hand, is ***internally focused***, and helps us sense what's going on in our bodies. It's more involved in the body-based aspects of emotions, like arousal.

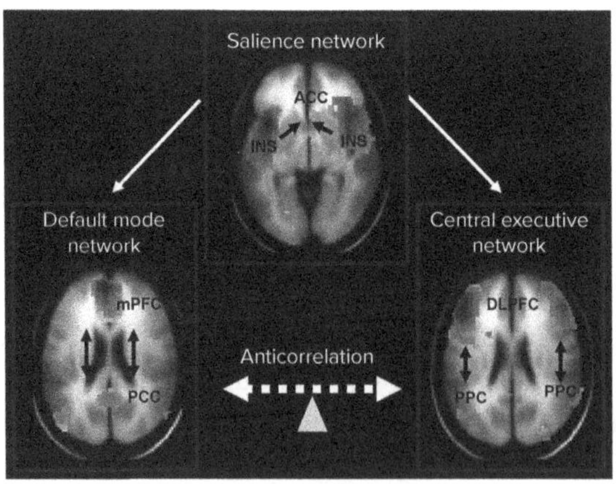

FIGURE 4.11: THE TRIPLE NETWORK MODEL VIA NEUROIMAGING

Nekovarova, Fajnerova, Horacek, Spaniel, Wikimedia Commons

Triple network model

CENTRAL EXECUTIVE NETWORK (CEN) "On task" Executive functioning and sensorimotor processing	↔	**SALIENCE NETWORK (SN)** "The switch" What is most important in this moment?	↔	**DEFAULT MODE NETWORK (DMN)** "Off task" Daydreaming, reflecting

The anchor structures of each network

Dorsolateral prefrontal cortex (dlPFC) Working memory and attention **Posterior parietal cortex (PPC)** Sensorimotor processing	**Anterior insula** Internally focused, "the feeling self," including pain **Dorsal anterior cingulate cortex (dACC)** Externally focused; helps amygdala to assess threat **Together, the insula and dACC guide action**	**Medial prefrontal cortex (mPFC)** Orchestrates thoughts, promotes embodied self-awareness, regulates emotions **Posterior cingulate cortex (PCC)** Self-reflection, daydreaming, integrates current internal experiences with past memory and future plans

FIGURE 4.12: THE ANCHOR STRUCTURES OF EACH NETWORK IN THE TRIPLE NETWORK MODEL

Based on Akiki et al. (2017); Bluhm et al. (2009); Lanius et al. (2015); Menon (2011); Patel et al. (2012); Sridharan et al. (2008); Sripada et al. (2012); Yehuda et al. (2015)

The two brain structures that anchor the SN work together to prioritize what's important in the moment and guide behavior accordingly. Shaw *et al.* (2021) provided evidence that the SN synchronizes its activity with the network it needs to activate through neuronal gating mechanisms. It is also theorized that the right anterior insula sends a gamma wave control signal to the PPC, which deactivates the DMN and activates the CEN involved in focused attention and learning (Sridharan *et al.* 2008). This process reflects the sensory integration theory proposed by Dr. Jean Ayres (1972), which suggests that areas of the brain involved in sensorimotor processes, like the PPC, have a strong influence over brain processes involved in focused attention and learning. Yoga, as a rich sensorimotor activity that promotes mindfulness, has already been found to improve cognitive function (Gothe and McAuley 2015), and may thus hold potential for cognitive development.

In PTSD, there is often impaired ability to shift between the on-task CEN and the off-task DMN, disrupting the functioning of all three networks, and leading to clinical symptoms like those listed (Akiki *et al.* 2017; Lanius *et al.* 2015). This can leave individuals with PTSD stuck in a state of chronic hyperarousal and hypervigilance, unable to disengage from the SN, particularly the amygdala and insula (Sripada *et al.* 2012). As a result, intrusive thoughts can disrupt concentration by making it difficult to transition from the DMN to the CEN. ***In children, these networks are still just developing, so when they experience a traumatic event, it can disrupt these networks even more dramatically.***

Initial studies suggest that traumatized children show a similar pattern to adults, in fitting with both the neurocircuitry model of PTSD and the triple network model of PTSD (Herringa 2017; Lei *et al.* 2015; Xu *et al.* 2018). Herringa's (2017) review of pediatric studies found that as children with PTSD age, the SN (dACC and amygdala) becomes hyperactive. It also becomes harder to engage the CEN, particularly the dmPFC and dlPFC, which play large roles in controlling our stream of thoughts and working memory, respectively. These findings reflect reduced top-down cortical control of the limbic structures, leading to inattention and emotional dysregulation.

RELATIONSHIP BETWEEN THE CORPUS CALLOSUM AND TRIPLE NETWORK SYSTEM

Most of the brain structures discussed thus far in this book consist primarily of **gray matter** (Siehl *et al.* 2018). The gray color of this tissue is due to the very high concentration of cell bodies and dendrites. In contrast, **white matter** consists of myelinated nerve axons that connect the gray matter regions, allowing them to communicate with one another. It is the myelin sheath (a protective layer around the axon that speeds impulse transmission) that creates the white appearance of these tracts. The largest white matter structure in the brain is the **corpus callosum**, which has frequently been found to be reduced in size in PTSD, particularly in children (De Bellis and Zisk 2014; Siehl *et al.* 2018). The primary purpose of the corpus callosum is to integrate sensory, motor, and cognitive information between the two hemispheres (see Figures 4.5 and 4.6).

While the corpus callosum is not directly part of the triple network model, it plays an important role in facilitating communication between the brain regions involved in these networks. Changes in white matter have been found to be connected with abnormalities in the triple network system in various mental health conditions, including borderline personality disorder (Quattrini *et al.* 2022), schizophrenia (Kang *et al.* 2020), and attention deficit hyperactivity disorder (ADHD) (Bu *et al.* 2022). Siehl *et al.* (2018) speculate that white matter changes in PTSD may reflect changes in functional connectivity between different brain regions just as gray matter changes do. As a matter of fact, one study showed a correlation between decreased corpus callosum size and intrusive, avoidant, and hyperarousal symptoms, childhood dissociation, and child internalizing behavior (De Bellis and Zisk 2014)—all of which are suggestive of network anomalies. Thus, it would be well worth investigating the relationship of this structure to network changes in PTSD to shed more light on how we can best address these symptoms.

We have just described a plethora of changes that can occur as a result of an unresolved stress response, all interrelated to each other. Brain chemistry changes create ***neurotransmitter imbalances*** that affect ***brain networks*** and lead to ***structural brain changes*** over time. You may be wondering why we have ventured in such detail to describe these changes, but this will all become clear in the next chapter, when we discuss brain changes that occur in yoga and other mindfulness-based practices, and the inverse relationship between these changes and those that occur in PTSD.

CHAPTER 5

The Inverse Relationship Between Toxic Stress/PTSD and Mindfulness

As fast as neuroimaging studies were revealing brain structures affected by trauma, other neuroimaging studies were implicating the same brain structures with regard to yoga and other mindfulness-based practices—but were showing a ***reverse pattern***! This makes perfect sense, as people who have PTSD are stuck in the "there and then," desperately trying to come back to the "here and now," which is the very definition of mindfulness. We are excited to share these findings with you, but in order for them to be fully meaningful, we first need to present Clancy *et al.*'s (2017) **Sensory Hypothesis of PTSD**, which goes a long way to explain ***why*** sensory and mindfulness-based practices can be so powerful in healing the condition.

THE SENSORY HYPOTHESIS OF PTSD

Clancy *et al.*'s (2017) **Sensory Hypothesis of PTSD** adds another piece to the neurocircuitry puzzle and, as was later discovered (Clancy *et al.* 2020; Clancy *et al.* 2022), helps to integrate it with the triple network model. This research team compared individuals with PTSD (n=25), generalized anxiety (n=24), and healthy subjects (n=20) to study the sensory pathology of PTSD using Granger causality analysis with electroencephalography (EEG), which is a type of analysis that identifies the "causal" direction of interactions between brain structures using time-series data. As you will recall, the Neurocircuitry Model of PTSD focuses on the problem of not enough top-down inhibition of lower brain structures by the mPFC and hippocampus. Clancy and his colleagues found that with PTSD, ***not only*** is the cortex not providing enough top-down inhibition, ***but also that sensory input is not being filtered on the way up to the cortex***.

Sensory filtering was measured in terms of **alpha power**, which is believed to play a key role in filtering and organizing the flow of sensory information to the brain (Kerr *et al.* 2013). So the problem is going both ways and is reinforcing its own loop (see Figure 5.1). Reduced bottom-up sensory filtering correlated with frontal overload, hypervigilance, and impulse control deficits (Clancy *et al.* 2017). ***By incorporating therapeutic sensory input into yoga, SMYLE™ aims to improve bottom-up filtering, which helps to correct the entire loop, both bottom-up and top-down.***

Interactions between the thalamus and cerebral cortex are required to generate alpha rhythms, which are brain waves in the frequency range of 8–12 Hz produced when in a relaxed and restful state (Abdou *et al.* 2006). Peak alpha frequency increases quickly in early childhood, attaining 8.4 Hz at five years, and leveling off at almost 10 Hz by early adolescence (Freschi *et al.* 2022). Several studies have found a correlation between alpha rhythms and levels of the inhibitory neurotransmitter GABA (Abdou *et al.* 2006; Jensen and Mazaheri 2010; Klimesch 2012). While both excitatory and inhibitory neurotransmitters help create alpha rhythms in our brain, GABA is particularly important because it helps control the activity between the thalamus and the cortex, and also promotes regular rhythmic patterns in our brain (Llinás *et al.* 2005).

One hypothesis suggests that alpha waves may reflect synchronized firing of certain groups of inhibitory GABA neurons, referred to as "pulsed inhibition" (Jensen and Mazaheri 2010; Sadaghiani *et al.* 2012). This hypothesis is supported by the observation that both alpha waves and GABA are involved in the filtering of sensory information, both bottom-up and top-down, and both are associated with a more relaxed state of mind (Abdou *et al.* 2006). However, more research is needed to fully clarify the relationship between alpha rhythms and GABA.

Alpha rhythms not only serve as a two-way information filter between the thalamus and cerebral cortex, but are also believed to help segregate the functional activity of different brain areas so each area can operate more efficiently (Huang *et al.* 2014). Additionally, alpha rhythms help to regulate activity within the DMN and SN (Clancy 2017; Clancy *et al.* 2022; Nicholson *et al.* 2020). There is a significant positive correlation between alpha rhythms and activity of the DMN, which makes sense as both are active in restful or reflective mind states (Clancy 2017; Clancy *et al.* 2022; Jann *et al.* 2009; Klimesch 2012; Mantini *et al.* 2007; Nicholson *et al.* 2020).

Clancy *et al.*'s (2017) Sensory Hypothesis of PTSD is bolstered by additional studies showing that PTSD is associated with significantly reduced alpha power, particularly in the DMN (Clancy *et al.* 2020; Nicholson *et al.* 2023). Low alpha power has been interpreted as an indication that there is less communication between the thalamus and cerebral cortex, which would explain why the SN, DMN, and CEN become hyperconnected in PTSD (Lanius *et al.* 2015; Sripada *et al.* 2012), causing the person to experience symptoms of hyperarousal, sensory sensitivity, re-experiencing, and dissociation (Clancy 2017; Lanius *et al.* 2014). Since alpha rhythms provide essential support to the functioning of the major brain networks, it is not surprising that alpha-targeted neurofeedback (a type of treatment that helps people consciously control their alpha brain waves) has been shown to significantly reduce symptoms of PTSD in adults (Nicholson *et al.* 2020, 2023; van der Kolk *et al.* 2016) and is also showing potential to do so in children (Rogel *et al.* 2020).

Recall that in children, the SN, DMN, and CEN are not yet fully formed and separated from one another to begin with; thus, severe stress and/or trauma can be surmised to seriously impact the maturation of these networks. So, when your students are acting up, having trouble attending, or demonstrating hyperactivity, do not rush to address it from a behavioral perspective. These changes that are going on deep in the brain, especially a developing brain, could be the root cause of these challenges. Therefore, it is important to keep in mind that these behaviors you are observing may be out of the student's control. We need to address these problems at their root cause instead of trying to mold the surface behaviors.

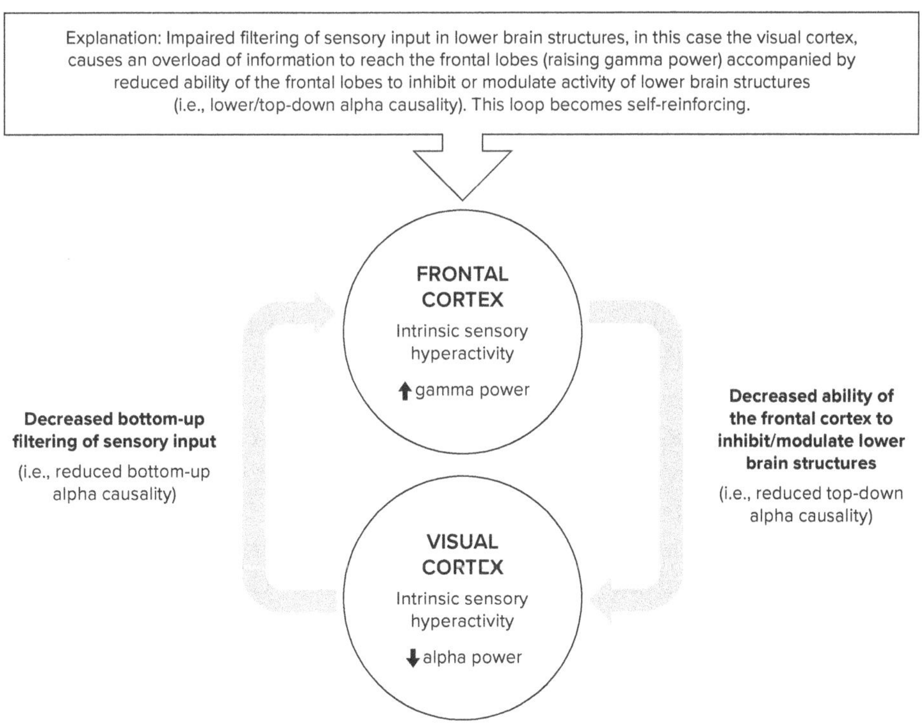

FIGURE 5.1: A NOVEL VISUAL DEPICTION OF CLANCY *ET AL.*'S *A SENSORY HYPOTHESIS OF PTSD* (2017)

HOW YOGA CAN POTENTIALLY REPAIR THESE PROCESSES

There is direct evidence to support the idea that yoga can help to repair these processes. Many studies have investigated the effects of yoga on brain wave activity, with two recent reviews arriving at the same conclusion: ***yoga, pranayama (breathing), and meditation practices enhance overall brain wave activity and are correlated with improvements in various cognitive functions, mood, and anxiety*** (De and Mondal 2020; Desai, Tailor, and Bhatt 2015). An increase in alpha power during meditative states is a particularly common finding in these studies (Cahn and Polich 2006; van Lutterveld *et al.* 2017).

In Kamei *et al.*'s (2000) EEG study, experienced yoga practitioners exhibited increased alpha power in the frontal areas, suggesting that yoga improved the inhibitory mechanisms in the brain. Kerr *et al.* (2013) discussed alpha rhythms in the context of a theoretical framework to explain the effectiveness of standardized traditional mindfulness practices (specifically mindfulness-based stress reduction [MBSR] and mindfulness-based cognitive therapy [MBCT]). They proposed that the somatic focus of the practices, especially the Body Scan meditations, helps to modulate the local alpha rhythm in the primary sensory cortex through attention to bodily sensation (subtle changes in tactile and interoceptive feedback) which then "bootstraps to other thalamic-cortical circuits" (2000, p.3) to enhance filtering and prioritization of information flow throughout the brain.

To provide some added context, when attention is externally directed to what is going on in the environment, the magnitude of alpha waves decreases, which is believed to reflect cortical excitability. Conversely, when attention is directed internally, such as when retaining the thread of working memory, alpha waves increase, which decreases excitability in the areas of the brain that are irrelevant to the task at hand (Bollimunta *et al.* 2011). Focusing on ***bodily sensation*** in particular, such as in the context of a Body Scan or mindful movement, could be especially powerful in generating alpha rhythms due to the activation of the sensory cortex. This is because ***the sensory cortex has been found to be a particularly strong cortical generator of alpha waves*** (Bollimunta *et al.* 2011).

Research suggests that yoga can increase levels of GABA, a neurotransmitter involved in the generation of alpha rhythms in the brain. Streeter and colleagues conducted studies showing that thalamic GABA levels increased significantly after yoga compared to reading (2007) or walking (2010). They also found that 90 minutes of Iyengar yoga and coherent breathing, plus homework, reduced depression and increased GABA levels in people with MDD (Streeter *et al.* 2020). The team also compared two of their studies with very similar interventions and found thalamic GABA levels normalized in the MDD group (Streeter *et al.* 2018). Symptoms of depression also decreased significantly in the MDD group while anxiety decreased in both groups. However, in at least one of their studies, they discovered the GABA benefits disappeared after eight days, suggesting that regular yoga practice may be necessary to maintain the effects (Streeter *et al.* 2020).

To summarize, we discussed how alpha rhythms and GABA levels reflect sensory filtering in the brain, and how increasing GABA and (related) alpha brain waves may thus promote healing from trauma and other related conditions. In addition, we presented evidence that yoga or mindfulness can strengthen GABA and alpha rhythms. Alpha rhythms support cortical networks and orchestrate long-range communications between them (Clancy 2017). By modulating alpha rhythms, we may improve regulation of the major large-scale neural networks, and thus positively influence cognition, emotion, and behavior. Improved functioning of cortical networks enables a person to better focus on sensation, movement, and breath without becoming distracted by irrelevant thoughts, thus promoting embodiment. This creates a positive, upward spiral, which, through yoga and mindfulness-based practices, we can strengthen over time (see Figure 5.2).

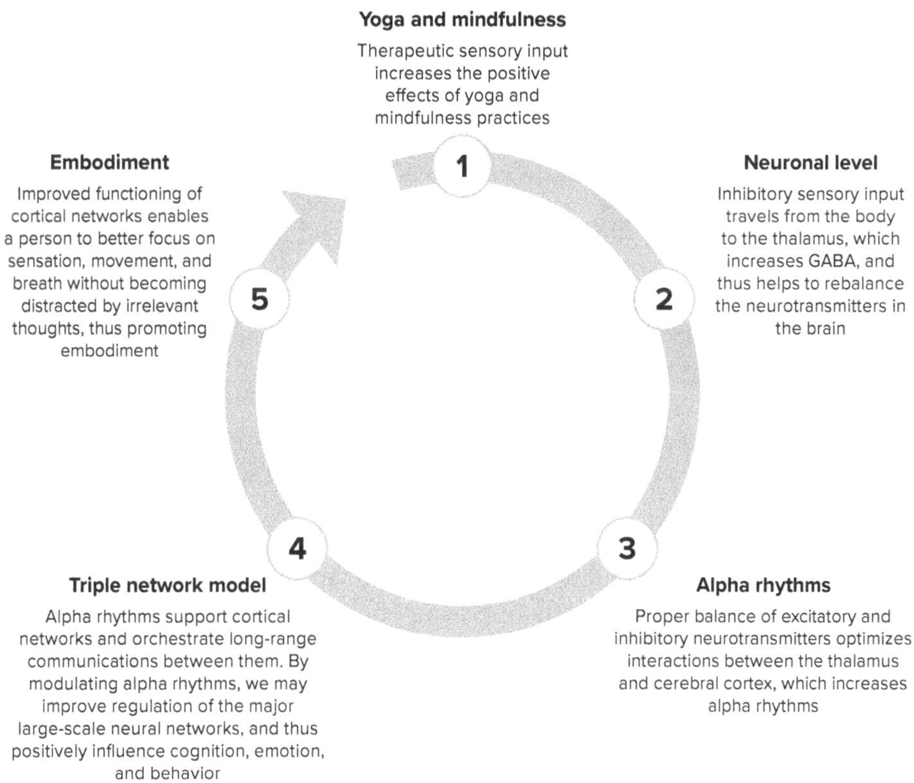

FIGURE 5.2: NEURAL PATH TO EMBODIMENT

Next, we will show how mindfulness-based practices can affect specific brain structures as well as networks. We will finish the chapter by summarizing how we can apply key brain findings (limbic, thalamic, insula, cortical) to yoga and mindfulness-based practices.

COMPARISON OF THE NEUROCIRCUITRY MODEL WITH MINDFULNESS-BASED FINDINGS

Among the first neuroimaging discoveries of mindfulness-based practices was the negative correlation between mindfulness and the early neurocircuitry model of PTSD. Figure 5.3 depicts the early findings regarding brain changes seen in PTSD (**black arrows**) and in mindfulness-based practices (**gray arrows**), illustrating this inverse relationship. Yoga and mindfulness practices were found to bring brain structures more into balance, which led trauma researchers to take a keen interest in their potential role as an adjunct treatment for PTSD (Hölzel *et al.* 2011).

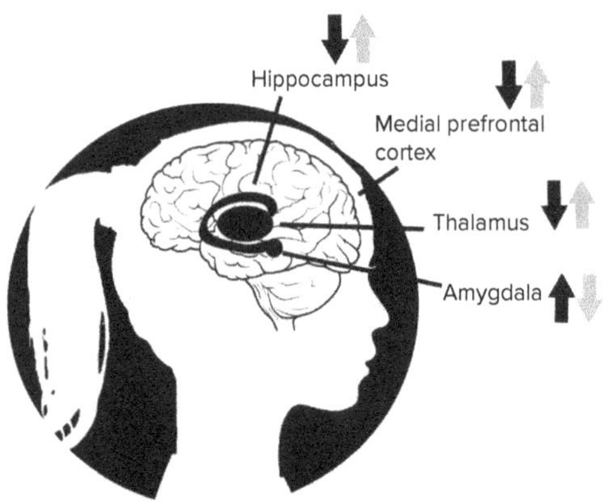

Black arrows represent results of neuroimaging studies of children or adults with histories of early life stress or childhood trauma. Hippocampus changes appear in adulthood.

Gray arrows represent results from neuroimaging studies of adults post yoga or related mindfulness-based practices (e.g., MBSR, which includes yoga).

FIGURE 5.3: SELECTED BRAIN CHANGES IN PTSD AND MINDFULNESS-BASED PRACTICES, THE EARLY FINDINGS

As more brain structures were implicated in PTSD, the two subtypes of hyperarousal/re-experiencing and hypoarousal/dissociation were identified, which are hypothesized to have mostly opposing effects on some brain structures, as previously discussed. In creating a new model (Figure 5.3), we accounted for these two subtypes of PTSD by planting an asterisk next to those brain structures to cue you to swing the black arrow 180 degrees when considering the hypoaroused/dissociated subtype. This model is highly simplified, as it does not distinguish between different parts of structures (which may have different responses) or under what circumstances/in what manner they become activated. Nonetheless, it is remarkable that *most* of the structures currently implicated in *most* studies of PTSD still typically show an *opposite activation pattern* in response to mindfulness-based practices (see Figure 5.4).

We should point out that almost all of these studies were conducted with ***adults***. While preliminary studies on yoga for children have shown many benefits, they typically relied on self-report measures (Hagen and Nayar 2014; Khalsa and Butzer 2016). In fact, there has only been one ***neuroimaging*** study conducted on the effects of mindfulness-based practices in children (Marusak *et al.* 2018), which will be discussed later on as it relates to network functioning, not brain structures.

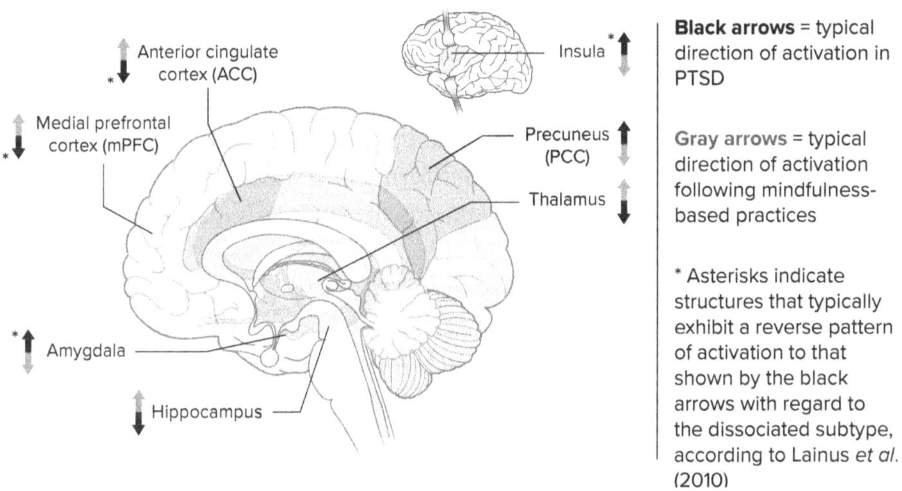

FIGURE 5.4: PTSD AND MINDFULNESS, THE INVERSE RELATIONSHIP
Reproduced from Stoller (2019)

The new brain structure model incorporates almost all of the key anchor structures from the triple network model, but it does not depict changes in functional connectivity between brain structures. Nonetheless, the mere fact of ***the inverse relationship between PTSD and mindfulness states in a multitude of brain structures*** adds strong support to the existing clinical research showing that mindfulness-based practices hold great healing power for PTSD. But not just any mindfulness practice, because the evidence is now pretty clear that, in PTSD, ***the road back to the "here and now" runs through the body***.

As has been stated by Dr. van der Kolk (2008, 2014), and in similar words by many other trauma experts, trauma is held in all cells of the body and must be released by the body for complete healing to occur. Meditation techniques that emphasize attention focusing through top-down cortical control without addressing the body are usually too difficult for those who have PTSD, and can be emotionally overwhelming. Yoga (or another appropriate mind–body modality) is often a necessary "stepping stone" to draw traumatized individuals away from their intrusive thoughts and back into fully sensing bodies and to the "here and now" of present moment awareness.

Table 4.2 from *Sensory-Enhanced Yoga for Self-Regulation and Trauma Healing* (Stoller 2019) presents many of the neuroimaging findings of PTSD related to specific brain structures, followed by findings from neuroimaging studies of mindfulness practices, most of which incorporated at least some yoga. The reader is encouraged to refer to that text for many details that cannot be provided here.

A high percentage of the neuroimaging studies investigated the effectiveness of the eight-week MBSR protocol, which includes a Body Scan, Hatha yoga, and seated meditation, and thus falls within the definition of a yoga program. The ***yoga practice portion*** of MBSR, specifically, was associated with several aspects of mindfulness as well as well-being, perceived stress levels, and several psychological symptoms, in a large participant rating study (Carmody and Baer 2008). Other studies investigated other forms of yoga and meditation, such as Kundalini yoga, Iyengar yoga, Trauma-sensitive Yoga, Vipassana meditation, and Insight meditation.

In full accordance with the Stoller chart (2019, Table 4.2), a recent and thorough review of existing (n=34) international peer-reviewed neuroimaging studies of yoga practitioners ***consistently found increased gray matter volume in the insula and hippocampus and increased activation of regions in the PFC*** (van Aalst *et al.* 2020). Decreases in density and volume of the ***amygdala*** were observed in two of the studies (Gotink *et al.* 2018; Hölzel *et al.* 2010). Van Aalst *et al.* (2020) hypothesized that a smaller amygdala and increased hippocampal volumes could be a result of experiencing less stress due to practicing yoga.

The results of the review provide strong supporting evidence for the idea that it is the full discipline of yoga—asana, breathing techniques, and meditation combined—and not simply one-pointed focus meditation that is the driving force of positive brain changes. The findings also reinforce the wisdom of the ancient yogis, who organized the discipline of yoga around Patanjali's Eight Limbs, which makes very clear that the purpose of asana is to ***prepare*** a person to meditate. Yoga (and the Eight Limbs specifically) would not have lasted for over 2000 years unless there was something to it!

EFFECTS OF MINDFULNESS ON BRAIN NETWORKS IN CHILDREN

We now also have some preliminary information on how mindfulness in children correlates with the large-scale networks. Marusak *et al.* (2018) conducted the only published neuroimaging study thus far of mindfulness in children by evaluating how it relates to the dynamics between the large-scale networks

(DMN, SN, and CEN). The study was conducted with a racially and economically diverse group of 42 children and adolescents. In self-report measures, 40 percent of the participants exceeded thresholds for anxiety; 45 percent for depression; and 62 percent of the total group for anxiety and/or depression. The researchers used an advanced functional magnetic resonance imaging (MRI) imaging technique that looked at dynamic connectivity in addition to conducting static scans that were used in most prior studies.

What is fascinating about this study is that it found that more mindful children demonstrate greater neural flexibility, that is, the ability to switch between different states of mind, involving different networks. The researchers explain their findings as follows:

> Greater neural flexibility associated with mindfulness may protect individuals against getting "stuck in a rut" of repetitive and uncontrollable worry about potential future threats, a hallmark of anxiety. More mindful individuals may be less prone to these anxious cognitions, more aware of or more able to challenge them, or better able to switch to another mode of awareness (e.g., present moment). (Marusak *et al.* 2018, p.10)

Hasenkamp *et al.* (2012) identified four neural states associated with mindful meditation in adults, which helps to make sense of Marusak and colleagues' findings with respect to mindfulness in children. You can easily see from this sequence of mental states how important it is for students to be able to easily switch between different brain networks to pay attention and effectively learn:

- ***Mind-wandering (DMN)***
- ***Attentional awareness of mind-wandering (SN)***
- ***Shift of attention back to present moment (CEN)*** and
- ***Focus on the present moment (CEN).***

When working with children and adolescents, step back for a minute and think about how much time you spend redirecting them to a learning task at hand. Do you help to prepare their entire body and mind to be ***able*** to pay attention, or do you rely on typical top-down strategies, such as "focus on your work?" Do you teach them how to become aware of their own mind wandering, or do your students rely on you to let them know their attention has drifted? Do you help your students sense their body and breath to help bring them back to the "here and now" and draw them away from their daydreams and worries?

Children and adolescents who are dealing with toxic stress, the after-effects of trauma, and/or who have special needs are much more likely to have difficulty switching gears either because their brain networks have not fully developed in the first place or because they are not working properly due to brain chemistry changes. It cannot be overstated how important it is to work at the body level, such as through the practice of yoga, to make lasting changes in the ability to independently draw the mind back to the present moment and to the task at hand.

According to Marusak *et al.* (2018, p.8), their findings suggest that "flexibility in transitioning between neural states bridges the well-established link between higher mindfulness and lower anxiety in children," so if we can help children to reduce their stress levels and relax, it should help to increase their mastery in employing brain network states to match the need of the moment. Supporting this hypothesis, the more mindful participants in the study showed less DMN connectivity with the right and left CEN components, suggesting less mind wandering when trying to attend to a task.

The more developed and separated the networks are, the more they can operate independently of one another to pay attention when necessary or to relax, reflect, or daydream when the time is appropriate. It is when the DMN intrudes on the operation of the CEN that children get stuck in ruminative states of mind, such as being hyperfocused on an upcoming test, whether it is time for lunch or gym yet, or whether their friend is mad at them. We have all experienced these states of mind, but typically can shift out of them at least after a short period of time. In the case of PTSD, it is the trauma itself that becomes stuck in the mind, and it is not uncommon for it to remain there for years (or even a lifetime).

IMPLICATIONS OF BRAIN STUDIES FOR YOGA PRACTICE

The implications of brain studies for children's yoga practice will be discussed based on the results of everything we have presented:

- Neuroimaging research on:
  - The brain effects of PTSD in children and adults
  - The development of brain networks in children
  - The effects of mindfulness-based practices in adults
  - The effects of mindfulness on the brains of children (one study).
- Non-imaging research on yoga and mindfulness conducted with children and adults.

Due to limited information on the effects of mindfulness on children's brain networks, we will organize our discussion primarily according to the brain structures affected by PTSD and mindfulness-based practices, and will infer how the inverse relationship between the two may affect the networks, based on the Marusak *et al.* study just discussed, and mindfulness studies conducted with adults.

Limbic findings

A yoga program carefully designed to reduce hyperarousal may help to repair the destructive neurochemical processes that are responsible for the structural and functional changes in the limbic system (i.e., "emotional brain"). The most powerful means of reducing hyperarousal is through control of the breath, since respiration is typically the only function of the ANS that can be controlled by the conscious mind. Yogic breathing practices have been shown to increase parasympathetic activation and heart rate variability. They are also theorized to improve GABA levels, which can influence brain structures implicated in PTSD to reduce symptoms of the condition (Streeter *et al.* 2012). Preliminary evidence also suggests that quiet, natural breathing actively promotes synchronous electrical brain rhythms in limbic areas, and may thus improve information processing in higher cortical brain areas (Zelano *et al.* 2016).

However, voluntarily controlling the breath can sometimes be challenging if the individual is in an acutely stressed state; combining breathwork with sensorimotor input can often be more accessible and particularly powerful—such as by coordinating simple movements with the breath. Carefully chosen sensory input (e.g., deep touch pressure, enhanced proprioceptive input, slow rhythmic movements, neutral warmth) within the context of yoga is theorized to significantly reduce hyperarousal by enhancing inhibitory mechanisms within the brainstem and thalamus. This, in turn, should help to normalize (reduce) the amount of sensory input reaching the amygdala and higher cortical centers, including the insular, sensory, and visual cortices, thereby reducing hypervigilance and sensory hypersensitivities, which drive hyperarousal. Through this process, the SN becomes disentangled from the DMN (resting state) and CEN (working state), thus helping to draw the mind back to the present moment.

Thalamic findings

The thalamus is the last relay station before sensory input reaches the higher cortical levels, and also plays a large role in orchestrating connectivity within and between brain regions (Hwang *et al.* 2017; Nakajima and Halassa 2017). It is not only important for vertical integration (between lower and higher brain centers), but also for horizontal integration of information between the two hemispheres of the brain. Although horizontal integration occurs at the level of the corpus callosum, the information must pass through the thalamus first (Lanius *et al.* 2014). Therefore, the thalamus needs to function properly for higher brain centers to effectively process information and do their jobs. As discussed in this chapter, alpha waves likely reflect inhibitory neural processes (usually involving

GABA as a transmitter), and are generated by cortico–thalamic interactions, so manipulating thalamic functioning via carefully controlled therapeutic sensory input may conceivably help to correct imbalances between excitatory and inhibitory mechanisms within brain structures and between global brain networks. Furthermore, when therapeutic sensory input is presented within the context of enhanced mindfulness to sensation, such as within Sensory-Enhanced Yoga®/SMYLE™, the therapeutic effects are accentuated through the combination of both bottom-up and top-down processes of integration. Finally, the thalamic link between the mPFC and hippocampus is crucial for the consolidation of memories into long-term storage, so improving function of the thalamus may conceivably facilitate the consolidation of fragmented traumatic memories into a cohesive whole "story" that can be appropriately filed into long-term memory.

Insula findings

Yoga practices that help traumatized individuals befriend their bodies can be expected to be particularly helpful for healing PTSD (van der Kolk 2008, 2014). Lanius *et al.* (2015) hypothesized that Body Scan meditations in particular, which are designed to increase interoceptive awareness (a primary role of the insula), could be especially beneficial for those who tend toward hypoarousal/dissociation; however, they caution that Body Scans need to be carried out in a trauma-sensitive manner so the individual does not become overwhelmed by the Body Scan practice. They hypothesize that there may be greater potential for this occurring in some individuals who demonstrate the hyperaroused subtype of PTSD.

Villemure and colleagues (2014) found in their study of the effect of yoga on pain that half of the treatment participants thought regular practice would increase *awareness* but also *tolerance* of pain, make the pain more neutral, and/or reduce reactivity to it, thus allowing more control over it. Gard and colleagues apparently agreed, explaining, "Mindfulness practice encourages practitioners to take a meta-cognitive view of their experience, to notice the experience without judging it or modifying it and is thus a form of self-regulation" (2014, p.7). They explained that yoga allows one to practice mindfulness in this manner, described as "witness consciousness."

In our own professional experience, Body Scans can help a person shift from an externally to a more internally oriented focus, thereby reducing hypervigilance to external stimuli. As mentioned in Chapter 2, traumatized individuals may be more oriented to external (environmental) or internal (bodily) cues depending on the nature of the trauma, so their experience of Body Scans may vary accordingly. Be observant and seek feedback from your students regarding their own experience. If any of your students has difficulty accessing a Body Scan, you might try having them coordinate simple movements with the breath, which can help quiet the mind so they can more easily focus on their breath and sensations they are experiencing.

Cortical findings

Yoga is a powerful mind–body discipline shown to help draw a person back into the **present moment**. This process involves activation of the PFC, which is often deactivated by trauma. The PFC also plays a large role in **top-down** processing, that is, it can powerfully regulate lower-level brain structures including the amygdala. Sensory-Enhanced Yoga®/SMYLE™ promotes "bottom-up" activation of the PFC, and simultaneously capitalizes on it using "top-down" strategies including positive suggestions and guided meditations, making the practice that much more powerful.

The imbalances often seen in the left and right hemispheres of individuals who have PTSD or related conditions may conceivably correct themselves in the process, since the enhanced inhibitory mechanisms (GABA/alpha power) generated by a carefully designed yoga program should help to disentangle the major brain networks. Thus, intrusive thoughts and memories (generated by a hyperactive right hemisphere) should interfere less often with working memory processes (in the left hemisphere). Luders *et al.* (2012) found thicker corpus callosum regions in meditators, supporting the idea that mindfulness may improve interhemispheric integration.

We now know that the human brain is highly plastic and changes in response to everything we say, do, feel, and experience. As fast as brain researchers are adding to the empirical knowledge base regarding how the brain works, therapists in the helping professions are learning how to manipulate brain processes to promote healing from a variety of conditions. Unfortunately, PTSD is one of the more debilitating mental health conditions and can affect the brain like a sledgehammer, while certain mindfulness-based practices, including yoga, can exert a highly positive influence on many of the same brain structures affected by PTSD. This points to the huge potential mindfulness-based practices hold for addressing this condition as well as related health conditions such as anxiety, attention deficit disorder, MDD, and bipolar disorder, which share some overlapping symptoms and neuropathology. We will discuss how to harness this potential in the chapters ahead.

References for Part 1

CHAPTER 1

Burke Harris, N. (2018) *The Deepest Well: Healing the Long-Term Effects of Childhood Adversity*. Boston, MA: Houghton Mifflin Harcourt.

Butzer, B., Bury, D., Telles, S., and Khalsa, S.B.S. (2016) "Implementing yoga within the school curriculum: A scientific rationale for improving social-emotional learning and positive student outcomes." *Journal of Children's Services 11*, 1, 3–24. doi: 10.1108/JCS-10-2014-0044.

Folleto, J.C., Pereira, K.R., and Valentini, N.C. (2016) "The effects of yoga practice in school physical education on children's motor abilities and social behavior." *International Journal of Yoga 9*, 2, 156–162. doi: 10.4103/0973-6131.183717.

Galantino, M.L., Galbavy, R., and Quinn, L. (2008) "Therapeutic effects of yoga for children: A systematic review of the literature." *Pediatric Physical Therapy 20*, 1, 66–80. doi: 10.1097/PEP.0b013e31815f1208.

Kessler, R.C., Petukhova, M., Sampson, N.A., Zaslavsky, A.M., and Wittchen, H.-U. (2012) "Twelve-month and lifetime prevalence and lifetime morbid risk of anxiety and mood disorders in the United States." *International Journal of Methods in Psychiatric Research 21*, 3, 169–184. https://doi.org/10.1002/mpr.1359

Khalsa, S.B.S., Cohen, L., McCall, T., and Telles, S. (2016) *The Principles and Practice of Yoga in Health Care*. Pencaitland: Handspring Publishing Limited.

Lewis, S.J., Arseneault, L., Caspi, A., Fisher, H.L., *et al.* (2019) "The epidemiology of trauma and post-traumatic stress disorder in a representative cohort of young people in England and Wales." *The Lancet. Psychiatry 6*, 3, 247–256. https://doi.org/10.1016/S2215-0366(19)30031-8

Miller, S., Mendelson, T., Lee-Winn, A., Dyer, N.L., and Khalsa, S.B.S. (2020) "Systematic review of randomized controlled trials testing the effects of yoga with youth." *Mindfulness 11*, 6, 1336–1353. https://doi.org/10.1007/s12671-019-01230-7

Nilsoge, D., Bagade, A., Tumbigeremutt, V., Kulkarni, P., *et al.* (2016) "Evaluation of attention and verbal memory in yoga practicing pre-adolescents: A cross-sectional study." *Journal of Restorative Medicine 5*, 1, 3–13. doi: 10.14200/jrm.2016.5.0112.

Razza, R.A., Bergen-Cico, D., and Raymond, K. (2013) "Enhancing preschoolers' self-regulation via mindful yoga." *Journal of Child and Family Studies 24*, 2, 372–385. doi: 10.1007/S10826-013-9847-6.

Rosenberg, M. (2018) "Reducing Anxiety in Elementary School Children by Implementing Yoga." The Eleanor Mann School of Nursing Undergraduate Honors Theses. http://scholarworks.uark.edu/nursuht/66

SAMHSA (Substance Abuse and Mental Health Services Administration) (2023) "Understanding child trauma." March 17. www.samhsa.gov/child-trauma/understanding-child-trauma

Triggle, N. (2021) "Covid: The devastating toll of the pandemic on children." BBC News, January 30. www.bbc.com/news/health-55863841

CHAPTER 2

Algoe, S.B., Kurtz, L.E., and Grewen, K. (2017) "Oxytocin and social bonds: The role of oxytocin in perceptions of romantic partners' bonding behavior." *Psychological Science 28*, 12, 1763–1772. https://doi.org/10.1177/0956797617716922

American Academy of Pediatrics (2016) *Helping Foster and Adoptive Parents Cope with Trauma.* Itasca, IL: American Academy of Pediatrics. https://downloads.aap.org/AAP/PDF/Foster%20Care/hfca_foster_trauma_guide.pdf

American Institute of Stress, The (2020) "What is stress?" www.stress.org/what-is-stress

American Psychological Association (2020) *Stress in America™ 2020: A National Mental Health Crisis.* Washington, DC: American Psychological Association. www.apa.org/news/press/releases/stress/2020/report-october

Arnsten, A.F., Raskind, M.A., Taylor, F.B., and Connor, D.F. (2015) "The effects of stress exposure on prefrontal cortex: Translating basic research into successful treatments for post-traumatic stress disorder." *Neurobiology of Stress 1*, 89–99. https://doi.org/10.1016/j.ynstr.2014.10.002

Barker, D.P. (1995) "Fetal origins of coronary heart disease." *BMJ 311*, 171. https://doi.org/10.1136/bmj.311.6998.171

BBC News (2019) "World is angry and stressed, Gallup report says." April 26. www.bbc.com/news/world-48063982

Bremner, J.D. (1999) "Does stress damage the brain?" *Biological Psychiatry 45*, 7, 797–805. https://doi.org/10.1016/s0006-3223(99)00009-8

Burke Harris, N. (2014) "How childhood trauma affects health across a lifetime." TED Talk. www.ted.com/talks/nadine_burke_harris_how_childhood_trauma_affects_health_across_a_lifetime/transcript?language=en

Burke Harris, N. (2019) *The Deepest Well: Healing the Long-Term Effects of Childhood Adversity.* San Francisco, CA: HMH Books.

Center on the Developing Child, Harvard University (no date-a) "Toxic stress." https://developingchild.harvard.edu/science/key-concepts/toxic-stress

Center on the Developing Child, Harvard University (no date-b) "Resilience." https://developingchild.harvard.edu/science/key-concepts/resilience

Cooper, O., Bonert, V., Moser, F., Mirocha, J., and Melmed, S. (2017) "Altered pituitary gland structure and function in posttraumatic stress disorder." *Journal of the Endocrine Society 1*, 6, 577–587. https://doi.org/10.1210/js.2017-00069

Donadon, M.F., Martin-Santos, R., and Osório, F.L. (2018) "The associations between oxytocin and trauma in humans: A systematic review." *Frontiers in Pharmacology 9*, 154. https://doi.org/10.3389/fphar.2018.00154

Franke, H.A. (2014) "Toxic stress: Effects, prevention and treatment." *Children 1*, 3, 390–402. https://doi.org/10.3390/children1030390

Herman, J.P. (2013) "Neural control of chronic stress adaptation." *Frontiers in Behavioral Neuroscience 7*, 61. https://doi.org/10.3389/fnbeh.2013.00061

Herman, J.P., McKlveen, J.M., Ghosal, S., Kopp, B., *et al.* (2016) "Regulation of the hypothalamic-pituitary-adrenocortical stress response." *Comprehensive Physiology 6*, 2, 603–621. https://doi.org/10.1002/cphy.c150015

Hopper, J.W., Frewen, P.A., van der Kolk, B.A., and Lanius, R.A. (2007) "Neural correlates of reexperiencing, avoidance, and dissociation in PTSD: Symptom dimensions and emotion dysregulation in responses to script-driven trauma imagery." *Journal of Traumatic Stress 20*, 5, 713–725. doi: 10.1002/jts.20284.

James-Palmer, A., Anderson, E.Z., Zucker, L., Kofman, Y., and Daneault, J.-F. (2020) "Yoga as an intervention for the reduction of symptoms of anxiety and depression in children and adolescents: A systematic review." *Frontiers in Pediatrics 8*. doi: 10.3389/fped.2020.00078.

Jänig, W. (2006) *Integrative Action of the Autonomic Nervous System: Neurobiology of Homeostasis*. Cambridge: Cambridge University Press. doi: 10.1017/CBO9780511541667.

Lanius, R.A., Bluhm, R., Lanius, U., and Pain, C. (2006) "A review of neuroimaging studies in PTSD: Heterogeneity of response to symptom provocation." *Journal of Psychiatric Research 40*, 709–729. doi: 10.1016/j.jpsychires.2005.07.007.

Lanius, R.A., Frewen, P.A., Vermetten, E., and Yehuda, R. (2010) "Fear conditioning and early life vulnerabilities: Two distinct pathways of emotional dysregulation and brain dysfunction in PTSD." *European Journal of Psychotraumatology 1*, 1. https://doi.org/10.3402/ejpt.v1i0.5467

Levine, P.A. (1997) *Waking the Tiger: Healing Trauma*. Berkeley, CA: North Atlantic Books.

McCorry, L.K. (2007) "Physiology of the autonomic nervous system." *American Journal of Pharmaceutical Education 71*, 4, 78. doi: 10.5688/aj710478.

McEwen, B.S. (2008) "Understanding the potency of stressful early life experiences on brain and body function." *Metabolism: Clinical and Experimental 57*, Suppl. 2, S11–S15. https://doi.org/10.1016/j.metabol.2008.07.006

Middlebrooks, J.S. and Audage, N.C. (2008) *The Effects of Childhood Stress on Health Across the Lifespan*. Atlanta, GA: Centers for Disease Control and Prevention, National Center for Injury Prevention and Control. https://stacks.cdc.gov/view/cdc/6978

Nappa, A. (2016) "Emotional regulation and executive function skills: A powerful link." Beyond Booksmart Blog, September 6. www.beyondbooksmart.com/executive-functioning-strategies-blog/emotional-regulation-and-executive-function-skills-a-powerful-link

National Scientific Council on the Developing Child (2005) *Excessive Stress Disrupts the Architecture of the Developing Brain*. Working Paper 3. Cambridge, MA: Center on the Developing Child, Harvard University. https://edn.ne.gov/cms/sites/default/files/u1/pdf/se05SE2%20Stress%20Disrupts%20Architecture%20Dev%20Brain%203.pdf

National Scientific Council on the Developing Child (2015) *Supportive Relationships and Active Skill-Building Strengthen the Foundations of Resilience*, Working Paper 13. Cambridge, MA: Center on the Developing Child, Harvard University. https://developingchild.harvard.edu/wp-content/uploads/2015/05/The-Science-of-Resilience.pdf

NIH (National Center for Complementary and Integrative Health) (2020) "Stress." www.nccih.nih.gov/health/stress

NIH (no date) "I'm so stressed out! Fact sheet." www.nimh.nih.gov/sites/default/files/documents/health/publications/stress/19-mh-8109-5-things-stress.pdf

Ogle, C.M., Rubin, D.C., and Siegler, I.C. (2015) "The relation between insecure attachment and posttraumatic stress: Early life versus adulthood traumas." *Psychological Trauma: Theory, Research, Practice and Policy 7*, 4, 324–332. https://doi.org/10.1037/tra0000015

Pascoe, M.C., Thompson, D.R., and Ski, C.F. (2017) "Yoga, mindfulness-based stress reduction and stress-related physiological measures: A meta-analysis." *Psychoneuroendocrinology 86*, 152–168. https://doi.org/10.1016/j.psyneuen.2017.08.008

Phillips, D.A., Hutchinson, J., Martin, A., Castle, S., and Johnson, A.D. (2022) "First do no harm: How teachers support or undermine children's self-regulation." *Science Direct 59*, 172–185. https://doi.org/10.1016/j.ecresq.2021.12.001

Porges, S.W. (2011) *The Polyvagal Theory: Neurophysiological Foundations of Emotions, Attachment, Communication, and Self-Regulation*. New York: W.W. Norton & Company.

Rainville, P., Bechara, A., Naqvi, N., and Damasio, A.R. (2006) "Basic emotions are associated with distinct patterns of cardiorespiratory activity." *International Journal of Psychophysiology 61*, 1, 5–18. https://doi.org/10.1016/j.ijpsycho.2005.10.024

Rajkumar, R.P. (2020) "Rapid Response, Re: Risks to children and young people during Covid-19 pandemic." *BMJ* 369, m1669, May 2. www.bmj.com/content/369/bmj.m1669/rapid-responses

Rogers, H.L. (2016) "Heart disease and the stress hypothesis in the mid-twentieth century: A historical review." *Psicologia: Reflexão e Crítica 29*, 47. https://dx.doi.org/10.1186/s41155-016-0053-5
Shenk, C.E. and Fruzzetti, A.E. (2011) "The impact of validating and invalidating responses on emotional reactivity." *Journal of Social and Clinical Psychology 30*, 2, 163–183. https://doi.org/10.1521/jscp.2011.30.2.163
Sherin, J.E. and Nemeroff, C.B. (2011) "Post-traumatic stress disorder: The neurobiological impact of psychological trauma." *Dialogues in Clinical Neuroscience 13*, 3, 263–278. doi: 10.31887/DCNS.2011.13.2/jsherin.
Siegel, D.J. (1999) *The Developing Mind: Toward a Neurobiology of Interpersonal Experience.* New York: Guilford Press.
Stoller, L. (2019) *Sensory-Enhanced Yoga for Self-Regulation and Trauma Healing.* Pencaitland: Handspring Publishing Limited.
Tan, S.Y. and Yip, A. (2018) "Hans Selye (1907–1982): Founder of the stress theory." *Singapore Medical Journal 59*, 4, 170–171. doi: 10.11622/smedj.2018043
van der Kolk, B.A. (2014) *The Body Keeps the Score: Brain, Mind, and Body in the Healing of Trauma.* New York: Viking (Penguin Random House).
Wadhwa, P.D., Sandman, C.A., and Garite, T.J. (2001) "The neurobiology of stress in human pregnancy: Implications for prematurity and development of the fetal central nervous system." *Progress in Brain Research 133*, 131–142. https://doi.org/10.1016/s0079-6123(01)33010-8
Wilbarger, P. and Wilbarger, J. (1990) "Sensory defensiveness and related social/emotional and neurological problems." Conference, October 13–14, Hartford, CT.
Wilbarger, P. and Wilbarger, J. (1997) *Sensory Defensiveness and Related Social/Emotional and Neurological Problems* [Self-published].
Yehuda, R., Hoge, C.W., McFarlane, A.C., Vermetten, E., *et al.* (2015) "Post-traumatic stress disorder." *Nature Reviews. Disease Primers 1*, 15057, 1–22. https://doi.org/10.1038/nrdp.2015.57

Figure attribution

Figure 2.5: CC BY-SA 3.0, https://commons.wikimedia.org/w/index.php?curid=30465526

CHAPTER 3

Agorastos, A., Pervanidou, P., Chrousos, G.P., and Baker, D.G. (2019) "Developmental trajectories of early life stress and trauma: A narrative review on neurobiological aspects beyond stress system dysregulation." *Frontiers in Psychiatry 10*, 118. doi: 10.3389/fpsyt.2019.00118.
APA (American Psychiatric Association) (2013) *Diagnostic and Statistical Manual of Mental Disorders (DSM-5)* (5th edn). Washington, DC: APA.
Ayres, A.J. (1972) *Sensory Integration and Learning Disorders.* Los Angeles, CA: Western Psychological Services.
Brewin, C.R., Lanius, R.A., Novac, A., Schnyder, U., and Galea, S. (2009) "Reformulating PTSD for DSM-V: Life after Criterion A." *Journal of Traumatic Stress 22*, 5, 366–373. http://dx.doi.org/10.1002/jts.20443
Briere, J. (2002) "Treating Adult Survivors of Severe Childhood Abuse and Neglect: Further Development of an Integrative Model." In J.E.B. Myers, L. Berliner, J. Briere, C.T. Hendrix, C. Jenny, and T.A. Reid (eds) *The APSAC Handbook on Child Maltreatment* (pp.175–203). Washington, DC: Sage Publications, Inc.
Bundy, A., Lane, S., and Murray, E. (2002) *Sensory Integration: Theory and Practice* (2nd edn). Philadelphia, PA: F.A. Davis Company.

Calati, R., Bensassi, I., and Courtet, P. (2017) "The link between dissociation and both suicide attempts and non-suicidal self-injury: Meta-analyses." *Psychiatry Research 251*, 103–114. https://doi.org/10.1016/j.psychres.2017.01.035

Cermak, S.A. and Daunhauer, L.A. (1997) "Sensory processing in the postinstitutionalized child." *The American Journal of Occupational Therapy 51*, 7, 500–507. https://doi.org/10.5014/ajot.51.7.500

Costanzo, M., Jovanovic, T., Norrholm, S.D., Ndiongue, R., Reinhardt, B., and Roy, M.J. (2016) "Psychophysiological investigation of combat veterans with subthreshold post-traumatic stress disorder symptoms." *Military Medicine 181*, 8, 793–802. https://doi.org/10.7205/MILMED-D-14-00671

Dohrenwend, B.P. (2010) "The Stressor Criterion A in Posttraumatic Stress Disorder: Issues, Evidence, and Implications." In H.B. Simpson, R. Lewis-Fernandez, Y. Neria, and F. Schneier (eds) *Anxiety Disorders: Theory, Research and Clinical Perspectives* (pp.216–226). Cambridge: Cambridge University Press.

Haradon, G., Bascom, B., Dragomir, C., and Scripcaru, V. (1994) "Sensory functions of institutionalized Romanian infants: A pilot study." *Occupational Therapy International 1*, 4, 250–260. https://doi.org/10.1002/oti.6150010405

Herman, J.P., Mueller, N.K., and Figueiredo, H. (2004) "Role of GABA and glutamate circuitry in hypothalamo-pituitary-adrenocortical stress integration." *Annals of the New York Academy of Sciences 1018*, 1, 35–45. https://doi.org/10.1196/annals.1296.004

Kendall-Tackett, K.A. (2000) "Physiological correlates of childhood abuse: Chronic hyperarousal in PTSD, depression, and irritable bowel syndrome." *Child Abuse & Neglect 24*, 6, 799–810. https://doi.org/10.1016/s0145-2134(00)00136-8

Koomar, J. (2009) "Trauma and attachment-informed sensory integration assessment and intervention." *Sensory Integration Special Interest Section Quarterly/American Occupational Therapy Association 32*, 4, 1–4.

Lanius, R.A., Frewen, P.A., Vermetten, E., and Yehuda, R. (2010) "Fear conditioning and early life vulnerabilities: Two distinct pathways of emotional dysregulation and brain dysfunction in PTSD." *European Journal of Psychotraumatology 1*, 1. https://doi.org/10.3402/ejpt.v1i0.5467

Lin, S., Cermak, S., Coster, W., and Miller, L. (2005) "The relation between length of institutionalization and sensory integration in children adopted from Eastern Europe." *American Journal of Occupational Therapy 59*, 2, 139–147. https://doi.org/10.5014/ajot.59.2.139

Newport, D.J. and Nemeroff, C.B. (2000) "Neurobiology of post traumatic stress disorder." *Current Opinions in Neurobiology 10*, 211–218.

Roberts, A.L., Dohrenwend, B.P., Aiello, A., Wright, R.J., *et al.* (2012) "The stressor criterion for posttraumatic stress disorder: Does it matter?" *The Journal of Clinical Psychiatry 73*, 2, e264–e270. http://doi.org/10.4088/JCP.11m07054

Robinson, C. and Brown, A.M. (2016) "Considering sensory processing issues in trauma affected children: The physical environment in children's residential homes." *Scottish Journal of Residential Child Care 15*, 1, 6–18. www.celcis.org/application/files/8316/2308/6835/002._2016_Vol_15_1_Robinson_Considering_Sensory_Processing.pdf

Rothschild, B. (1997) "Post-traumatic stress disorder: Identification and diagnosis." *Soziale Arbeit Schweiz (The Swiss Journal of Social Work)*. www.healing-arts.org/tir/n-r-rothschild.htm

Rothschild, B. (2000) *The Body Remembers: The Psychophysiology of Trauma and Trauma Treatment*. New York: W.W. Norton & Company.

Schore, A.N. (2012) *The Science of the Art of Psychotherapy*. New York: W.W. Norton & Company.

Siegel, D. and Buczynski, R. (no date) "Rethinking trauma: How to use brain science to heal after trauma." Main session. National Institute for the Clinical Application of Behavioral Medicine (NICABM) [Seminar transcript]. https://s3.amazonaws.com/nicabm-stealthseminar/Rethinking-trauma-new/Dan/NICABM-DanSiegel_Part5-Transcript2.pdf

Stewart, L.P. and White, P.M. (2008) "Sensory filtering phenomenology in PTSD." *Depression and Anxiety 25*, 1, 38–45. https://doi.org/10.1002/da.20255

Stoller, L. (2019) *Sensory-Enhanced Yoga for Self-Regulation and Trauma Healing*. Pencaitland: Handspring Publishing Limited.

Thayer, J.F. and Lane, R.D. (2000) "A model of neurovisceral integration in emotion regulation and dysregulation." *Journal of Affective Disorders 61*, 3, 201–216. doi: 10.1016/s0165-0327(00)00338-4.

Thayer, J.F. and Lane, R.D. (2009) "Claude Bernard and the heart–brain connection: Further elaboration of a model of neurovisceral integration." *Neuroscience & Biobehavioral Reviews 33*, 2, 81–88. doi: 10.1016/j.neubiorev.2008.08.004.

van der Kolk, B.A. (1997) "The psychology of posttraumatic stress disorder." *Journal of Clinical Psychiatry 58*, 16–24.

van der Kolk, B.A. (2004) "Psychobiology of Posttraumatic Stress Disorder." In J. Panksepp (ed.) *Textbook of Biological Psychiatry* (pp.319–344). New York: Wiley-Liss.

van der Kolk, B.A. (2014) *The Body Keeps the Score: Brain, Mind, and Body in the Healing of Trauma.* New York: Viking (Penguin Random House).

Wilbarger, J., Gunnar, M., Schneider, M., and Pollak, S. (2010) "Sensory processing in internationally adopted, post-institutionalized children." *Journal of Child Psychology and Psychiatry, and Allied Disciplines 51*, 10, 1105–1114. doi: 10.1111/j.1469-7610.2010.02255.x.

Yehuda, R., Hoge, C.W., McFarlane, A.C., Vermetten, E., *et al.* (2015) "Post-traumatic stress disorder." *Nature Reviews. Disease Primers 1*, 15057, 1–22. https://doi.org/10.1038/nrdp.2015.57

CHAPTER 4

Agorastos, A., Pervanidou, P., Chrousos, G.P., and Baker, D.G. (2019) "Developmental trajectories of early life stress and trauma: A narrative review on neurobiological aspects beyond stress system dysregulation." *Frontiers in Psychiatry 10*, 118. doi: 10.3389/fpsyt.2019.00118.

Akiki, T., Averill, C., and Abdallah, C. (2017) "A network-based neurobiological model of PTSD: Evidence from structural and functional neuroimaging studies." *Current Psychiatry Reports 19*, 11, 81. doi: 10.1007/s11920-017-0840-4.

Anda, R.F., Felitti, V.J., Bremner, J.D., Walker, J.D., *et al.* (2006) "The enduring effects of abuse and related adverse experiences in childhood: A convergence of evidence from neurobiology and epidemiology." *European Archives of Psychiatry and Clinical Neuroscience 256*, 3, 174–186. https://doi.org/10.1007/s00406-005-0624-4

Andrewes, D.G. and Jenkins, L.M. (2019) "The role of the amygdala and the ventromedial prefrontal cortex in emotional regulation: Implications for post-traumatic stress disorder." *Neuropsychological Review 29*, 220–243. https://doi.org/10.1007/s11065-019-09398-4

Averill, L.A., Purohit, P., Averill, C.L., Boesl, M.A., Krystal, J.H., and Abdallah, C.G. (2016) "Glutamate dysregulation and glutamatergic therapeutics for PTSD: Evidence from human studies." *Neuroscience Letters 649*, 147–155. doi: 10.1016/j.neulet.2016.11.064.

Ayres, A.J. (1972) *Sensory Integration and Learning Disorders*. Los Angeles, CA: Western Psychological Services.

Bergmann, U. (2008) "The neurobiology of EMDR: Exploring the thalamus and neural integration." *Journal of EMDR Practice and Research 2*, 4, 300–314. http://dx.doi.org/10.1891/1933-3196.2.4.300

Bilimoria, P.M. and Bonni, A. (2013) "Molecular control of axon branching." *The Neuroscientist 19*, 1, 16–24. https://doi.org/10.1177/1073858411426201

Bluhm, R.L., Williamson, P.C., Osuch, E.A., Frewen, P.A., *et al.* (2009) "Alterations in default network connectivity in posttraumatic stress disorder related to early-life trauma." *Journal of Psychiatry & Neuroscience 34*, 3, 187–194.

Bremner, J. (2007) "Neuroimaging in posttraumatic stress disorder and other stress-related disorders." *Neuroimaging Clinics of North America 17*, 4, 523–538. doi: 10.1016/j.nic.2007.07.003.

Bremner, J., Staib, L., Kaloupek, D., Southwick, S., Soufer, R., and Charney, D. (1999) "Neural correlates of exposure to traumatic pictures and sound in Vietnam combat veterans with and without posttraumatic stress disorder: A positron emission tomography study." *Biological Psychiatry 45*, 7, 806–816. https://doi.org/10.1016/S0006-3223(98)00297-2

Bu, X., Gao, X., Liang, K., Chen, Y., Guo, L., and Huang, X. (2022) "Investigation of white matter functional networks underlying different behavioral profiles in attention-deficit/hyperactivity disorder." *Psychoradiology 2*, 3, 69–77. https://doi.org/10.1093/psyrad/kkac012

Coulon, P., Budde, T., and Pape, H.-C. (2012) "The sleep relay—The role of the thalamus in central and decentral sleep regulation." *Pflügers Archiv – European Journal of Physiology 463*, 53–71. https://doi.org/10.1007/s00424-011-1014-6

Courtiol, E. and Wilson, D. (2015) "The olfactory thalamus: Unanswered questions about the role of the mediodorsal thalamic nucleus in olfaction." *Frontiers in Neural Circuits 9*, 49. doi: 10.3389/fncir.2015.00049.

De Bellis, M.D. and Zisk, A. (2014) "The biological effects of childhood trauma." *Child and Adolescent Psychiatric Clinics of North America 23*, 2, 185–222. doi: 10.1016/j.chc.2014.01.002.

Etkin, A. and Wager, T.D. (2007) "Functional neuroimaging of anxiety: A meta-analysis of emotional processing in PTSD, social anxiety disorder, and specific phobia." *American Journal of Psychiatry 164*, 10, 1476–1488. doi: 10.1176/appi.ajp.2007.07030504.

Fanselow, M.S. and Dong, H. (2010) "Are the dorsal and ventral hippocampus functionally distinct structures?" *Neuron 65*, 1, 7–19. doi: 10.1016/j.neuron.2009.11.031.

Flory, J.D. and Yehuda, R. (2015) "Comorbidity between post-traumatic stress disorder and major depressive disorder: Alternative explanations and treatment considerations." *Dialogues in Clinical Neuroscience 17*, 2, 141–150. https://doi.org/10.31887/DCNS.2015.17.2/jflory

Fogel, A. (2009) *Body Sense: The Science and Practice of Embodied Self-Awareness*. New York: W.W. Norton & Company.

Funahashi, S. (2017) "Working memory in the prefrontal cortex." *Brain Sciences 7*, 5, 49. http://doi.org/10.3390/brainsci7050049

Goldman-Rakic, P.S., Selemon, L., and Schwartz, M.L. (1984) "Dual pathways connecting the dorsolateral prefrontal cortex with the hippocampal formation and parahippocampal cortex in the rhesus monkey." *Neuroscience 12*, 3, 719–743. https://doi.org/10.1016/0306-4522(84)90166-0

Gothe, N.P. and McAuley, E. (2015) "Yoga and cognition: A meta-analysis of chronic and acute effects." *Psychosomatic Medicine 77*, 7, 784–797. https://doi.org/10.1097/PSY.0000000000000218

Hare, B.D. and Duman, R.S. (2020) "Prefrontal cortex circuits in depression and anxiety: Contribution of discrete neuronal populations and target regions." *Molecular Psychiatry 25*, 11, 2742–2758. doi: 10.1038/s41380-020-0685-9.

Harricharan, S., Nicholson, A.A., Thome, J., Densmore, M., *et al.* (2020) "PTSD and its dissociative subtype through the lens of the insula: Anterior and posterior insula resting-state functional connectivity and its predictive validity using machine learning." *Psychophysiology 57*, 1, e13472. https://doi.org/10.1111/psyp.13472

Hayes, J.P., Hayes, S.M., and Mikedis, A.M. (2012a) "Quantitative meta-analysis of neural activity in posttraumatic stress disorder." *Biology of Mood & Anxiety Disorders 2*, 9. https://doi.org/10.1186/2045-5380-2-9

Herringa, R.J. (2017) "Trauma, PTSD, and the developing brain." *Current Psychiatry Reports 19*, 10, 69. https://doi.org/10.1007/s11920-017-0825-3

Hopper, J.W., Frewen, P.A., van der Kolk, B.A., and Lanius, R.A. (2007) "Neural correlates of reexperiencing, avoidance, and dissociation in PTSD: Symptom dimensions and emotion dysregulation in responses to script-driven trauma imagery." *Journal of Traumatic Stress 20*, 5, 713–725. doi: 10.1002/jts.20284.

Hwang, K., Bertolero, M.A., Liu, W.B., and D'Esposito, M. (2017) "The human thalamus is an integrative hub for functional brain networks." *Journal of Neuroscience 37*, 23, 5594–5607. doi: 10.1523/JNEUROSCI.0067-17.2017.

Jin, J. and Maren, S. (2015) "Prefrontal-hippocampal interactions in memory and emotion." *Frontiers in Systems Neuroscience 9*, 170. http://doi.org/10.3389/fnsys.2015.00170

Kang, Y., Huang, K., Lin, Y., Xu, H., *et al.* (2020) "Abnormalities of effective connectivity and white matter microstructure in the triple network in patients with schizophrenia." *Psychiatry Research 290*, 113019. https://doi.org/10.1016/j.psychres.2020.113019

Kim, S.J., Lyoo, I.K., Lee, Y.S., Kim, J., *et al.* (2007) "Decreased cerebral blood flow of thalamus in PTSD patients as a strategy to reduce reexperience symptoms." *Acta Psychiatrica Scandinavica 116*, 2, 145–153. https://doi.org/10.1111/j.1600-0447.2006.00952.x

Koomar, J. (2009) "Trauma and attachment-informed sensory integration assessment and intervention." *Sensory Integration Special Interest Section Quarterly/American Occupational Therapy Association 32*, 4, 1–4.

Kuhn, G., Toda, T., and Gage, F.H. (2018) "Adult hippocampal neurogenesis: A coming-of-age story." *Journal of Neuroscience 38*, 49, 10401–10410.

Lanius, R.A., Frewen, P.A., Tursich, M., Jetly, R., and McKinnon, M.C. (2015) "Restoring large-scale brain networks in PTSD: A proposal for neuroscientifically-informed treatment interventions." *European Journal of Psychotraumatology 6*, 27313. doi: 10.3402/ejpt.v6.27313.

Lanius, R.A., Vermetten, E., Loewenstein, R.J., Brand, B., *et al.* (2010) "Emotion modulation in PTSD: Clinical and neurobiological evidence for a dissociative subtype." *American Journal of Psychiatry 167*, 6, 640–647. doi: 10.1176/appi.ajp.2009.09081168.

Lanius, R.A., Williamson, P.C., Bluhm, R.L., Densmore, M., *et al.* (2005) "Functional connectivity of dissociative responses in posttraumatic stress disorder: A functional magnetic resonance imaging investigation." *Biological Psychiatry 57*, 8, 873–884. https://doi.org/10.1016/j.biopsych.2005.01.011

Lanius, R.A., Williamson, P.C., Boksman, K., Densmore, M., *et al.* (2002) "Brain activation during script-driven imagery induced dissociative responses in PTSD: A functional magnetic resonance imaging investigation." *Biological Psychiatry 52*, 4, 305–311. https://doi.org/10.1016/S0006-3223(02)01367-7

Lanius, R.A., Williamson, P.C., Densmore, M., Boksman, K., *et al.* (2001) "Neural correlates of traumatic memories in posttraumatic stress disorder: A functional MRI investigation." *American Journal of Psychiatry 158*, 11, 1920–1922. doi: 10.1176/appi.ajp.158.11.1920.

Lanius, R.A., Williamson, P.C., Hopper, J., Densmore, M., *et al.* (2003) "Recall of emotional states in posttraumatic stress disorder: An fMRI investigation." *Biological Psychiatry 53*, 3, 204–210. https://doi.org/10.1016/s0006-3223(02)01466-x

LeDoux, J. (2015) *Anxious: Using the Brain to Understand and Treat Fear and Anxiety*. New York: Penguin, Random House LLC.

Lei, D., Li, L., Li, L., Suo, X., *et al.* (2015) "Microstructural abnormalities in children with post-traumatic stress disorder: A diffusion tensor imaging study at 3.0T." *Scientific Reports* 5, 8933. doi: 10.1038/srep08933.

Lenroot, R.K. and Giedd, J.N. (2006) "Brain development in children and adolescents: Insights from anatomical magnetic resonance imaging." *Neuroscience & Biobehavioral Reviews 30*, 6, 718–729. doi: 10.1016/j.neubiorev.2006.06.001.

Liu, W., Ge, T., Leng, Y., Pan, Z., *et al.* (2017) "The role of neural plasticity in depression: From hippocampus to prefrontal cortex." *Neural Plasticity* 6871089. doi: 10.1155/2017/6871089.

Madonna, D., Delvecchio, G., Soares, J.C., and Brambilla, P. (2019) "Structural and functional neuroimaging studies in generalized anxiety disorder: A systematic review." *Brazilian Journal of Psychiatry/Revista brasileira de psiquiatria 41*, 4, 336–362. https://doi.org/10.1590/1516-4446-2018-0108

Marsh, R., Gerber, A.J., and Peterson, B.S. (2008) "Neuroimaging studies of normal brain development and their relevance for understanding childhood neuropsychiatric disorders." *Journal of the American Academy of Child and Adolescent Psychiatry 47*, 11, 1233–1251. https://doi.org/10.1097/CHI.0b013e318185e703

McEwen, B.S. (2008) "Understanding the potency of stressful early life experiences on brain and body function." *Metabolism: Clinical and Experimental 57*, Suppl. 2, S11–S15. https://doi.org/10.1016/j.metabol.2008.07.006

Menon, B. (2019) "Towards a new model of understanding—The triple network, psychopathology and the structure of the mind." *Medical Hypotheses 133*, 109385. doi: 10.1016/j.mehy.2019.109385.

Menon, V. (2011) "Large-scale brain networks and psychopathology: A unifying triple network model." *Trends in Cognitive Sciences 15*, 10, 483–506. https://doi.org/10.1016/j.tics.2011.08.003

Menon, V. (2013) "Developmental pathways to functional brain networks: Emerging principles." *Trends in Cognitive Sciences 17*, 12, 627–640. https://doi.org/10.1016/j.tics.2013.09.015

Menon, V. and Uddin, L.Q. (2010) "Saliency, switching, attention and control: A network model of insula function." *Brain Structure & Function 214*, 5–6, 655–667. http://doi.org/10.1007/s00429-010-0262-0

Nakajima, M. and Halassa, M.M. (2017) "Thalamic control of functional cortical connectivity." *Current Opinion in Neurobiology 44*, 127–131. https://doi.org/10.1016/j.conb.2017.04.001

Paivio, S.C. and McCulloch, C.R. (2004) "Alexithymia as a mediator between childhood trauma and self-injurious behaviors." *Child Abuse & Neglect 28*, 3, 339–354. https://doi.org/10.1016/j.chiabu.2003.11.018

Patel, R., Spreng, R.N., Shin, L.M., and Girard, T.A. (2012) "Neurocircuitry models of posttraumatic stress disorder and beyond: A meta-analysis of functional neuroimaging studies." *Neuroscience & Biobehavioral Reviews 36*, 9, 2130–2142. doi: 10.1016/j.neubiorev.2012.06.003.

Patriquin, M.A. and Mathew, S.J. (2017) "The neurobiological mechanisms of generalized anxiety disorder and chronic stress." *Chronic Stress 1*, 2470547017703993. doi: 10.1177/2470547017703993.

Philip, N.S., Tyrka, A.R., Albright, S.E., Sweet, L.H., *et al.* (2016) "Early life stress predicts thalamic hyperconnectivity: A transdiagnostic study of global connectivity." *Journal of Psychiatric Research 79*, 93–100. doi: 10.1016/j.jpsychires.2016.05.003.

Quattrini, G., Magni, L.R., Lanfredi, M., Pedrini, L., *et al.* (2022) "Aberrant structural connectivity of the triple network system in borderline personality disorder is associated with behavioral dysregulation." *Journal of Clinical Medicine 11*, 7, 1757. http://dx.doi.org/10.3390/jcm11071757

Radley, J.J. and Sawchenko, P.E. (2011) "A common substrate for prefrontal and hippocampal inhibition of the neuroendocrine stress response." *The Journal of Neuroscience 31*, 26, 9683–9695. https://doi.org/10.1523/JNEUROSCI.6040-10.2011

Rauch, S.L., Shin, L.M., and Phelps, E.A. (2006) "Neurocircuitry models of posttraumatic stress disorder and extinction: Human neuroimaging research—past, present, and future." *Biological Psychiatry 60*, 4, 376–382. https://doi.org/10.1016/j.biopsych.2006.06.004

Riccomagno, M.M. and Kolodkin, A.L. (2015) "Sculpting neural circuits by axon and dendrite pruning." *Annual Review of Cell and Developmental Biology 31*, 779–805. https://doi.org/10.1146/annurev-cellbio-100913-013038

Rinne-Albers, M.A., van der Wee, N.J., Lamers-Winkelman, F., and Vermeiren, R.R. (2013) "Neuroimaging in children, adolescents and young adults with psychological trauma." *European Child & Adolescent Psychiatry 22*, 12, 745–755. https://doi.org/10.1007/s00787-013-0410-1

Roxo, M.R., Franceschini, P.R., Zubaran, C., Kleber, F.D., and Sander, J.W. (2011) "The limbic system conception and its historical evolution." *The Scientific World Journal 11*, 2428–2441. http://doi.org/10.1100/2011/157150

Roy, A. (2005) "Reported childhood trauma and suicide attempts in schizophrenic patients." *Suicide and Life-Threatening Behavior 35*, 6, 690–693. https://doi.org/10.1521/suli.2005.35.6.690

Roy, M., Shohamy, D., and Wager, T.D. (2012) "Ventromedial prefrontal-subcortical systems and the generation of affective meaning." *Trends in Cognitive Sciences 16*, 3, 147–156. http://doi.org/10.1016/j.tics.2012.01.005

Saalmann, Y.B. and Kastner, S. (2015) "The cognitive thalamus." *Frontiers in Systems Neuroscience 9*, 39. https://doi.org/10.3389/fnsys.2015.00039

Sakai, J. (2020) "Core concepts: How synaptic pruning shapes neural wiring during development and, possibly, in disease." *Proceedings of the National Academy of Sciences of the United States of America 117*, 28, 16096–16099. https://doi.org/10.1073/pnas.2010281117

Seeley, W.W., Menon, V., Schatzberg, A.F., Keller, J., *et al.* (2007) "Dissociable intrinsic connectivity networks for salience processing and executive control." *The Journal of Neuroscience 27*, 9, 2349–2356. http://doi.org/10.1523/JNEUROSCI.5587-06.2007

Shaw, S.B., McKinnon, M.C., Heisz, J., and Becker, S. (2021) "Dynamic task-linked switching between brain networks - A tri-network perspective." *Brain and Cognition 151*, 105725. https://doi.org/10.1016/j.bandc.2021.105725

Shin, L.M. and Liberzon, I. (2010) "The neurocircuitry of fear, stress, and anxiety disorders." *Neuropsychopharmacology 35*, 1, 169–191. doi: 10.1038/npp.2009.83.

Shin, L.M., Rauch, S.L., and Pitman, R.K. (2005) "Structural and Functional Anatomy of PTSD." In B. Vasterling (ed.) *Neuropsychology of PTSD* (Chapter 3). New York: Guilford Press.

Shin, L.M., Rauch S.L., and Pitman, R.K. (2006) "Amygdala, medial prefrontal cortex, and hippocampal function in PTSD." *Annals of the New York Academy of Sciences 1071*, 67–79. https://doi.org/10.1196/annals.1364.007

Shonkoff, J.P. and Phillips, D.A. (eds) (2000) *The Science of Early Childhood Development*. Washington, DC: National Research Council and Institute of Medicine, National Academy Press.

Siehl, S., King, J.A., Burgess, N., Flor, H., and Nees, F. (2018) "Structural white matter changes in adults and children with posttraumatic stress disorder: A systematic review and meta-analysis." *NeuroImage. Clinical 19*, 581–598. doi: 10.1016/j.nicl.2018.05.013.

Sripada, R.K., King, A.P., Welsh, R.C., Garfinkel, S.N., *et al.* (2012) "Neural dysregulation in posttraumatic stress disorder: Evidence for disrupted equilibrium between salience and default mode brain networks." *Psychosomatic Medicine 74*, 9, 904–911. http://doi.org/10.1097/PSY.0b013e318273bf33

Sridharan, D., Levitin, D.J., and Menon, V. (2008) "A critical role for the right fronto-insular cortex in switching between central-executive and default-mode networks." *Proceedings of the National Academy of Sciences of the United States of America 105*, 34, 12569–12574. doi: 10.1073/pnas.0800005105.

Stark, E.A., Parsons, C.E., Van Hartevelt, T.J., Charquero-Ballester, M., *et al.* (2015) "Post-traumatic stress influences the brain even in the absence of symptoms: A systematic, quantitative meta-analysis of neuroimaging studies." *Neuroscience & Biobehavioral Reviews 56*, 207–221. https://doi.org/10.1016/j.neubiorev.2015.07.007

Stephens, M.A. and Wand, G. (2012) "Stress and the HPA axis." *Alcohol Research 34*, 4, 468–483.

Stoller, L. (2019) *Sensory-Enhanced Yoga for Self-Regulation and Trauma Healing.* Pencaitland: Handspring Publishing Limited.

Thompson, P.M., Giedd, J.N., Woods, R.P., MacDonald, D., Evans, A.C., and Toga, A.W. (2000) "Growth patterns in the developing brain detected by using continuum mechanical tensor maps." *Nature 404*, 6774, 190–193. doi: 10.1038/35004593.

Toga, A.W., Thompson, P.M., and Sowell, E.R. (2006) "Mapping brain maturation." *Trends in Neurosciences 29*, 3, 148–159. https://doi.org/10.1016/j.tins.2006.01.007

Torre, J.B. and Lieberman, M.D. (2018) "Putting feelings into words: Affect labeling as implicit emotion regulation." *Emotion Review 10*, 2, 116–124. https://doi.org/10.1177/1754073917742706

TUM (Technical University of Munich) (2016) "Sensory function: Thalamus enhances, stores sensory information: Important brain network for processing sensory perceptions elucidated." *ScienceDaily*, January 21. www.sciencedaily.com/releases/2016/01/160121110929.htm

Tyborowska, A., Volman, I., Niermann, H., Pouwels, J.L., *et al.* (2018) "Early-life and pubertal stress differentially modulate grey matter development in human adolescents." *Scientific Reports 8*, 1, 9201. doi: 10.1038/s41598-018-27439-5.

van der Kolk, B.A. (2014) *The Body Keeps the Score: Brain, Mind, and Body in the Healing of Trauma*. New York: Viking (Penguin Random House).

van der Kolk, B.A., Perry, C., and Herman, J.L. (1991) "Childhood origins of self-destructive behavior." *The American Journal of Psychiatry 148*, 12, 1665–1671. doi: 10.1176/ajp.148.12.1665.

van der Werff, S.J.A., van den Berg, S.M., Pannekoek, J.N., Elzinga, B.M., and van der Wee, N.J.A. (2013) "Neuroimaging resilience to stress: A review." *Frontiers in Behavioral Neuroscience 7*, 39. http://doi.org/10.3389/fnbeh.2013.00039

VanElzakker, M.B., Dahlgren, M.K., Davis, F.C., Dubois, S., and Shin, L.M. (2014) "From Pavlov to PTSD: The extinction of conditioned fear in rodents, humans, and in anxiety disorders." *Neurobiology of Learning and Memory 113*, 3–18. http://doi.org/10.1016/j.nlm.2013.11.014

Wang, X., Wu, Q., Egan, L., Gu, X., *et al.* (2019) "Anterior insular cortex plays a critical role in interoceptive attention." *eLife 8*, e42265. https://doi.org/10.7554/eLife.42265

Wijesinghe, R., Protti, D.A., and Camp, A.J. (2015) "Vestibular interactions in the thalamus." *Frontiers in Neural Circuits 9*, 79. http://doi.org/10.3389/fncir.2015.00079

Wimmer, R.D., Schmitt, L.I., Davidson, T.J., Nakajima, M., Deisseroth, K., and Halassa, M.M. (2015) "Thalamic control of sensory selection in divided attention." *Nature 526*, 705–709. doi: 10.1038/nature15398.

Xu, J., Chen, F., Lei, D., Zhan, W., *et al.* (2018) "Disrupted functional network topology in children and adolescents with post-traumatic stress disorder." *Frontiers in Neuroscience 12*, 709. doi: 10.3389/fnins.2018.00709.

Yehuda, R., Hoge, C.W., McFarlane, A.C., Vermetten, E., *et al.* (2015) "Post-traumatic stress disorder." *Nature Reviews. Disease Primers 1*, 15057, 1–22. https://doi.org/10.1038/nrdp.2015.57

Zeidman, P. and Maguire, E.A. (2016) "Anterior hippocampus: The anatomy of perception, imagination and episodic memory." *Nature Reviews. Neuroscience 17*, 3, 173–182. https://doi.org/10.1038/nrn.2015.24

Figure attributions

Figure 4.2: http://training.seer.cancer.gov/module_anatomy/unit5_3_nerve_org1_cns.html, CC BY-SA 3.0, https://commons.wikimedia.org/w/index.php?curid=29055751

Figure 4.3: This file was derived from: Brain human sagittal section.svg, Brain bulbar region.svg, CC BY-SA 4.0, https://commons.wikimedia.org/w/index.php?curid=85747830

Figure 4.4: Modified version of Basal Ganglia and Related Structures.svg, which, in turn, was based on Brain structure.gif from Henkel, John (July–August 1998). "Parkinsons Disease: New Treatments Slow Onslaught of Symptoms," FDA Consumer: p.17. ISSN 0362-1332. Retrieved on 2009-07-23, Public Domain, https://commons.wikimedia.org/w/index.php?curid=23221891

Figure 4.5: From Anatomography website maintained by Life Science Databases (LSDB), CC BY-SA 2.1 jp, https://commons.wikimedia.org/w/index.php?curid=7762044

Figure 4.6: "Magnetic Resonance Imaging of the Living Brain: Evidence for Brain Degeneration Among Alcoholics and Recovery With Abstinence;" Alcohol Research; Health Volume 31, Number 4 (2008), pp.362–376, Public Domain, https://commons.wikimedia.org/w/index.php?curid=8138147

Figure 4.7a: From Anatomography, website maintained by Life Science Databases (LSDB), CC BY-SA 2.1 jp, https://commons.wikimedia.org/w/index.php?curid=7894800

Figure 4.7b: Polygon data are from BodyParts3D, CC BY-SA 2.1 jp, https://commons.wikimedia.org/w/index.php?curid=32490636

Figure 4.7c: From Anatomography, website maintained by Life Science Databases (LSDB), CC BY-SA 2.1 jp, https://commons.wikimedia.org/w/index.php?curid=7887124

Figure 4.8: From Anatomography, website maintained by Life Science Databases (LSDB), CC BY-SA 2.1 jp, https://commons.wikimedia.org/w/index.php?curid=7845016

Figure 4.11: Bridging disparate symptoms of schizophrenia: a triple network dysfunction theory, CC BY 3.0, https://commons.wikimedia.org/w/index.php?curid=62546913

CHAPTER 5

Abdou, A.M., Higashiguchi, S., Horie, K., Kim, M., Hatta, H., and Yokogoshi, H. (2006) "Relaxation and immunity enhancement effects of gamma-aminobutyric acid (GABA) administration in humans." *BioFactors 26*, 3, 201–208. https://doi.org/10.1002/biof.5520260305

Bollimunta, A., Mo, J., Schroeder, C.E., and Ding, M. (2011) "Neuronal mechanisms and attentional modulation of corticothalamic α oscillations." *The Journal of Neuroscience 31*, 13, 4935–4943. https://doi.org/10.1523/JNEUROSCI.5580-10.2011

Cahn, B.R. and Polich, J. (2006) "Meditation states and traits: EEG, ERP, and neuroimaging studies." *Psychological Bulletin 132*, 2, 180–211. doi: 10.1037/0033-2909.132.2.180.

Carmody, J. and Baer, R.A. (2008) "Relationships between mindfulness practice and levels of mindfulness, medical and psychological symptoms and well-being in a mindfulness-based stress reduction program." *Journal of Behavioral Medicine 31*, 1, 23–33. https://doi.org/10.1007/s10865-007-9130-7

Clancy, K.J. (2017) "Assessing the Clinical Utility of Non-Invasive Brain Stimulation in the Treatment of Anxious Arousal and Sensory Hypersensitivity: A Targeted Transcranial Alternating Current Stimulation Study." Thesis. http://purl.flvc.org/fsu/fd/FSU_FALL2017_Clancy_fsu_0071N_14146

Clancy, K.J., Andrzejewski, J.A., Simon, J., Ding, M., Schmidt, N.B., and Li, W. (2020) "Post-traumatic stress disorder is associated with α dysrhythmia across the visual cortex and the default mode network." *eNeuro 7*, 4. https://doi.org/10.1523/ENEURO.0053-20.2020

Clancy, K.J., Andrzejewski, J.A., You, Y., Rosenberg, J.T., Ding, M., and Li, W. (2022) "Transcranial stimulation of alpha oscillations up-regulates the default mode network." *Proceedings of the National Academy of Sciences of the United States of America 119*, 1, e2110868119. https://doi.org/10.1073/pnas.2110868119

Clancy, K.J., Ding, M., Bernat, E., Schmidt, N.B., and Li, W. (2017) "Restless 'rest': Intrinsic sensory hyperactivity and disinhibition in post-traumatic stress disorder." *Brain 140*, 7, 2041–2050. https://doi.org/10.1093/brain/awx116

De, A. and Mondal, S. (2020) "Yoga and brain wave coherence: A systematic review for brain function improvement." *Heart Mind 4*, 33–39.

Desai, R., Tailor, A., and Bhatt, T. (2015) "Effects of yoga on brain waves and structural activation: A review." *Complementary Therapies in Clinical Practice 21*, 2, 112–118. https://doi.org/10.1016/j.ctcp.2015.02.002

Freschi, J., Azizi, L.A., Balboa, L., Kaldy, Z., and Blaser, E. (2022) "The development of peak alpha frequency from infancy to adolescence and its role in visual temporal processing: A meta-analysis." *Developmental Cognitive Neuroscience 57*, 101146. https://doi.org/10.1016/j.dcn.2022.101146

Gard, T., Noggle, J.J., Park, C.L., Vago, D.R., and Wilson, A. (2014) "Potential self-regulatory mechanisms of yoga for psychological health." *Frontiers in Human Neuroscience 8*, 770. https://doi.org/10.3389/fnhum.2014.00770

Gotink, R.A., Vernooij, M.W., Ikram, M.A., Niessen, W.J., *et al.* (2018) "Meditation and yoga practice are associated with smaller right amygdala volume: The Rotterdam study." *Brain Imaging and Behavior 12*, 1631–1639. https://doi.org/10.1007/s11682-018-9826-z

Hagen, I. and Nayar, U.S. (2014) "Yoga for children and young people's mental health and well-being: Research review and reflections on the mental health potentials of yoga." *Frontiers in Psychiatry 5*, 35. https://doi.org/10.3389/fpsyt.2014.00035

Hasenkamp, W., Wilson-Mendenhall, C.D., Duncan, E., and Barsalou, L.W. (2012) "Mind wandering and attention during focused meditation: A fine-grained temporal analysis of fluctuating cognitive states." *NeuroImage 59*, 1, 750–760. doi: 10.1016/j.neuroimage.2011.07.008.

Hölzel, B.K., Carmody, J., Evans, K.C., Hoge, E.A., *et al.* (2010) "Stress reduction correlates with structural changes in the amygdala." *Social Cognitive and Affective Neuroscience 5*, 1, 11–17. https://doi.org/10.1093/scan/nsp034

Hölzel, B.K., Carmody, J., Vangel, M., Congleton, C., *et al.* (2011) "Mindfulness practice leads to increases in regional brain gray matter density." *Psychiatry Research 191*, 1, 36–43. doi: 10.1016/j.pscychresns.2010.08.006.

Huang, M.-X., Yurgil, K.A., Robb, A., Angeles, A., *et al.* (2014) "Voxel-wise resting-state MEG source magnitude imaging study reveals neurocircuitry abnormality in active-duty service members and veterans with PTSD." *NeuroImage. Clinical 5*, 408–419.

Hwang, K., Bertolero, M.A., Liu, W.B., and D'Esposito, M. (2017) "The human thalamus is an integrative hub for functional brain networks." *The Journal of Neuroscience 37*, 23, 5594–5607. doi: 10.1523/JNEUROSCI.0067-17.2017.

Jann, K., Dierks, T., Boesch, C., Kottlow, M., Strik, W., and Koenig, T. (2009) "BOLD correlates of EEG alpha phase-locking and the fMRI default mode network." *NeuroImage 45*, 3, 903–916. doi: 10.1016/j.neuroimage.2009.01.001.

Jensen, O. and Mazaheri, A. (2010) "Shaping functional architecture by oscillatory alpha activity: Gating by inhibition." *Frontiers in Human Neuroscience 4*, 186. https://doi.org/10.3389/fnhum.2010.00186

Kamei, T., Toriumi, Y., Kimura, H., Ohno, S., Kumano, H., and Kimura, K. (2000) "Decrease in serum cortisol during yoga exercise is correlated with alpha wave activation." *Perceptual and Motor Skills 90*, 1027–1032. doi: 10.2466/pms.2000.90.3.1027.

Kerr, C.E., Sacchet, M.D., Lazar, S.W., Moore, C.I., and Jones, S.R. (2013) "Mindfulness starts with the body: Somatosensory attention and top-down modulation of cortical alpha rhythms in mindfulness meditation." *Frontiers in Human Neuroscience 7*, 12. http://doi.org/10.3389/fnhum.2013.00012

Khalsa, S.B.S. and Butzer, B. (2016) "Yoga in school settings: A research review." *Annals of the New York Academy of Sciences 1373*, 1, 45–55. https://doi.org/10.1111/nyas.13025

Klimesch, W. (2012) "Alpha-band oscillations, attention, and controlled access to stored information." *Trends in Cognitive Sciences 16*, 12, 606–617. http://doi.org/10.1016/j.tics.2012.10.007

Lanius R.A., Vermetten, E., Loewenstein, R.J., Brand, B., Schmahl, C., Bremner, J.D. *et al.* (2020) "Emotion modulation in PTSD: clinical and neurobiological evidence for a dissociative subtype." *American Journal of Psychiatry 167*, 6, 640–7. doi: 10.1176/appi.ajp.2009.09081168.

Lanius, R.A., Frewen, P.A., Tursich, M., Jetly, R., and McKinnon, M.C. (2015) "Restoring large-scale brain networks in PTSD: A proposal for neuroscientifically-informed treatment interventions." *European Journal of Psychotraumatology 6*, 27313. doi: 10.3402/ejpt.v6.27313.

Lanius, U.F., Paulsen, S.L., and Corrigan, F.M. (2014) "Dissociation: Cortical Deafferentation and the Loss of Self." In U.F. Lanius, S.L. Paulsen, and F.M. Corrigan (eds) *Neurobiology and Treatment of Traumatic Dissociation: Towards an Embodied Self* (Chapter 1). New York: Springer Publishing Co.

Llinás, R.A., Urbano, F.J., Leznik, E., Ramírez, R.R., and van Marle, H.J. (2005) "Rhythmic and dysrhythmic thalamocortical dynamics: GABA systems and the edge effect." *Trends in Neurosciences 28*, 6, 325–333. https://doi.org/10.1016/j.tins.2005.04.006

Luders, E., Phillips, O.R., Clark, K., Kurth, F., Toga, A.W., and Narr, K.L. (2012) "Bridging the hemispheres in meditation: Thicker callosal regions and enhanced fractional anisotropy (FA) in long-term practitioners." *NeuroImage 61*, 1, 181–187. https://doi.org/10.1016/j.neuroimage.2012.02.026

Mantini, D., Perrucci, M.G., Del Gratta, C., Romani, G.L., and Corbetta, M. (2007) "Electrophysiological signatures of resting state networks in the human brain." *Proceedings of the National Academy of Sciences of the United States of America 104*, 32, 13170–13175. doi: 10.1073/pnas.0700668104.

Marusak, H.A., Elrahal, F., Peters, C.A., Kundu, P., *et al.* (2018) "Mindfulness and dynamic functional neural connectivity in children and adolescents." *Behavioural Brain Research 336*, 211–218. https://doi.org/10.1016/j.bbr.2017.09.010

Nakajima, M. and Halassa, M.M. (2017) "Thalamic control of functional cortical connectivity." *Current Opinion in Neurobiology 44*, 127–131. https://doi.org/10.1016/j.conb.2017.04.001

Nicholson, A.A., Densmore, M., Frewen, P.A., Neufeld, W.J., *et al.* (2023) "Homeostatic normalization of alpha brain rhythms within the default-mode network and reduced symptoms in post-traumatic stress disorder following a randomized controlled trial of electroencephalogram neurofeedback." *Brain Communications 5*, 2, fcad068. https://doi.org/10.1093/braincomms/fcad068

Nicholson, A.A., Ros, T., Densmore, M., Frewen, P.A., *et al.* (2020) "A randomized, controlled trial of alpha-rhythm EEG neurofeedback in posttraumatic stress disorder: A preliminary investigation showing evidence of decreased PTSD symptoms and restored default mode and salience network connectivity using fMRI." *NeuroImage. Clinical 28*, 102490. https://doi.org/10.1016/j.nicl.2020.102490

Rogel, A., Loomis, A., Hamlin, E., Hodgdon, H., Spinazzola, J., and van der Kolk, B. (2020) "The impact of neurofeedback training on children with developmental trauma: A randomized controlled study." *Psychological Trauma: Theory, Research, Practice, and Policy 12*, 8, 918–929. doi: 10.1037/tra0000648.

Sadaghiani, S., Scheeringa, R., Lehongre, K., Morillon, B., *et al.* (2012) "Alpha-band phase synchrony is related to activity in the fronto-parietal adaptive control network." *Journal of Neuroscience 32*, 41, 14305–14310.

Sripada, R.K., King, A.P., Welsh, R.C., Garfinkel, S.N., *et al.* (2012) "Neural dysregulation in posttraumatic stress disorder: Evidence for disrupted equilibrium between salience and default mode brain networks." *Psychosomatic Medicine 74*, 9, 904–911. http://doi.org/10.1097/PSY.0b013e318273bf33

Stoller, L. (2019) *Sensory-Enhanced Yoga for Self-Regulation and Trauma Healing*. Pencaitland: Handspring Publishing Limited.

Streeter, C.C., Gerbarg, P.L., Brown, R.P., Scott, T.M., *et al.* (2020) "Thalamic gamma aminobutyric acid level changes in major depressive disorder after a 12-week Iyengar yoga and coherent breathing intervention." *Journal of Alternative and Complementary Medicine (New York) 26*, 3, 190–197. https://doi.org/10.1089/acm.2019.0234

Streeter, C.C., Gerbarg, P.L., Nielsen, G., Brown, R., Jensen, J.E., and Silveri, M.M. (2018) "Effects of yoga on thalamic gamma-aminobutyric acid, mood and depression: Analysis of two randomized controlled trials." *Neuropsychiatry (London) 8*, 6, 1923–1939. https://www.jneuropsychiatry.org/peer-review/effects-ofyoga-on-thalamic-gammaaminobutyric-acid-mood-anddepression-analysis-of-two-randomized-controlled-trials-12856.html

Streeter, C.C., Gerbarg, P.L., Saper, R.B., Ciraulo, D., and Brown, R.P. (2012) "Effects of yoga on the autonomic nervous system, gamma-aminobutyric-acid, and allostasis in epilepsy, depression, and post-traumatic stress disorder." *Medical Hypotheses 78*, 5, 571–579. doi: 10.1016/j.mehy.2012.01.021.

Streeter, C.C., Jensen, J.E., Perlmutter, R.M., Cabral, H.J., *et al.* (2007) "Yoga Asana sessions increase brain GABA levels: A pilot study." *Journal of Alternative and Complementary Medicine 13*, 4, 419–426. doi: 10.1089/acm.2007.6338.

Streeter, C.C., Whitfield, T.H., Owen, L., Rein, T., *et al.* (2010) "Effects of yoga versus walking on mood, anxiety, and brain GABA levels: A randomized controlled MRS study." *Journal of Alternative and Complementary Medicine (New York) 16*, 11, 1145–1152. https://doi.org/10.1089/acm.2010.0007

van Aalst, J., Cessarini, J., Demyttenaere, K., Sunaert, S., and Van Laere, K. (2020) "What has neuroimaging taught us on the neurobiology of yoga? A review." *Frontiers in Integrative Neuroscience 14*. www.frontiersin.org/article/10.3389/fnint.2020.00034

van der Kolk, B. (2008) "Affect regulation." Pre-conference Institute, 19th Annual International Trauma Conference, June 25, Boston, MA.

van der Kolk, B.A. (2014) *The Body Keeps the Score: Brain, Mind, and Body in the Healing of Trauma*. New York: Viking (Penguin Random House).

van der Kolk, B.A, Hodgdon H., Gapen, M., Musicaro, R., Suvak, M.K, Hamlin, E., and Spinazzola, J.A. (2016) "Randomized Controlled Study of Neurofeedback for Chronic PTSD." *PLoS One 11*, 12. e0166752. doi: 10.1371/journal.pone.0166752.

van Lutterveld, R., van Dellen, E., Pal, P., Yang, H., Stam, C.J., and Brewer, J. (2017) "Meditation is associated with increased brain network integration." *NeuroImage 158*, 18–25. https://doi.org/10.1016/j.neuroimage.2017.06.071

Villemure, C., Čeko, M., Cotton, V.A., and Bushnell, M.C. (2014) "Insular cortex mediates increased pain tolerance in yoga practitioners." *Cerebral Cortex (New York) 24*, 10, 2732–2740. https://doi.org/10.1093/cercor/bht124

Zelano, C., Jiang, H., Zhou, G., Arora, N., *et al.* (2016) "Nasal respiration entrains human limbic oscillations and modulates cognitive function." *The Journal of Neuroscience 36*, 49, 12448–12467. https://doi.org/10.1523/JNEUROSCI.2586-16.2016

PART 2

The Theory

CHAPTER 6

The Yogic Perspective

HEALING TRAUMA THROUGH THE KOSHAS

In Part 1, we provided objective research evidence to support our claim that yoga is one of the best adjunct treatments for PTSD and related mental health conditions. However, we still haven't explained what yoga actually is, as that can only be accurately described from the perspective of its traditional Eastern origins. Thus, in this chapter, we will reintroduce yoga from the ancient yogic perspective of the kosha model that provides the foundation for the Sensory-Enhanced Yoga® methodology used in the SMYLE™ program. We will specifically discuss how this model applies to children.

This discussion will lead directly into the ***Transdisciplinary Model for Post-Traumatic Growth for Children*** and the definition, purpose, and guiding principles of ***Sensory-Enhanced Yoga®***. The program synthesizes Western theoretical concepts and research findings with traditional Eastern yogic philosophy to produce a cogent practice model for healing symptoms of toxic stress, PTSD, anxiety, or other unresolved trauma or ANS conditions.

A PATH TO SELF-AWARENESS AND INTEGRATION

Yoga is a mindfulness-based practice that has evolved over the past 5000 years or even longer, and has its roots in ancient India. The word "yoga" is derived from the Sanskrit (ancient Indian) word "yuj," which means "yoking." Its most common contemporary translation is "union," which has most frequently been interpreted to mean the union of mind, body, and spirit. Yoga has easily transcended its Eastern cultural origins because the practice helps to bring individuals home to themselves, wherever they are located on this planet, and whatever their faith or lack thereof. Patanjali, author of the *Yoga Sutras* (circa 400 CE), writes in *Yoga Sutra* 1.2: *Yoga is the cessation of the fluctuations of the mind.* By clearing the mind of the clutter created by the sensory world and our resulting conditioning, a person comes to better understand their own true nature.

THE KOSHA MODEL

Around 3000 years ago, the yogic sages organized the practice of yoga around a model they created to describe the different layers, sheaths, or "bodies" of a person, which they called the "koshas." They consist of the ***annamaya kosha*** (physical body), ***pranamaya kosha*** (energy body), ***manomaya kosha*** (mental body), ***vijnanamaya kosha*** (wisdom body), and ***anandamaya kosha*** (bliss body). These five parts of our being were first documented in writing in the *Taittiriya Upanishad*, a Vedic text composed in approximately 6 BCE (Sharvananda 1921). The following briefly reviews the five koshas, and describes how they can be affected by trauma. Each of the treatment principles of Sensory-Enhanced Yoga® (and SMYLE™) is associated with a koshic level, which is listed along with the kosha.

Annamaya kosha (physical body)

The ***annamaya kosha*** refers to the skin, flesh, bones, and all of the other material of the physical body made from the food that we eat. The annamaya kosha provides the solid form of our existence, the foundation, and physical boundary within which the other elements of our being reside. Our survival depends most of all on the integrity of the annamaya kosha, without which the other four layers of our being could not exist. It is thus the annamaya kosha that is most closely tied to our sense of safety in the world. When children are feeling unsafe due to abuse, neglect, witnessing the abuse of other family members, living in an unsafe neighborhood, or living through a man-made or natural disaster (such as genocide, or displacement to a refugee camp), they often become hyperaroused, hypervigilant, and fearful. When left unresolved, they are at high risk for developing PTSD. Furthermore, many trauma victims dissociate from the annamaya kosha in order to numb difficult emotions associated with the trauma, since we largely identify our emotions from the sensations we feel in our bodies. And as we know, many people, including children, are physically injured during a traumatic event, which obviously violates the annamaya kosha.

Annamaya kosha guiding treatment principle:
A sense of safety is essential to healing.

Pranamaya kosha (energy body)

The ***pranamaya kosha*** is the "life energy" that fills the physical body and is most obviously manifested by the breath, which draws in oxygen, revitalizing the blood and thus all of the cells of the body. Our life energy pulsates throughout the body with each beat of the heart. It flows through our arteries, air passages, nerves, and lymph system, and is essential to the functioning of every organ. The ANS strongly influences the flow of our life energy. When we are relaxed, our life energy is focused on homeostatic functions such as digestion, tissue repair, and immune functions. However, when we are under threat, or under stress, our life energy is diverted from these functions. Our heart beats faster, our breath becomes shallow, and blood is shunted to our extremities in a classic "fight or flight" reaction, or a subtler version of it. When a person becomes chronically stuck in such an altered energy state, or becomes overwhelmed and energetically shuts down, it compromises the ability to self-regulate emotional states. Thus, the pranamaya kosha has a huge influence on the manomaya kosha (mental body).

Children are initially dependent on their primary caregivers to help them co-regulate their ANS (and thus, pranamaya kosha), and it is through these attachment relationships that they gradually learn to ***self***-regulate. The quality of caregiving therefore has a significant effect on the functioning of the child's energetic state. As children become more independent from their caregivers, other social relationships fill the void to help them stay regulated (Porges and Furman 2011). Thus, the "social engagement system," that is, the ventral vagal branch of the PNS, has a huge influence on the functioning of the pranamaya kosha. In addition to these ***co***-regulating forces, children need to learn to develop their own internal resources to stay regulated. The most powerful way to ***self***-regulate is through control of the breath, as respiration is the only direct control we have over the ANS, and specifically the ventral vagal branch of the PNS.

Pranamaya kosha guiding treatment principle:
The most direct and powerful way to self-regulate is through control of the breath.

Manomaya kosha (mental body)

The ***manomaya kosha*** consists of the emotions and reflexive mental chatter that typically fill our waking moments. It is said to be composed of the mind and the sensory organs. The manomaya kosha is reflected in our underlying emotional tone, passing emotional states, and the reflexive attitudes and thoughts that are influenced by these emotions and other mostly unconscious processes as we go about our day-to-day lives. The manomaya kosha also controls our sensorimotor system in our everyday actions, such as brushing our teeth, driving to work, or typing on the computer. These mental processes work together to enable us to do what we need and want to do in our daily lives, and largely consist of instinctual, conditioned thought and action patterns. This is certainly true of children who are concrete thinkers by nature and learn by doing. Since the PFC does not fully mature until the mid-20s, the more emotional areas of the brain "rule the roost," responding to situations and the environment in a more reactive style.

Children are also mostly "here and now" creatures who are not yet able to make complex future plans or reflect deeply on past events. This is because the "stories" of our lives (episodic memories) rely on the functioning of the hippocampus, which undergoes developmental and volume changes throughout childhood. As a child develops, the hippocampus becomes more integrated with the PFC and other cortical areas as these, too, mature. This explains why, as children get older, they can better remember the location, action, and timing of the events in their lives (Riggins *et al.* 2015).

However, making sense of ***traumatic*** events in narrative form can be difficult for a person of any age, since the hippocampus goes offline during these events. Instead, these memories will be held in the body as implicit (unconscious) memories. ***So, with trauma, the disruption to the manomaya kosha frequently bubbles up through the annamaya and pranamaya koshas.*** The undischarged residue of energy from the traumatic event often creates uncomfortable bodily sensations and associated emotions. Some dissociate from the body to numb the emotions, while others become hyperaroused by the emotions and inappropriately act on them, such as by rising easily to anger. The sensorimotor system is impacted as well. When a healthy connection to the body is lost, postures and movements can become more restricted, or can seem to occur out of the individual's control.

Numbing symptoms compound the problem for the manomaya kosha, as they cause the person to not only lose their connection with the body, but also to the "here and now" of the present moment, affecting their ability to effectively engage in daily life tasks. Normal "mental chatter," such as "I need to do my homework before soccer practice" or "I should ask my friend at lunch if she wants to come over to my house after school," as well as the correlating action impulse to perform those tasks, can become totally knocked out by the numbness and intrusive thoughts about the traumatic event. Thus, the person becomes emotionally and mentally "stuck"—like a car stuck in the mud. And just as a car stuck in the mud can be more easily released when people are pushing rhythmically from both the front and the back of the car, the manomaya kosha can more easily be released by approaching it through adjacent koshas—and the "art" of it becomes a rhythm as well. That is, we artfully combine "bottom-up" (i.e., the body affecting the mind) and "top-down" (i.e., the mind affecting the body) approaches when treating the emotional wounds of traumatized individuals using yoga therapy.

Manomaya kosha guiding treatment principle:
Yoga can promote effective sensory, motor, and cognitive processing of traumatic experiences, and thus aid healing.

Vijnanamaya kosha (wisdom body)

The ***vijnanamaya kosha*** is known as the "wisdom body" and encompasses the functions of the higher mind, including conscience, judgment, morality, and will. It is the part of our being that allows us to stand back and become a "witness" to the "mental chatter" of the manomaya kosha (which is largely conditioned based on our everyday experiences) so we can begin to see the larger picture of who we are and make more insightful choices in our actions.

The vijnanamaya kosha is also the part of our being that forms our ethics, which lie at the very foundation of yoga practice. In fact, Patanjali's *Yoga Sutras* places yoga's ethical guidelines—the Yamas and Niyamas—at the very forefront of the Eight Limbs of Yoga (see Table 6.1).

Table 6.1: Patanjali's Eight Limbs of Yoga

1	Yamas (restraints, i.e., what not to do)
2	Niyamas (observances, i.e., what to do)
3	Asana (postures)
4	Pranayama (control of the breath)
5	Pratyahara (withdrawal of the senses)
6	Dharana (concentration, i.e., one-pointed attention)
7	Dhyana (meditation, i.e., keen awareness without focus)
8	Samadhi (bliss, i.e., non-duality, experiencing the interconnection of all living things)

From Stoller (2019)

The ethical guidelines presented in the first two limbs are divided into the **yamas**, or restraints, and the **niyamas**, or observances, and are briefly listed in Table 6.2. It is thought that Patanjali positioned these yogic "dos" and "don'ts" prior to the asana (postures) and pranayama (breathwork) limbs, because working at the physical and energy levels can draw out emotions, and we need to know how to handle these emotions in an ethical manner when they arise. Thus, the ethical guidelines provide a "top-down" wisdom-based approach to managing potential emotional abreactions that may be elicited from the "bottom-up" effects of the yoga movements and breathwork, in addition to more generally guiding our actions in our everyday lives.

Table 6.2: Yamas and niyamas

Yamas (Things not to do)	Niyamas (Things to do)
Ahimsa (non-violence)	***Sancha*** (cleanliness)
Satya (non-lying, i.e. truthfulness and authenticity)	***Santosha*** (contentment)
Asteya (non-stealing)	***Tapas*** (self-discipline, perseverance)
Brachmacharya (non-excess, i.e., of sensual pleasures, including sexual energy)	***Svadhyaya*** (study of one's self, i.e., self-awareness; self knowledge)
Aparigraha (non-possessiveness; non-greed)	***Ishvara pranidhana*** (devotion, i.e., surrendering the fruit of one's actions to a higher power)

From Stoller (2019)

The ethical guidelines of yoga (yamas) need to be approached with sensitivity with trauma survivors as they are at particular risk for developing symptoms of "moral injury." According to Maguen and Litz (2012, p.1), moral injury is "an act of serious transgression that leads to serious inner conflict because the experience is at odds with core ethical and moral beliefs." The core belief here is, *it is my fault and I am a bad person.* Moral injury events may include situations where the individual was the agent of a harmful action; caused harm due to failure to act; witnessed a harmful action or inaction; or felt betrayed by someone they trusted who they think did something really wrong (Chaplo, Kerig, and Wainryb 2019).

Moral injury has been most frequently studied in military personnel, since combat involves harming or killing another human being, violating the usual moral codes (Maguen and Litz 2012). However, it is now recognized that even children may experience moral injury. Those who are at particular risk include children who have been maltreated, are in the juvenile justice system, are/were exposed to gang and community violence, or are/were child soldiers (Chaplo *et al.* 2019). However, various degrees of moral injury occur among teens, such as "romantic relationship infidelities or break-ups, betrayal by friends, academic or work-related cheating, witnessing bullying or hazing, and harm to others caused by excessive alcohol or substance use" (Chaplo *et al.* 2019, p.449). Moral injury shares PTSD-like symptoms (such as intrusions, avoidance, and numbing), but also includes symptoms of shame, guilt, demoralization, self-handicapping behaviors, and self-harm (Maguen and Litz 2012). Hyperarousal is not considered a symptom of moral injury; thus, moral injury and PTSD are two different but related conditions (see Figure 6.1). However, someone can certainly suffer from both. In the case of PTSD specifically, underlying core beliefs can generally be sorted into two major categories: "the world is dangerous" (hyperarousal) and/or "the world is meaningless" (dissociation). There are often others, such as "I can't trust you," "I don't care about you," "My life will never get better," "My mind can never heal," or "No one cares about me," any of which can lead someone to compromise their ethics. In particular, those who feel their life has hit rock bottom and have nothing more to lose may be less apt to restrain their impulses.

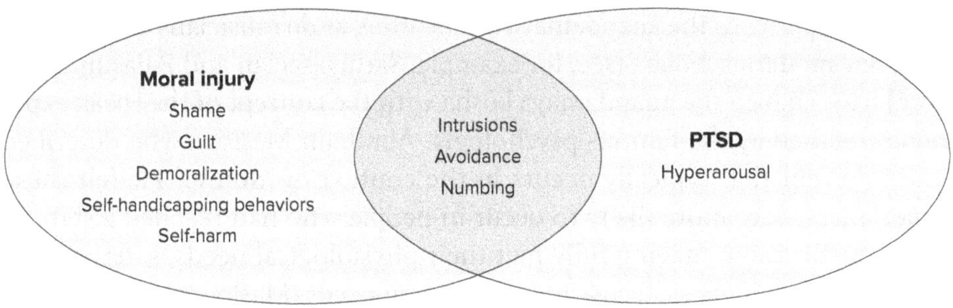

FIGURE 6.1: SYMPTOM OVERLAP BETWEEN PTSD AND MORAL INJURY
Based on Maguen and Litz (2012)

Individuals suffering from moral injury require very special care. Due to the depth and complexity of the injury, we can't simply ask a child or adolescent to forgive themself for their transgressions. We also can't address moral injury using strategies to reduce hyperarousal, as moral injury is shame-based, not fear-based (Maguen and Litz 2012)—addressing hyperarousal will not address the shame. However, as with all deeply held emotions, the moral injury is carried in the body, and will likely remain there until it is safely released from the body, and not simply through an act of intellectual rationalization. Yoga and breathwork combined with careful use of language—together with professional counseling—can help to safely release these difficult emotions and thoughts and allow space for more positive attitudes and beliefs to take hold.

Vijnanamaya kosha guiding treatment principle:
New beliefs and attitudes more easily take hold when we first prepare the body to receive and accept them.

Anandamaya kosha (bliss body)

The ***anandamaya kosha***, known as the "bliss body," is a transcendent state of consciousness characterized by a feeling of deep peace, joy, and love, achieved when we are "one" with the experience of being fully immersed in what we are doing. It is often discussed in the context of a deep state of meditation, but can also be experienced when actively engaged in a task to the point where the person loses their sense of separation from it. Unlike the vijnanamaya kosha, which steps back from an experience to "witness" it, at the level of the anandamaya kosha you don't witness the bliss—you "are" the bliss. You're not "*doing*" skiing, you are "skiing *itself*." Once you stop to contemplate it, you're no longer experiencing the anandamaya kosha but have instead dropped back down to the vijnanamaya kosha as the "witness." As Shiva Rea (2007) points out, children typically experience the anandamaya kosha often, as do musicians and dancers.

A few modern scholars (see, for example, Sathiyaseelan and Balasundaram 2016) have aligned the anandamaya kosha with the concept of the "peak experience" coined by the famous psychologist Abraham Maslow, who described it as an event that typically occurs in the context of "doing." He felt these experiences were more likely to occur in people who had reached a state of "self-actualization," having fully met their physiological needs, safety needs, love and belongingness needs, and self-esteem needs (Maslow 1962).

Whether intended by the ancient text or not, with respect to PTSD it seems most appropriate to describe the "bliss body" as *both* a state of "optimal being" and "optimal doing," particularly since PTSD is a mental condition in which an impairment in occupational functioning, that is, "doing," is a diagnostic requirement. States of "being" and "doing" usually do go hand-in-hand and relate to the concepts of spirit and self-empowerment respectively. Since we are ultimately concerned with helping our students achieve both happy and productive lives, we believe it is important to look at trauma, toxic stress, and related conditions from this wider lens. This is reflected in the fifth guideline to practice.

Anandamaya kosha guiding treatment principle:
Self-empowerment is born on the wings of the spirit rising from the mind-body connection.

Table 6.3 depicts a healing process through the koshas according to PTSD subtype (Bremner 1999; Lanius *et al.* 2010). Many people who have been traumatized will experience symptoms in both columns (Lanius *et al.* 2010, 2015). For example, it is common to experience intrusive thoughts of trauma and at the same time experience poverty of thought, that is, a reduction in the typical "mental chatter" that normally occurs as the person goes about their daily life. In a similar vein, someone may be hypersensitive to certain types of sensory input, such as sound or visual stimuli, at the expense of registering other types of input, such as bodily sensations—or conversely, be preoccupied by internal bodily sensations at the expense of noticing what is happening around them in the environment. You will notice that the guiding principles for treatment are the same for both subtypes of PTSD.

Table 6.3: Healing trauma through the koshas

<table>
<tr><th>Kosha</th><th>Hyperarousal/ re-experiencing</th><th>Hypoarousal/ dissociation</th><th>Sensory-Enhanced Yoga® guiding principle</th></tr>
<tr><td>Annamaya kosha (physical body)</td><td>Lost sense of bodily safety</td><td>Lost sense of bodily safety</td><td>A sense of safety is essential to healing</td></tr>
<tr><td>Pranamaya kosha (energy body)</td><td>Hyperarousal</td><td>Hypoarousal</td><td>The most direct and powerful way to self-regulate is through control of the breath</td></tr>
<tr><td>Manamaya kosha (emotional/ mental body)</td><td>Sensory sensitivity
Rigid movements
Intrusive thoughts</td><td>Low registration
Dissociated movements
Poverty of thought</td><td>Yoga can promote effective sensory, motor, and cognitive processing of traumatic experiences, and thus aid healing</td></tr>
<tr><td rowspan="2">Vijnanamaya kosha (wisdom body)</td><td>“The world is a dangerous place”</td><td>“The world is a meaningless place”</td><td rowspan="2">New beliefs and attitudes more easily take hold when we first prepare the body to receive and accept them</td></tr>
<tr><td colspan="2">In the case of moral injury: “It is all my fault and I am a bad person.”</td></tr>
<tr><td>Anandamaya kosha (bliss body)</td><td>Too hypervigilant to relax into joy</td><td>Too numbed out to feel joy</td><td>Self-empowerment is born on the wings of the spirit rising from the mind-body connection</td></tr>
</table>

SENSORY-ENHANCED YOGA®

Thus, we have arrived at the very heart of the book, the description of Sensory-Enhanced Yoga®, which is the methodology of the SMYLE™ program. The kosha model, and all of the Western science information presented in the chapters leading up to this one, closely inform this method. The program is intended for use by yoga therapists and yoga teachers, allied and mental health professionals, and licensed educators who serve individuals who have experienced trauma or toxic stress and/or who suffer from related conditions such as high anxiety, ADHD, sensory processing disorder, bipolar disorder, or mixed anxiety-depression.

Here is the definition and purpose of the program:

Definition: Sensory-Enhanced Yoga® incorporates carefully selected sensory input, breathing techniques, and language into yoga practice, within the context of a safe container, in order to address issues related to hyperarousal, hyperactivity, hypervigilance, dissociation, and/or sensory sensitivities.

Purpose: The purpose of Sensory-Enhanced Yoga® is to help individuals manage (and hopefully eventually resolve) these symptoms and be able to self-regulate, that is, conduct their daily lives in a calm, centered, focused, and productive manner.

The program is designed to help participants meet the following goals:

- Effectively manage stress before it leads to emotional imbalance and/or inappropriate behaviors.
- Develop emotional resiliency, that is, the ability to rise to meet a challenge or threat as well as easily calm once it has passed.
- Decrease hypervigilance and overreaction to sensory input (e.g., visual, crowds, touch, noise, movement).
- Improve quality of sleep and energy levels to support wellness and enhance daily productivity.
- Decrease intrusive thoughts by learning to become present through breath and body awareness.
- Enhance someone's sense of self-worth and personal empowerment.

Sensory-Enhanced Yoga®/SMYLE™ incorporates principles and techniques from sensory integration theory and neurorehabilitation practice to reduce symptoms of toxic stress, PTSD, or other mental health conditions. As examples, the yoga sessions are especially designed to provide enhanced proprioceptive (muscle) input, deep touch pressure, some slow rhythmical movement, carefully selected pranayama (breathing) techniques that promote calming, and a series of asanas that are chosen to balance the nervous system toward a more relaxed and steady state. Special care is taken to help students coordinate movements with the breath, which is especially powerful in reducing hyperarousal and drawing the mind back into the body and the present moment.

The movement and breathwork of Sensory-Enhanced Yoga®/SMYLE™ helps to safely release body-stored tensions, trauma, and negative attitudes, thus preparing the body to more readily respond to positive suggestions and guided meditations, which are also incorporated into the program. These verbal elements of the program promote a sense of self-worth and personal empowerment, which support health, well-being, and achieving a person's goals. Thus, Sensory-Enhanced Yoga®/SMYLE™ uses the *power of the mind to influence the body.* Great care is also taken to create a "safe container" for students, both physically and psychologically, in which healing can occur. Students' abreactions (purging of emotional tensions) are welcomed and responded to skillfully and with compassion, and a range of precautions is followed in working with traumatized individuals.

The ***Transdisciplinary Model for Post-Traumatic Growth in Children*** and the Sensory-Enhanced Yoga®/SMYLE™ ***guiding principles of Sensory-Enhanced Yoga®*** inform the implementation of a SMYLE™ program. These are discussed in the remainder of this chapter.

A TRANSDISCIPLINARY MODEL FOR POST-TRAUMATIC GROWTH IN CHILDREN

Figure 6.2 presents a theoretical framework for addressing mind–body health and quality of life for children who suffer from PTSD, other forms of toxic stress, and related mental health conditions. It summarizes the underlying theory for Sensory-Enhanced Yoga® through a wide lens, showing how carefully designed mind–body modalities may help someone heal from PTSD, regain a positive outlook, and develop a sense of self-empowerment that will facilitate successful re-engagement in valued occupational activities and roles in society. When used within a therapeutic setting, mind–body modalities should ideally be presented in concert with an articulated plan for meeting client-set goals in order to capitalize on the person's physiological readiness for psychological change.

The ***Transdisciplinary Model for Post-Traumatic Growth in Children*** is a lightly edited version of the ***Transdisciplinary Model for Post-Traumatic Growth*** created by Lynn Stoller (2019). The new version is a joint effort by Lynn Stoller, Meg Hennessey Schofield, and Dr. Erin O'Neill. Lynn created the original version to explain the likely reasons why the Iraq Yoga Study treatment protocol worked and the treatment implications; she later added the kosha language at the top of the model. This model was written entirely from a Western science perspective, incorporating research and concepts from the fields of occupational therapy and trauma psychology, before Lynn even realized how well it fit in with the kosha model. Many experts have identified and developed important concepts for healing trauma, and these were simply woven together, effectively "recreating the (ancient) wheel." As we delve into the model, we hope to impress upon readers that some of the perceived discrepancy between Eastern philosophy and Western science is simply due to the language barrier, and that Western science is quickly validating what the ancient yogis have theorized all along. A brief summary of the model is presented, following which we will introduce the Sensory-Enhanced Yoga®/SMYLE™ ***guidelines for practice***.

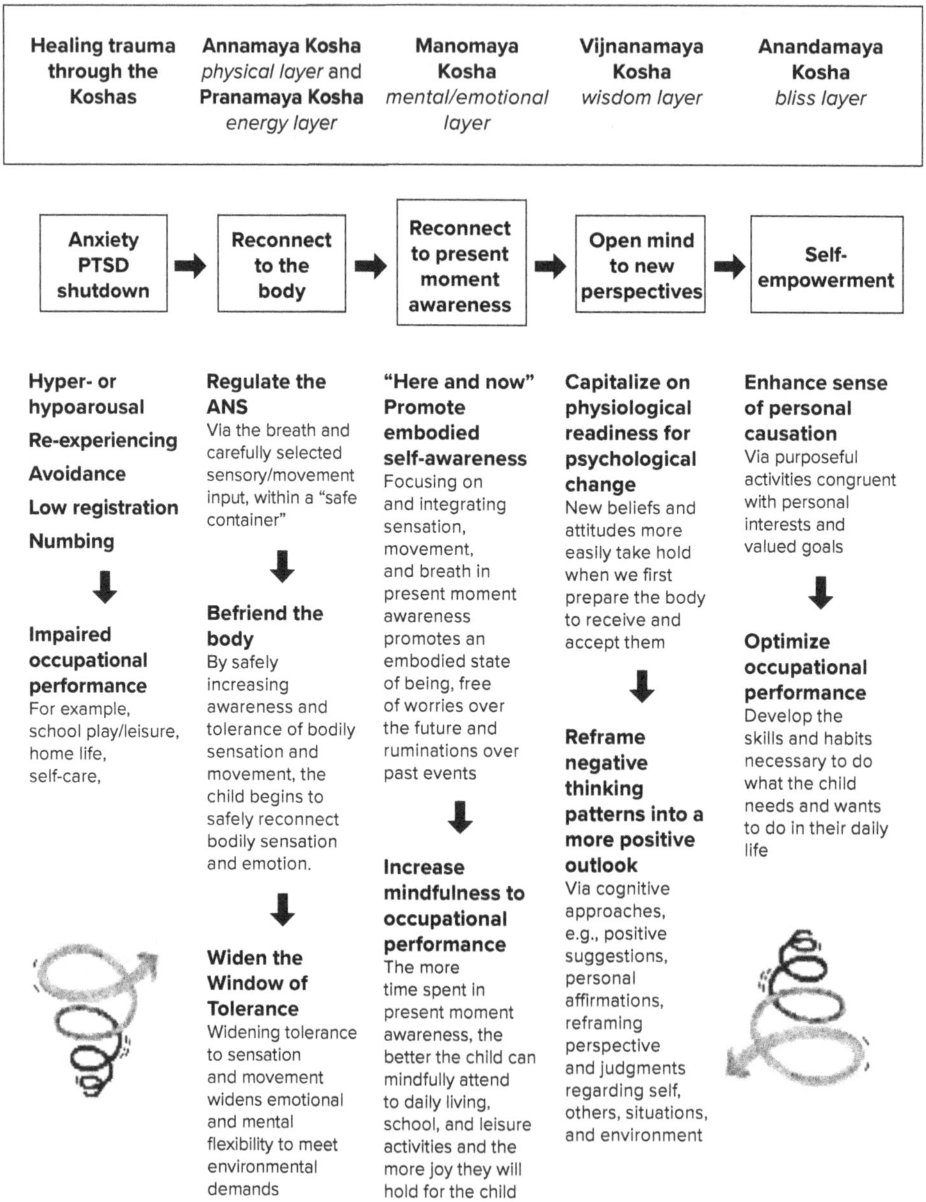

FIGURE 6.2: A TRANSDISCIPLINARY MODEL FOR POST-TRAUMATIC GROWTH IN CHILDREN

This model includes concepts introduced by others: "befriend the body" by van der Kolk (2008); Window of Tolerance by Siegel (1999), based on the concept by Wilbarger and Wilbarger (1990, 1997); "personal causation" component of Model of Human Occupation developed by Keilhofner (1980, 2008); link between the "here and now" and opening the mind to new perspectives neurophysiologically explained by Fogel (2009)

To help children heal from trauma, toxic stress, or related mental health conditions, the first step is to ***help them safely reconnect to their body, aka the annamaya kosha***, and to do that, we need to help them to ***self-regulate***. We can do this pretty effectively through the use of carefully selected sensory input and breathing techniques designed to rebalance the ANS (at the level of the ***pranamaya kosha***), as described earlier, and by helping them to release trauma-based muscular tension. These techniques must be provided within a "safe container," which is a term used in trauma work that means attending to the environmental qualities of the setting as well as the interpersonal relationship between therapist/teacher and student. We can't guarantee "safety" for our students, but we can control the variables that influence it (see Chapter 7).

By safely increasing awareness and tolerance of bodily sensation and movement, one begins to ***safely reconnect bodily sensation and emotion—at the level of the manomaya kosha, or mental/emotional body***. This helps the child to develop the emotional and mental flexibility to more effectively adapt to social and environmental demands, thus widening their window of tolerance.

Focusing on and integrating sensation, movement, and breath in ***present moment awareness*** promotes an embodied state of being, free from worries over the future and ruminations about the past. The more time spent in the "here and now," the better the child can mindfully attend to school, play, and daily living tasks, and the more value these tasks will hold for the child. When a child is fully embodied and their mind is clear, they can also better connect with others.

Through this process, the mind becomes more open to new perspectives—at the level of the vijnanamaya kosha, or wisdom body. New beliefs and attitudes more easily take hold when we first prepare the body to receive and accept them. If a child is tense with anxiety or slumped in a depression, they are literally not in a position to take the good advice of their teacher or therapist to heart. Talk therapies may thus be more effective when paired with yoga, and combining top-down and bottom-up approaches within yoga—such as through Sensory-Enhanced Yoga®—can be especially therapeutic.

Reframing negative thinking patterns into a more positive outlook helps to promote a sense of self-empowerment, which is associated with the bliss body, or anandamaya kosha. It is by working through the other layers that a child achieves an optimal sense of "well-being" ***and*** an optimal sense of "well-doing," as the two go hand in hand. This can be further promoted through a variety of purposeful activities congruent with someone's personal interests and valued goals. Through this process, the child develops the neurophysiological readiness and the intrinsic motivation to address the skills and habits necessary to meet daily living needs and school demands, and to pursue play or leisure activities, enabling them to live a fully engaged life.

GUIDING PRINCIPLES OF SENSORY-ENHANCED YOGA®/SMYLE™

Here are the guiding principles of Sensory-Enhanced Yoga®, which are closely informed by the ***Transdisciplinary Model for Post-Traumatic Growth in Children***:

1. A sense of safety is essential to healing

The hyperarousal symptoms are rooted in an unresolved "fight–flight" reaction that occurs in response to what may be perceived as a safety threat. Many children with a wide range of disabilities may show symptoms of hyperarousal due to disruptions in sensory processing. In order to resolve these symptoms, it is necessary to restore a sense of safety within the body. Toward this end, great care is taken to create a "safe container" for students within a SMYLE™ class. Among the variables to consider are the setting and timing of classes, choice of yoga forms and other techniques, and the interactions between the teacher and the student. Classes are conducted at a quiet time and place to reduce the possibility of interruption and distraction. Efforts are made to reduce visual clutter and environmental noise as much as possible to promote calming. If music is used, instrumentals are chosen that are soothingly melodic and/or have a slow, even rhythm, and high-pitched or low, threatening sounds are particularly avoided. Special care is taken before introducing any scents (such as incense) into the environment as olfactory nerves synapse directly on the emotional center of the brain (amygdala) and can potentially trigger hyperarousal (Vermetten and Bremner 2003). SMYLE™ instructors recognize that there are a variety of ability levels in students and meet them where they are to ensure students are not over-challenged by the demands of the activity and feel safe in the situation. They also help to foster the student's sense of control in the session, through the use of invitational language and by presenting choices. SMYLE™ instructors offer physical assists very judiciously, if at all, and always ask first. If used, they use a firm, "whole hand" touch rather than a light feathery touch. In order to gain the full benefit of the practice tools for the other guidelines, a strong sense of safety must be established.

2. The most direct and powerful way to self-regulate is through control of the breath

Breathing, or respiration, is the only function of the ANS that humans can intentionally influence and control. Other functions of the ANS, such as heart rate, blood pressure, and digestion, occur without conscious control. Pranayama is the yogic word for breathing techniques. These techniques can either be excitatory or calming, depending on the technique used. Excitatory techniques stimulate the SNS (the "fight or flight" system), whereas calming techniques stimulate the PNS (the "rest and digest" system). To achieve a "just right" state of arousal, the breathing methods most typically recommended are calming techniques to reduce hyperarousal and sensory overload, and thereby increase the ability to self-regulate. Children tend to be highly reactive to environmental input, and have limited awareness of their arousal states and how they are affected by sensory stimulation in their environments. Breathwork, coordinated with movement, is utilized as a tool to bring attention to the present moment, and helps to reconnect children to their bodies. Linking breath with movement in yoga allows for deeper, longer diaphragmatic breathing, which stimulates the calming PNS. However, breathing techniques alone have been found to have positive effects on arousal, self-regulation, and systems of the ANS that we do not have conscious control over, such as blood pressure and heart rate.

3. Yoga can promote effective sensory, motor, and cognitive processing of stressful or traumatic experiences, and thus aid healing

SMYLE™ incorporates principles from sensory integration theory and neurorehabilitation into the yoga sessions to maximize the innate benefit of yoga for reducing symptoms of trauma or extreme stress. Yoga sessions are especially designed to provide enhanced proprioceptive (muscle) input, deep touch pressure, some slow rhythmical movement, carefully selected pranayama (breathing) techniques that promote calming, and a series of yoga forms that are chosen to balance the nervous system toward a more relaxed and steady state. Generally speaking, a SMYLE™ session will have a greater predominance of forward bends, twists, and/or forward inversions, and will take special care to provide effective counterforms to balance the potentially arousing effects of backbends. Backward inversions (with the head strongly tipped backward) are either avoided altogether or presented with extreme caution. Balance forms are also included to promote sensory integration on many levels, and are especially powerful for helping to improve focus, bringing the mind back to the present moment.

4. New beliefs and attitudes more easily take hold when we first prepare the body to receive and accept them

When a student is struggling with anxiety, a trauma, stressors, or other difficult situations, the mind often develops negative thinking patterns, which can become reinforced over time, leading to an increased sense of insecurity or loss of control. This negative mindset often expresses itself in the body in a myriad of ways, and is further reinforced by that expression. For example, anxiety is frequently accompanied by an increase in heart rate and muscle tension, while depression tends to be accompanied by lethargy or fatigue. Mind states also affect and are further reinforced by the manner in which someone holds and moves their body, such as through protective posturing (e.g., hunched shoulders, aversive gaze, stiff movements). By helping to safely release these body-stored emotions, and by calling the mind back to the present moment, yoga clears space to allow new positive beliefs and attitudes to take hold. SMYLE™ capitalizes on this opportunity by pairing positive suggestions with specific yoga forms that embody their essence in order to bring the power of the thought into the full "mind–body" experience. These suggestions are carefully worded to increase awareness of and validate the student's own inner experiences.

5. Self-empowerment is born on the wings of the spirit rising from the mind–body connection

Children cannot function very well in life if their spirit has been broken by trauma, toxic stress, or depression. In many cases, everyday tasks become more of an effort, and there is no motivation to socialize, play, academically perform, or care for themselves. When the spirit plummets, so does the sense of self-empowerment. But when we address the stress or trauma by carefully choosing and integrating bottom-up and top-down approaches, as described by the other guidelines, we provide the right conditions for the spirit to lift again. Life regains meaning and motivates the child to identify and pursue interests, hobbies, dreams, and goals. Teachers, occupational therapists, mental health professionals, and certified yoga therapists are especially qualified to facilitate the life re-engagement process using the tools of their respective trades. Building partnerships between various professions, schools, and organizations can help to form the necessary referral networks—essentially, "safety nets"—to ensure that those children in need are fully supported along their journey to reconnect body, mind, and spirit and to find renewed meaning in their lives.

This chapter has provided an overview of the Sensory-Enhanced Yoga® methodology used by the SMYLE™ program and the ***Transdisciplinary Model for Post-Traumatic Growth in Children***, which provides its foundation. This model synthesizes the ancient kosha model with current treatment concepts from the fields of trauma psychology and occupational therapy in order to support clinical decision-making when working with traumatized individuals. The remaining chapters of Part 2 will provide detailed information on each of the guidelines, and then, in Part 3, we will put the whole practice together.

CHAPTER 7

Guideline #1: A Sense of Safety Is Essential to Healing

In her groundbreaking book *Trauma and Recovery*, psychiatrist Judith Herman (1997) declared that the first central task of healing from trauma is to ***establish a sense of safety***, a belief that continues to be strongly echoed by many renowned trauma experts (Ogden, Minton, and Pain 2006; Porges 2011; van der Kolk 2014). In yogic philosophy, a sense of safety has traditionally been linked with the ***annamaya kosha***, that is, the physical layer of one's being, since without a physical body a person cannot survive. Proper diet, exercise, and sanitation practices all have an important role in the health of the annamaya kosha. However, there is also a large psychological component to our sense of bodily safety, especially for those who have been traumatized. As Dr. van der Kolk explains:

> Traumatized people chronically feel unsafe inside their bodies: The past is alive in the form of gnawing interior discomfort. Their bodies are constantly bombarded by visceral warning signs, and, in an attempt to control these processes, they often become expert at ignoring their gut feelings and in numbing awareness of what is played out inside. They learn to hide from their selves. (2014, p.97)

The psychological aspect of bodily safety is acknowledged in the meaning of ***embodiment***—a term frequently used in the trauma field referring to our sense of self as safely and fully inhabiting our bodies. Arielle Schwartz explains (2017, para. 6), "Embodiment is an integration of three sensory feedback systems—exteroception, proprioception, and interoception." Our ***exteroceptors***—eyes, ears, nose, tongue, skin—receive information from the external environment and contribute to our sense of connection to our surroundings. ***Proprioceptors*** receive information from our muscles, joints, and inner ear to let us know how our body is positioned in space relative to gravity, and how separate body parts are positioned relative to other body parts. Our ***interoceptors*** alert our brain to what is happening within our viscera (internal organs; fleshy parts of our body), which the brain then interprets as hunger, thirst, sleepiness, alertness, body temperature, tension, pain, restlessness, and so on (Schwartz 2017).

The integration of sensory input originating from both outside and inside our bodies gives rise to our emotions, thoughts, and memories, which, in their totality, produce a felt sense of our "self." When sensory, cognitive, and memory processing are impacted by a traumatic event, the lost sense of psychological safety, deeply felt in the ***body***mind, can be almost as devastating as actual loss of life because it can leave a person feeling dead on the "inside." In some cases, a person may lose their sense of personal identity (depersonalization) and sense of presence in the world (derealization).

As you will recall, the insula plays a large role in integrating bodily sensations with emotions, and thus contributes enormously to the felt sense of our self. It tends to be overly active in people who are in hyperaroused states and underactive in people who have numbed out the messages from their body due to feeling overwhelmed by them (Lanius *et al.* 2015). The insula works closely with the ventrolateral prefrontal cortex (vlPFC), which labels these feelings. Lieberman *et al.* (2007) found that labeling feelings not only lit up the vlPFC, but that it also showed an inverse relationship with the amygdala, that is, ***labeling our feelings can reduce our distress***.

There is just one problem: while it is true that we learn to identify emotions from the various sensations experienced in our body (Nummenmaa *et al.* 2018), many young children, including those with developmental challenges, do not yet have the language skills to label their emotions. When these children experience toxic stress, anxiety, or trauma, they may notice a swamp of uncomfortable or even intolerable bodily sensations and do not know what to make of them. Some great ways caregivers are helping children with this skill is by reading story books, using visual aids, and creating "social stories" that help them understand events, label emotions associated with the events, and identify strategies to deal with these emotions. All of these practices fall within the first guideline for practice as they help to create a perception of safety in the body and in the world.

The development of psychosocial skills is strongly dependent on a sense of safety, and can thus be particularly impacted by trauma and other forms of toxic stress. Erik Erikson's (1950, 1963) theory of psychosocial development describes specific age ranges, from birth through adulthood, during which the person will encounter a stage-specific crisis, which can have a positive or negative outcome for personality development. The first six stages occur from birth to young adulthood (see Figure 7.1). In trauma, a sense of safety is significantly lacking, and so these capacities are damaged (Herman 1998). Since they were originally ***developed*** through social relationships with other people, they must be ***repaired*** through social relationships with other people. Furthermore, these relationships must help to "restore power and control to the survivor" (Herman 1998, para. 2).

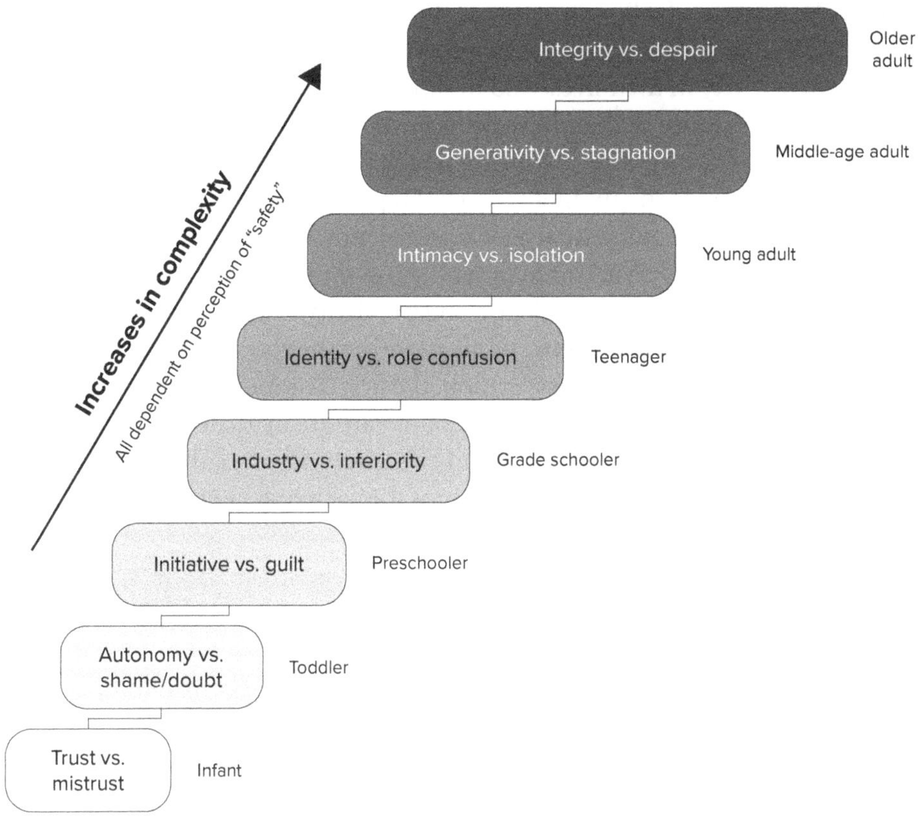

FIGURE 7.1: A PERCEPTION OF SAFETY IS CRUCIAL FOR PSYCHOSOCIAL DEVELOPMENT
Based on Erik Erikson's (1950, 1963) theory of psychosocial development and Herman (1998)

DEVELOPMENTAL FACTORS INFLUENCING A PERCEPTION OF SAFETY

A child's sense of safety is also affected by their sensory/perceptual and cognitive skills. One child may feel nervous or even overwhelmed walking along a busy city street, with cars and buses whipping by, while another child may walk right into the street without any thought for their safety. A child may use hand sanitizer until their hands get raw to cope with an excessive fear of germs, while another child may start eating their sandwich with dirt-covered hands. And we all have likely known a child who refuses to socially engage with unfamiliar people as well as a child who will readily walk off with strangers without a second thought. It can be a fine balance to teach children how to stay safe in their environment, relationships, and in their bodies without evoking hypervigilance or even fear!

Although we may have little influence over a child's situations outside of our settings, we can still have a strong influence on how safe they feel during our time with them. If a feeling of safety and relaxation is sufficiently soaked into their bodyminds during the yoga session, they may go home with an enhanced ***perception*** of safety in their lives. And in cases where this goal may be too incongruent with the reality of their life or circumstances (see Burstow 2003), we can nevertheless provide a pocket of time in which the ANS has a chance to learn to relax and feel safe for the moment. As Dr. Stephen Porges (2011, p.250) pointed out, "The human nervous system evolved efficiently to shift between conditions of safety and danger." It is in this manner that we promote greater ***resilience***, that is, the ability to rise to meet a challenge, and the ability to calm once the challenge has passed—thus mastering a sense of safety within the context of time and space.

So, taking all of this into consideration, the first treatment goals are to ensure, as far as possible, that the children under our care are in a safe environment; to surround them with safe people who can effectively promote their psychosocial development; and to help modulate the sensations they are experiencing so they feel safe in their own body.

THREE THINGS TO CONSIDER

In order to meet these goals, we need to ask ourselves three questions:

- ***Environmental safety:*** What is the child's perception of safety within the environmental setting, and how can we modify the setting to positively influence that perception?
- ***Social safety:*** What is the child's perception of safety with respect to their relationship with us (parent, teacher, caregiver, or therapist), and how can we modify our behavior and/or attitude to positively influence that perception?
- ***Bodily safety:*** What is the child's felt sense of safety (or lack thereof) regarding being in their body, and how can we modify the practice to positively influence that perception?

When providing yoga to highly stressed or traumatized students, it is ideal to design an optimal environment; develop a healing relationship with the child within that environment; and then help the child gradually and safely reconnect with their bodymind within this safe space. But an ideal environment is not always available: a child may live in a war zone, a refugee camp, a high crime neighborhood, or with a mentally ill parent. So again, it is helpful to consider the concept of safety in relative terms, and to set aside a special space in whatever environment the child finds themselves, which, over time, they begin to associate with healing, and which inspires them to let down their guard for even just moments of time.

CREATE A HEALING SPACE

We start by attending to the qualities of the environmental setting. We need to create a space for practice that allows children to deeply heal. We modify the environment to reduce stimuli that may reinforce hyperarousal or hypervigilance or possibly trigger an abreaction. We also remove any objects or symbols that could be construed to promote a certain religion or culture, such as statues of Buddha or Hindu gods or goddesses, or artifacts of Western religions for that matter.

Yoga and mindfulness practices can occur anywhere—classrooms, gymnasiums, libraries, auditoriums, courts, fields, bedrooms, church halls, community centers, counselor's offices, etc. If it is a community space, such as a gym or park, it is important to pick a time with minimal distractions from other people or activities. No matter what spaces are chosen, the key is to transform each setting into a welcoming, safe, and relaxing learning environment. This can be done by making purposeful, yet subtle, changes that focus on calming every sense.

When setting up the yoga space, we also must consider the needs of those who have been sexually abused. Sadly, it is estimated that one in four girls and one in six boys under the age of 18 have been sexually abused (Townsend and Rheingold 2013), so it is quite possible that this includes one or more children in any given yoga group. It is important to modify yoga practice to be sensitive to the needs of these students. For example, the term "yoga form" is used instead of "yoga pose," because the word "pose" is used in the sex trade. We take care in choosing and sequencing yoga forms, while providing choices, to reduce students' sense of vulnerability in various forms. We also use invitational language to give the children the onus of control for their own yoga practice. We discuss these concepts further throughout the book.

Not all settings are conducive to spreading out yoga mats. The reality is that in some settings, yoga mats may need to be positioned into "nooks and crannies" between desks, tables, or other furniture due to space limitations. Even so, it is important that there is sufficient space between yoga mats, and that they're not lined up one behind the other, in order to avoid awkward lines of vision. It is also advisable to remind children, adolescents especially, to wear clothing that will not inadvertently expose body parts during yoga forms (e.g., forward fold or downward-facing dog).

We suggest not separating yoga classes by gender. We may not be aware of which possible gender(s) a child is identifying themselves with, and nor which gender(s) they are sexually oriented to. Therefore, we feel the best approach is to simply be careful in setting up yoga mats, and to clearly identify and enforce clothing rules in a supportive and inclusive manner. Even given the rules, some children may forget or may not have access to appropriate clothing. In these circumstances, chair yoga forms can be substituted for mat practice so everyone can still participate, but from the chair position. You could also keep a supply of extra pants, shirts, and/or blankets in your room for children to borrow when needed. We never want to embarrass anyone, but instead, always encourage their participation in whatever form that may be.

Now we will go into our SMYLE™ recommendations for how to calm each sense.

Visual sense

In order to relax the visual sense, efforts should be made to reduce clutter on the walls, arrange furniture and materials in an organized manner, display relaxing images around the room, attend to the quality of lighting, and create a "relaxation space" that students can easily see and go to if they need a break. What follows are some important considerations in these areas:

Lighting: The lighting in a room significantly impacts how a person feels, thinks, and works in that environment. Finding balance is key, as going too far in either direction of the brightness spectrum can dramatically disrupt someone's attention, sense of safety, and performance. It cannot be too dark, or the person will feel less energized, and may even become sleepy. And while bright light in general has been shown to have a positive effect on feelings of alertness and vitality (Smolders and de Kort 2014), too much light—especially *artificial* light—has been associated with headaches, stress, anxiety, and other ill health conditions (Burks 1994; Khorshid *et al.* 2021).

Finally, the optimal lighting at any given moment will also depend on the ***activity*** being conducted. When offering yoga or mindfulness activities, it is best to adjust the lights to help reduce arousal levels by turning off the artificial lights to let some, or all, of the natural lighting stream through the windows. However, it is important to "read" the children you are working with; if they are all looking like they are falling asleep, you may want to increase the brightness level in the room and present a more energetic mindfulness practice that day. Dimmer switches are very helpful to control brightness levels, and even shaded lamps can be used to adjust lighting levels in different settings.

Offer views of nature: Window views of nature as well as videos and photographs of nature scenes have also been shown to enhance mood, reduce stress, and promote quality of life (Brown, Barton, and Gladwell 2013; Singh 2013). Meg "sets the scene" for her own students so that from the first moment they enter the classroom each morning they are greeted with dimmed lights, a meditation music video (such as the 24Relax or Yellow Brick music station on YouTube) with a soothing nature scene showing on the SmartBoard, alongside a consistent four-step morning arrival routine: 1) unpack your things; 2) greet teachers and friends; 3) check schedule for the day; 4) relax until yoga starts at 8.15am. Students have expressed the immediate sense of relaxation when they walk through the threshold of her door. By having the consistent, calm environment awaiting them daily, in combination with the clear expectations of their routine visually displayed, students' anticipatory anxiety is decreased.

Other visual considerations: Shabha and Gaines (2013) surveyed teachers to inquire which visual triggers in their classroom caused sensory sensitivity and stereotypic behaviors in students with autism. They discovered that it wasn't just the number of objects and decorations that could be visually overstimulating, but also the patterns and colors of the decor, furniture, flooring, and materials. Even covering bookshelves with solid fabric can give a room a cleaner look. Creating a serene, unified background helps center the attention on the important things. So, when designing a yoga setting, remember that "less is more."

Auditory sense

With regard to auditory sense, environmental noise should be reduced as much as possible to promote low stress emotional states. Tennis balls placed on chair feet are very effective in eliminating the irritating noise of chairs scraping along the floor. Playing calming music in the background is a subtle sensory strategy that helps block out distracting noises. White noise sound makers and water fountains are other great ways to block out external sound stimuli.

Music: If music is used, choose instrumentals that are soothingly melodic and/or have a slow, even rhythm. Native American flute, acoustic guitar, or soft piano music tends to be calming for many students. Meditation music in particular was shown to reduce state anxiety in a group of 70 Indian army recruits as compared to controls (Telles *et al.* 2012). As a general rule, the more predictable and rhythmic the music, the more calming it is to the listener (Porges 2011). In addition, songs with words can distract someone from the mental process of entering an embodied state. Even in instrumental form, popular music can distract students, causing them to only focus on the song melody rather than the task at hand. When music is chosen properly and played regularly, the calming music will subconsciously be paired with an increase in their relaxation response.

Sound signals: Some yoga instructors incorporate soothing sounds into sessions including singing bowls and chimes to draw attention to the present moment. When introducing routines, it is best to warn in advance that you will be using a particular sound at a specific point in time, and invite feedback. It should be noted that any high-pitched or low aggressive-sounding tones are to be avoided, as humans are innately wired to respond to these tones as indicating danger (Porges 2011).

Unexpected noises: There can also be unusual sounds, such as from plumbing pipes, heating systems, a vacuum, someone working in an adjacent room, or a creaky staircase. It is best to point out the source of these sounds when they occur, to reduce any fearful reactions. It also helps participants process these sounds when instructors make connections to their lives, such as "the heating system just turned on to keep us warm" or "that's the water rushing to the sink so we can wash our hands." For moments when the background music or sounds are not enough to block out certain sounds in the room or building, it is helpful to have soundproof headphones readily available to use when needed.

Tactile sense

We also promote calming through the tactile sense, which includes attending to the temperature and humidity of the room and any other sensation that we feel through our skin. Tactile stimulation occurs every time we touch something or something touches us.

Furniture: In any setting, it is helpful to have a dedicated relaxation space. This space should be all about comfort, so equip it with soft upholstered furniture such as a loveseat, cushy armchair, bean bag chair, and/or a *comfortable* rocking chair that is well fitted for the children to rock in it. A yoga mat could be left open on the floor, and blankets and other props, such as bolsters and pillows, could be stashed nearby.

Room temperature and humidity: One thing we do not often consider is how the air on someone's skin affects their functioning. Many studies have been conducted on the relationship of room temperature or humidity on school or work performance (Singh 2013). The general consensus appears to be that people perform best in rooms with moderate humidity and temperatures between 68°F and 74°F (Schneider 2002). When the body is too hot or too cold, the brain is focusing all of its attention and energy on fixing the problem, which makes it extremely difficult to focus on the task at hand.

Fidgets and weighted objects: One way to promote calming through the tactile sense is to provide weighted lap pillows and eye pillows (or eye masks) for students to use during meditation. Subtle tactile fidgets, like stress balls, silly putty, stretchy bracelets or rings, pop it toys, kinetic sand, and palm weights, that are non-distracting to others, are great for providing the sensory input needed to relax the rest of the body. These fidgets and weighted pillows are extremely helpful in quieting body movements and redirecting "busy hands" from compulsive tendencies such as picking, scratching, tapping, etc. They provide deep touch pressure input, which is known to inhibit the "fight–flight" response in the nervous system.

Physical assists: Always ask first before physically assisting in any activity, including yoga, and if you receive permission to assist, always use a "firm touch," using the whole hand, rather than a light or feathery fingertip touch. The setting may influence whether and to what degree physical assists are used. Participants who have mobility impairments may need physical assistance for some of the yoga forms. Even though they may be used to being touched, it is still important to ask first.

Keep in mind that as soon as you touch someone, body and mind become separated: whatever level of bodymind integration had been achieved will be disrupted as they switch back on the thinking, judging mind. Physical assists may also make the recipient feel that they are performing a yoga form incorrectly. It also reinforces the idea that the instructor is an authority figure, taking the control away from the student. Also, traumatized individuals are at greater risk of experiencing sensitivity to touch than the general population. Finally, keep in mind that the purpose of a yoga class for self-regulation and trauma healing is to support psychological (and brain rebalancing) as opposed to physical goals. We are not looking for perfect alignment in the yoga forms, although safe alignment is imperative. Careful verbal instruction and demonstration—repeated if necessary to the entire group (vs. singling out a participant)—would usually meet the latter criteria. Incorporating visual targets (e.g., feet/hand markers, yoga blocks) can be a less invasive and subtler way to achieve safe alignment without embarrassing anyone.

Olfactory sense

Smell (olfaction) is the only sense that synapses directly on the amygdala (and also connects rapidly to the hippocampus), making it a very powerful sensory stimulus for better or for worse (Mouly and Sullivan 2010). All other senses are filtered through the brainstem and thalamus before reaching other areas of the brain, lessening their impact. The amygdala is the center for emotional memories, which is why certain smells can trigger vivid memories of people, places, or things (Vermetten and Bremner 2003). The response to olfactory input is quite subjective and can carry strong emotional associations, positive or negative, and we usually don't know what those are for a given person. It can be extremely calming for some, while triggering hyperarousal for others. Therefore, it is important to find out from your participants (or their parents) whether they have any sensitivity to different types of smell before introducing any scents into the setting.

Sensory conclusions

Relaxing every sense invites the bodymind to let down its "guard" and function at a more calm and stable state. These more *passive* sensory methods help participants develop the fortitude, patience, and open-mindedness necessary to engage in the *active* mindfulness practices (i.e., yoga, breathing, and meditation), which enable them to exert control over their own "relaxation response," that is, to *self*-regulate. When participants operate within their window of tolerance, they are better able to listen, learn, socialize, and engage in all areas of their lives.

ATTEND TO THE TEACHER–STUDENT RELATIONSHIP

We create a space that is psychologically safe by interacting with participants in a manner that respects boundaries and welcomes whatever arises in them. SMYLE™ instructors need to feel grounded so they can respond to situations with self-awareness, rather than fear. If someone has an emotional catharsis, we support them in an authentic, trusting, and unconditionally accepting manner, to allow it to complete the process and serve as a healing experience. We communicate our confidence that they have the inner resources that will allow them to process their trauma the way they need to process it. However, we don't play the role of a counselor unless we *are* a licensed counselor; instead, we refer to someone who is, if the participant starts to confide personal issues beyond the domain of our profession.

Above all, we place participants—not the instructor or the therapist—in full control of their own yoga and mindfulness experiences. We do this by encouraging them to listen to their own bodymind, and to get out of a yoga form or to stop a breathing or meditation practice if it causes discomfort or distress, and also by giving them a *choice* in every aspect of the yoga practice. As Emerson and Hopper (2011) have emphasized, this is especially vital when working with individuals who have been traumatized.

PROMOTE SAFETY IN THE BODYMIND

Once the environmental and interpersonal factors are addressed, the instructor can begin to help the participant foster a sense of safety in the body, or, as Dr. Bessel van der Kolk put it, to "befriend the body" (2008, 2014). Dr. van der Kolk points out that, "In order to change, people need to become aware of their sensations and the way that their bodies interact with the world around them. Physical self-awareness is the first step in releasing the tyranny of the past" (2014, p.101). Attending to bodily sensation is a hallmark of a mindful yoga practice. However, with trauma survivors, this process needs to proceed in a careful manner in order to avoid becoming inundated by these sensations. Babette

Rothschild (2009), renowned trauma social worker, famously used the analogy of a pressurized soda bottle to drive this point home: the safest way to release the pressure is to open and close the cap in a slow, cautious, and intentional manner, so as to prevent an explosion.

How does this translate to yoga practice? Each participant brings to class their own personal experiences, which can be expressed by the body in a myriad of ways. For example, someone who is depressed may demonstrate a slouched or low tone posture, while another person who is highly anxious may present with arms pulled in protectively to the chest. Depending on many varying factors, how the bodymind presents can change day to day. So it is important for the instructor to constantly be reading the room in order to pick up on the subtle or more obvious cues participants are exhibiting, in order to best support them.

It is impossible for instructors to know every adverse experience each of their participants has had. That is why we recommend teaching in a manner that is sensitive to all experiences. In respect for those who have been sexually traumatized, when presenting hip-opener yoga forms, instructors should provide an alternative choice that does not open the hips, such as keeping legs straight and together. Additionally, a blanket can be offered to all participants during more vulnerable yoga forms, such as Bridge. Use of a blanket not only fosters a sense of safety within the practice, but also provides neutral warmth to the body, which promotes calming and the release of muscle tension.

Some experts feel that yoga straps might be triggering for sexual trauma or domestic violence survivors, and should be avoided in yoga classes. For this reason, when we offer the choice to use this prop, we refer to it as a "band" and not a "strap." Although we have not personally witnessed hesitation in using a band, the belief does seem intuitive. Certainly every yoga class should present yoga bands as a ***choice***, and not a requirement. All yoga forms and moves performed with a yoga band can also be easily performed without one, and this should be stated. However, banning yoga bands from a program altogether would eliminate a particularly rich form of proprioceptive input that can promote embodiment in a sensorially comfortable and integrating manner. Observing and soliciting feedback from our participants can help us make the best decisions with regard to these types of dilemmas. Other substitute props that may be less triggering than yoga bands include: t-shirts, towels, scarves, foam pipe insulation, or pool noodles.

Some of the yoga forms that appear to be the most innocuous on the surface can actually be among the most challenging for people who have been traumatized. For example, while most participants may look forward to the moments when they are invited to simply rest supine on their mats, this position can feel particularly vulnerable for those who have PTSD. Again, offering choices is important, such as Crocodile, in which the person is prone rather than supine, with the chest raised a bit and the head resting on the forearms. Other options include Child, or a side-lying position. Some participants may simply choose to remain seated during times when others are lying on their mats—not so much due to mobility issues, but simply because it feels safer to them.

One thing to keep in mind when offering choices in positioning is that someone is likely to take you up on the alternative offer, and when they do, you need to be prepared to instruct them on what to do next. This takes some advanced planning and choreography so the person who decides to assume Crocodile isn't just lying there the whole time while you are moving others through supine Leg Stretches. In this example, we simply wouldn't offer that particular combination of choices, but instead might offer the choice of doing the Leg Stretches on the mat or sitting in a chair.

INTRODUCE THE INNER RESOURCE

Another technique that helps to build a "safe container" is the ***Inner Resource***, developed by Dr. Richard Miller as a component of his Integrative Restoration (iRest®) program, which has been used at military and veteran facilities around the country. The Inner Resource is a somatically (body-based) felt state of well-being produced by the pure, present-moment awareness of the unchanging qualities of "being" itself. Initially, people tend to find it easier to access this state using sensory imagery, although this is simply a portal to the Inner Resource and not the Inner Resource itself. Dr. Miller emphasizes the importance not only of developing the imagery but also of letting it fall away in order to rest in the feeling state itself.[1]

What follows is one example of an Inner Resource script that comes from the iRest tradition. The language is more advanced, so is best used with teens and young adults—advanced training is suggested in order to use iRest techniques skillfully.[2]

> Take time now to develop your Inner Resource. A feeling of well-being in your body where you feel totally at ease and secure... You might imagine a special, peaceful place that you've visited...or a beautiful scene from a movie...or a place entirely in your imagination...one that makes you feel safe, relaxed, and comfortable. It could be in an outdoor setting, or in a special room, or may be the image of a special person or pet that helps you experience the feeling of well-being in your body... Allow your senses to come into play...the sights...sounds...smells... and tastes...or other resources that evoke the feelings of deep peace...comfort... and ease... Then allow these images to completely fade away while you remain

1 www.irest.org/system/files/2023-03/2023-03-21%20L1%20LIV%20Reference%20Guide.pdf
2 Please go to www.irest.org to learn more.

> with the felt sense of well-being in your body...a Being aware and awake to Itself...this is your Inner Resource...[long pause]...
>
> ...During practice, or during your daily life, should you feel distressed, you can return to your Inner Resource and feel at ease, secure, and comfortable.

Meg created this next example for the students in her classroom. She found that they needed a longer, more detailed journey, at a slower pace, with more concrete language, so they could experience their Inner Resource, or, as she calls it, their "safe place."

> When you are ready, meet me in a comfortable position.
> Close your eyes or keep your eyes just open a little...whatever feels right to you.
> Imagine you are walking down a hallway full of doors of all different colors.
> Look at the red door, blue, purple, green, and they keep going on...
> Find the door that is your favorite color.
> Look, it has your name on it, too.
> Reach out and turn the knob on the door.
> Open it and step through the doorway.
> Ahhh *[let out a relaxing sigh]*...you entered into your safe place.
> Where are you?
> Maybe you're at a place you've been to on vacation,
> Or a place you've always dreamed of going.
> Maybe you're in a beautiful scene from a movie you watched.
> A special spot in your house.
> Or even somewhere you totally made up in your imagination.
> Try to imagine different details that help relax each sense in your body.
> What do you see?... What do you hear?... What do you feel on your skin?
> What do you smell?... What do you taste?
> The more details you can think of, the stronger you can imagine this safe place.
> Now try to focus on how you feel in this safe place.
> Do you feel calm...comfortable...relaxed...at ease...or something different?
> Where in your body do you feel this feeling?
> Sit with that feeling for a moment... This feeling you get here is your true safe place.
> [Sit quietly for 15 seconds to 3 minutes—whatever is best for your group.]
> Remember this place is always here for you,
> No matter where you are or what you're doing.
> All you have to do is close your eyes and picture these details..."voila!" you're here!
> Maybe you want to stay a little longer or maybe you're ready to go back to class.
> You do what's right for you.
> Before you leave, take one more look around at your amazing, safe place.

You can say to yourself "I'll be back!"
Slowly...walk back to the door of your favorite color.
Turn the doorknob and push open the door.
Walk back through the doorway into that hallway of colorful doors.
This time please find the door back to the classroom.
Come in when you are ready.
Bring in with you that calm...safe...comfortable feeling.
[Take a slow, deep breath in through your nose and let it out.]
Optional: Listen for the three bells ending our meditation.
Ding... Ding... Ding...
Slowly bring your attention back to your body in the room.
Wiggle your toes and fingers,
Turn your head from side to side,
Move the muscles in your face.
If you want, put a big smile on your face.
Open your eyes when you're ready.
Take a moment to smile and wave to your friends and teachers,
Sending your good feelings to them and wishing them a good day ahead.
When you're ready you can sit up and get ready for ....

The imagery of a concrete object—the door—as a portal to the "safe place" can make it easier for participants to figure out how to mentally "get there." The use of the bell or chimes can be helpful to signal that the meditation is coming to an end, but should only be used if students associate it with relaxation and are not auditorily sensitive to it.

AVOID COMMON TRIGGERS

To foster a sense of safety, the instructor needs to carefully evaluate all aspects of the environmental setting, to reduce the potential for triggering flashbacks or states of dissociation. A trigger is a troubling reminder of a traumatic event, and may consist of just about anything: certain people, places, noises, music, images, candles, smells, tastes, objects, emotions, animals, scenes within movies or TV shows, certain dates or other time events, tones of voice, body positions, bodily sensations, certain words (e.g., relax, test, fire alarm, hospital, doctor, certain commands), or even weather conditions. Many adolescents and adults with PTSD typically avoid triggers that they are aware of, which may affect daily functioning and restrict their lifestyle (Hirsch and Holmes 2007).

Children, on the other hand, have less control of what they do in their lives, so can be forced into triggering situations and not have the awareness or emotional regulation skills to properly deal with it. Also, many children or young adults with disabilities do not have the language skills to express what is triggering to them, which is unfortunate since, as you will recall, labeling feelings can reduce distress. Often when children have tantrums, act overly silly, or do not pay attention, it's judged to be a maladaptive behavior that requires disciplinary action, when really it could be their only way of signaling discomfort due to the presence or anticipation of a trigger.

Those individuals, young and old, who are able to identify and avoid triggers in their lives, do so in order to stay within their window of tolerance. Some common situations that they avoid include noisy and/or crowded places such as large gatherings, school assemblies, school dances, and restaurants; certain smells (or situations that involve certain smells); 4th of July firework displays, and so on. Making minor environmental modifications can be a positive adaptation in someone's life. However, when a person's world becomes so restrictive that it impacts their ability to function, it can affect all areas of development, especially in children. You may have heard that some combat veterans who suffer from PTSD exhibit a "bunker mentality" by bolting their doors shut and/or rarely leaving the home. A similar level of avoidance can be seen in students who refuse to go to school in the morning.

Triggers can be difficult to anticipate. In any setting, it is helpful to try to eliminate the most common triggers (e.g., vulnerable body positions, loud noises, busy environments, certain words); however, it is usually impossible as well as unnecessary to eliminate everything that has ever been a trigger for someone, as most triggers are highly unique to each particular individual. After reducing or eliminating the most common triggers, the best approach is to simply be observant to the verbal and bodily reactions of your participants, such as a hesitancy to assume certain yoga forms or commenting on certain words, and, if reasonable, make adjustments accordingly.

EFFECTIVELY MANAGE EMOTIONAL ABREACTIONS

It is also important to be observant for signs of dissociation and flashbacks, both of which were described in Chapter 3. Flashbacks tend to be more obvious than states of dissociation, and can involve acting out the trauma. In the case of children, flashbacks may be demonstrated differently, including experiencing a repetitive nightmare, re-enacting the traumatic event through pretend play using toys or with their friends, or even just blurting out statements that are irrelevant to the current topic but that carry very strong emotional content, such as "A car is coming!" (when a child got hit by a car) or "Get the belt!" (repeating what they hear prior to being beaten).

In contrast, signs of dissociation tend to be more subtle. Some examples that you may notice include staring off into space, talking to themself, grimacing or making other facial expressions that do not match the present situation, twitching, self-soothing behaviors such as rocking, missing conversation or being slow to respond, darting eyes or far-away gaze, memory lapses, flat affect, and over- or underactivity (Schiraldi 2000). In contrast to flashbacks and dissociated states, outpourings of deep mourning are healthy reactions and are best allowed to unfold and process through the system. Flashbacks and dissociated states may or may not be triggered by something happening in the present moment. Here are some suggestions for how to handle the situation when these states occur.

HOW TO HANDLE FLASHBACKS AND DISSOCIATED STATES

Grounding techniques are considered to be the most important for helping someone handle dissociation or flashbacks. These are designed to help the person come back to their present surroundings by engaging the senses. There are two basic types of grounding techniques: sensory awareness techniques and cognitive techniques. ***Sensory awareness techniques*** use the senses to draw the person back into their body and present surroundings. ***Cognitive techniques*** involve asking questions to orient the individual to place and time. Both of these techniques are demonstrated below.

Rothschild (2000) also discusses the importance of developing "dual awareness" of the ***experiencing self*** and the ***observing self***, concepts she learned from Dr. van der Kolk, McFarlane, and Weisaeth (1996). When someone is having a flashback, they are completely immersed in the experiencing self, and the observing self needs to be re-awakened. Here are some ideas for doing that:

- Go over to the person, and using a firm, but soothing, voice, ask them to sit up and look around the room.
- If it seems that touch would be helpful, *ask* them if you can touch their shoulder or arm (to help with grounding, and so they know you are there to care for them).
- Ask the person to:
    - Describe objects or other details in the room, such as the color of the walls
    - Press their feet into the floor or stomp the feet
    - Rub the mat, rub their hands together, or rub another object.

In Meg's classroom, she sometimes has her students do a "Mindfulness Moment" as a group exercise or a 1:1 technique to help them come back into their window of tolerance. In a group mindfulness moment, the students are asked to describe something in the current location for each of the five senses. She welcomes them to participate in a quiet, calm voice: "Let's take a mindfulness moment together. Try to describe something for each sense. What do you see?... What do you hear?... What do you feel?... What do you smell?... What do you taste?..." She finds that sometimes if she provides examples of her own, it can help the students through the practice. If she notices the students need a deeper sensory grounding experience, she will extend the practice by asking for a specific quantity of observations for each sense. Figure 7.2 shows the visual Meg displays on the projection or interactive whiteboard (such as a SmartBoard) as she teaches the practice: "Tell me three things you see... Tell me two things you hear... Tell me one thing you feel."

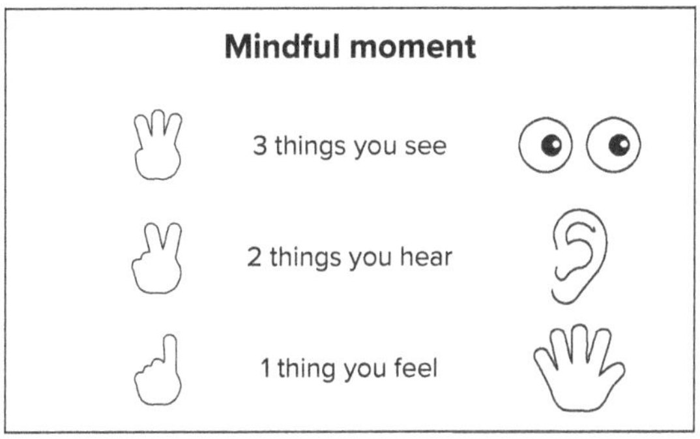

FIGURE 7.2: MINDFUL MOMENT 3–2–1

Recommended protocols for managing flashbacks

Rothschild (2000) developed a flashback halting protocol for when a person's ***observing self*** is again online, which we believe is most suitable for adolescents and adults who have sufficient cognitive skills to use it. She intended it for use in clinical settings or for self-use, but we believe it can be used in a yoga class or other setting if the instructor is in consultation with a mental health professional. We have adapted it for younger children to better meet their language and sensory awareness abilities (see "A grounding exercise for managing negative feelings and experiences"). From our perspective, the most important parts of this protocol are putting words to the feelings; matching feelings to bodily sensations; and directing the person's attention to concrete evidence that they are now safely in the "here and now," and not the "there and then." This exercise applies the findings from Lieberman *et al.* (2007), showing that labeling feelings and associated bodily sensations inhibits the amygdala and reduces emotional reactivity.

A GROUNDING EXERCISE FOR MANAGING NEGATIVE FEELINGS AND EXPERIENCES

(Adapted from Rothschild 2000)

Teacher: How do you feel?

Student: I feel . . . . [describe emotion].

Teacher: What sensations do you feel in your body?

Student: I sense in my body . . . . [describe bodily sensations].

Teacher: What are you remembering?

Student: I am remembering . . . . [name difficult event/memory].

Teacher: Where are you?

Student: I am at . . . . [place where you are/location].

Teacher: What do you see around you?

Student: I see . . . . [describe what you see right *now*, in *this* place].

Teacher: Is the . . . . [name difficult event/memory] happening now?

Student: No... . . . . [name difficult event/memory] is not happening now/anymore.

Teacher: Let's focus on . . . . [current activity].

Keep in mind when working with your participants that there is no objective measure that determines whether an event is traumatic or not, as each person perceives the world around them in their own unique way. It's important to validate their feelings about any situation and to meet them where they are to help them process what they are going through.

SUICIDAL REMARKS

The Center for Suicide Prevention (2017, para. 2) stated that "unresolved trauma in childhood and adolescence is linked to an increased risk of suicide ideation and if unaddressed, can escalate with age—potentially leading to suicide attempts or death by suicide. Early intervention post-trauma is crucial." Therefore, if a student makes a suicidal remark during a session, inform them that you take it seriously. Listen attentively, supportively, and without placing blame.

Gently ask probing questions, such as: "Is this something you have been thinking about a lot?" "Are you afraid for your own safety?" "Have you thought about how you would take your own life?" Through sensitive questioning and listening, you can determine whether they have a plan, a time frame, and access to methods for taking their life (such as a weapon or pills). It may seem counterintuitive and frightening to invite people to talk about suicidal thoughts, but it is necessary for assessing the level of seriousness of the threat. Also, offering the opportunity to talk about the feelings can reduce the risk of acting on them. The Mayo Clinic (2022) suicide guidelines echo this philosophy.

If a participant responds to your questions in a way that leads you to believe that they are suicidal, don't leave them alone—wait with them until there is a mental health professional or a family member to help them. If they ask you to not tell anyone, explain that you can't make that promise if you think their life is in danger. If the situation happens in a school or health setting, you can call or walk them to a mental health professional, if one is in the same building. If it occurs in the community during a club, yoga class, sporting event, private session, or other location where you don't have access to a mental health professional, ask the participant if they have a counselor and/or family member you can call to help them. As a best practice, having emergency contact information on hand is important before engaging anyone in a yoga session. If you can't locate a mental health professional or emergency contact person, you should call the national emergency or suicide hotline (see the box below).

Personal crisis helplines

US: Call 988, which is the Suicide & Crisis Lifeline number. To reach the Veterans Crisis Line, call 988, then press "1" to chat live or text 838255.

UK: Call 999 or the European emergency number, 112. The Samaritans[3] suicide hotline number in the UK is 116 123.

Australia: Call 000 or Lifeline at 13 11 14.

Despite these recommendations, we don't always know how we will react if such a situation actually arises. A statement such as "I don't know how I can go on living like this" can be taken as an off-the-cuff, innocuous remark about a temporary life situation and not as a literal statement; however, people have taken their lives soon after making such a remark, so it is important to clarify

3 www.samaritans.org

its meaning. More strongly worded remarks of suicidal ideation can feel disorienting and surreal for the listener, and can even be blocked from consciousness if they threaten the safety of their own psyche. We can't help our participants feel safe if what they are telling us makes us feel unsafe. We need to have the presence of mind to do the right thing to handle the situation. Yoga techniques, especially the breathing and grounding practices, are among the best tools to help us with that. So, as you help to ground your participant in such crises, remember to ground yourself as well.

CHAPTER 8

Guideline #2: The Most Direct and Powerful Way to Self-Regulate is Through Control of the Breath

You may already be familiar with the idea that focusing on your breath can help to sink the mind back into the body and draw awareness to the present moment. However, no amount of cuing to "breathe down into the bottom of the lungs" will make it so; this is a skill that evolves in developmental stages. Most young children have only a "surface" understanding of their human body as having a head, torso, limbs, and some additional details, like facial features, fingers, and toes. They do not have a strong grasp of how their bodies work from the inside. They may hear their heartbeat at times and know they have bones and muscles that enable them to move as well as a stomach that their food gets dumped into after they eat. That is about the extent of it. So, while we would love nothing better than for some of the children we work with to use breathing techniques to slow themselves down or help them to self-regulate their emotions, we can't expect them to fully grasp a discussion about the diaphragm or intercostal muscles and to willfully control the breath from the "inside out." They need to be developmentally ready to do so, and will likely require some extra tools from our toolbox.

THE EMERGENCE OF BREATH CONTROL

From a young age, and without knowing much about their internal body, children learn how to control their breath in order to make things happen in their ***external world***, such as:

- Smell a flower or candle
- Smell food cooking
- Blow out birthday candles

- Blow your nose
- Blow up a balloon
- Swim underwater
- Blow bubbles
- Cool off a cup of hot cocoa
- Play a musical instrument
- Blow the seeds off a dandelion
- Blow a pinwheel
- Suck through a straw.

Yet very rarely are children taught how to use their breath to control their ***internal sense of well-being***. This is a lost opportunity, as the breath is the most direct way for humans to control their own ANS, which powerfully influences a person's level of stress, state of arousal, mood, and behavior (Zaccaro *et al.* 2018). In fact, the breath is the only voluntary control we have over the ANS; all other functions are involuntary, such as heart rate, blood pressure, sweating, eye dilation, digestion, and so on.

Respiration is unique in that we need to be able to voluntarily control our breath at times to eat, speak, or perform the activities listed above, while at other times the breathing muscles are controlled automatically from the brainstem (Butler 2007). This dual neuronal wiring of the breath makes it an especially valuable self-regulation tool when the child is developmentally ready to harness it. We will show you how to teach students to do that, but let's first revisit the more primal pathway through which children learn to regulate their level of arousal, emotions, and behavior.

FROM CO-REGULATION TO SELF-REGULATION

As discussed in earlier chapters, children typically learn to ***self***-regulate through the process of ***co***-regulating with others. The attachment bonds that develop through this process stimulate the release of oxytocin, which regulates the HPA axis (hormonal response to stress) by reducing the activity of the amygdala (threat detector) and the fear response (Kovalchick 2015). In fact, attachment theory (Bowlby 1969; Saunders *et al.* 2015) is a prominent theory in the mental health field due to the powerful effects caregiver attachment has on child development and well-being.

When attachments to caregivers do not develop properly or are broken, it can have a highly deleterious effect on children, including dysregulating the HPA axis (Cavanaugh *et al.* 2016; Kovalchick 2015). Outside of the home setting, teachers and therapists assume the caregiving role for the child, especially at school. As discussed in the previous chapter on Guideline #1, the SMYLE™

program recognizes and supports the critical role supportive adults play in fostering a child's sense of safety, well-being, and empowerment.

As children grow, however, they need to learn to develop their own internal resources to stay regulated. The activities bulleted at the beginning of this chapter can be used either directly or through the imagination to help children develop awareness and control of their breath. Once a degree of control is established through these basic breath awareness activities, we teach children specific breathing practices that activate the parasympathetic ("rest and digest") branch of the ANS to help decrease the sympathetic branch ("fight–flight" response).

HARNESSING THE BREATH FOR SELF-REGULATION

Preliminary studies suggest that harnessing the power of the breath is both feasible for children and can be effective for regulating the ANS (Veerman 2017). However, most of what we know about the power of the breath is derived from studies of adults. Breathing interventions for adults have found reduced blood pressure, reduced heart rate, and improved vagal tone, which is a sign of PNS activation (Veerman 2017). All are indicators of stress reduction. Numerous studies have shown that heart rate variability and respiratory sinus arrhythmia, which are measures of vagal tone (a good thing!), are maximized at approximately six breaths per minute in adults (Russo, Santarelli, and O'Rourke 2017).

Saoji, Raghavendra, and Manjunath (2019) recently reviewed studies on breathing practices showing positive changes in neurocognitive, psychophysiological, respiratory, biochemical, and metabolic functions. Again, most breathing practices were found to demonstrate highly significant effects on autonomic functions. In Saoji *et al.*'s study, the vast majority of yoga breathing practices produced a parasympathetic shift in the balance of the ANS, while high frequency breathing techniques, such as Kapalabhati (Skull-Shining Breath), produced a sympathetic shift. They reported that, in general, yoga breathing practices can be considered safe when practiced under the supervision of a teacher who has received professional training in the techniques, although further studies are warranted.

Frequency, dosage, intensity, and duration of intervention significantly influence the size of the effects of breathing practices. Veerman (2017) presents an interesting discussion on this topic, contrasting the findings from adults with suggested modifications for children. Adult studies suggest that a minimum of three to four weeks' duration is necessary to obtain maximum benefits from the practices (Veerman 2017). While breathing sessions for adults can last 15–40 minutes, Semple, Reid, and Miller (2005) found that seven- to eight-year-olds could comfortably engage in breathing practices for only 3–5 minutes.

Suggesting breathing exercise parameters for children is challenging as studies of children have rarely investigated breathing practices in isolation. Rather, they are usually just one component of a broader treatment protocol of body-mind practices, such as MBSR (Veerman 2017). However, studies have been located that investigated the effects of isolated breathing practices on test anxiety, pain control, ADHD, respiratory dysfunction, and reaction times in children, all showing positive results (see Table 8.1).

Table 8.1: Selected breath studies

Author(s) and date	Study focus	Study methods	Participants and ages	Results
Breathing and pain control in children				
Bagheriyan *et al.* (2011)	Effects of breathing exercise and making bubbles on catheter insertion pain	Divided into two experimental groups (breathing exercise and bubble making) and a control group	60 children (ages 6–12) diagnosed with thalassemia (an inherited blood disorder)	Both methods were effective in reducing pain compared with controls. No significant differences were found between the treatment groups, suggesting children should decide for themselves which method to use
Pourmovahed, Dehghani, and Sherafat (2013)	Effects of Hey-Hu breathing on perception of pain during spinal injection	Children alternated uttering "Hey" and "Hu" with each exhalation while guided through a slow and deep breathing exercise	100 children diagnosed with leukemia between the ages of 6 and 15	Mean pain score was significantly lesser in the regular breathing (Hey-Hu) group than the control group, at the 0.001 level of significance
Breathing and childhood test anxiety				
Khng (2017)	Effects of deep (diaphragmatic) breathing on anxiety and test performance	Pre-test/post-test; controlled design To increase anxiety, students were told they would be given a timed test on math and attention skills, and that their results would be openly compared with other students	122 fifth grade students	Deep breaths taken just prior to a timed math test significantly reduced anxiety and improved performance on the test Reduction in state anxiety Significantly predicted state-of-mind improvement, which predicted math improvement

Su *et al.* (2010)	Effectiveness of: Relaxation, Breathing, Training (RBT)	Performed the RBT two times per week for two months prior to a performance examination to take place for a jury of their music teachers at the end of the semester	59 student musicians in grades 3–6	Significant reduction in music performance anxiety when anxiety levels were compared 30 minutes and 5 minutes prior to the performance exam However, anxiety had increased during those two months of breathing training until it reached a peak of 30 minutes prior to performance
Breath-controlled biofeedback games for ADHD				
Sonne and Jensen (2016)	The effects of a biofeedback game, ChillFish, on calming compared to a breathing exercise	Heart rate variability was monitored while playing a stressful activity (Pacman) followed by breathing exercises or the ChillFish biofeedback game	12 children with ADHD between the ages of 8 and 13	Positive tendency that playing ChillFish produces a similar calming experience as a traditional breathing exercise
Amon and Campbell (2008)	Breath-controlled biofeedback games for managing symptoms of inattention in children with ADHD	Children played the "Journey to Wild Divine" video game by manipulating their heart rate using breathing techniques taught in the game, measured through three finger sensors	24 children participated in the treatment group for this controlled study; 17 received biofeedback sessions once per week for 12 weeks and 7 attended sessions three times per week for 8 weeks	Biofeedback video games were effective for teaching breathing and relaxation techniques in children who have ADHD Children could manipulate their heart rates (measured through three finger sensors) using breathing techniques taught in the game They found that the video game, the "Journey to Wild Divine," has the potential to improve symptoms of ADHD as well as disruptive behaviors

cont.

Breathing and reaction times in children[1]				
Bhavanani and Madanmohan (2003)	Visual reaction time (VRT) and auditory reaction time (ART)	Measured VRT and ART following nine rounds of Mukha Bhastrika (Bellows Breath)	22 healthy schoolboys	Significant ($p<0.01$) reduction in both VRT and ART, indicating improved sensorimotor performance and processing ability of the central nervous system Authors theorize this may be due to increased arousal, rate of information processing, concentration, and/or ability to ignore irrelevant stimuli
Bhavanani, Ramanathan, and Harichandrakumar (2012)	Immediate effect of Mukha Bhastrika (a bellows-type pranayama) on reaction time	VRT and ART was measured before and after nine rounds of Mukha Bhastrika and a control period of 10 minutes of normal activities	34 adolescents with intellectual challenges who received yoga instruction once per week for more than three years	Significant ($p<0.0001$) reduction in VRT and ART following nine rounds of Mukha Bhastrika (Bellows Breath) Authors theorize that Mukha Bhastrika may alter afferent sensory input from abdominal and thoracic regions causing a modulation of neuronal activity in the reticular activation system and thalamic-cortical levels of the brain

RESPIRATORY RATE

The respiratory rate of children is markedly different from adults and declines over time, from infancy to adulthood. However, studies examining respiration rate by age have found varying results. Table 8.2 compares numbers from two sources, showing differences that are only partially explained by the different age range cut-offs (please only use these as "ballpark" numbers).

Table 8.2: Respiration rates decrease with age, but vary between individuals

Mersch (2020)		**Eldridge (2021)**	
Age range	**Breaths per minute**	**Age range**	**Breaths per minute**
Preschool (3–5 years)	20–25	Preschooler (3–5 years)	22–34
School-aged child (6–11 years)	14–22	School-aged child (6–12 years)	18–30
Adolescent (12–15 years)	12–18	Adolescent (13–17 years)	12–16

1 The SMYLE™ program does not teach Bellows Breath because it can activate the SNS.

"START WHERE THE CHILD IS AT"

The second guiding principle of Sensory-Enhanced Yoga®/SMYLE™ speaks to the energy layer of a person's being in general, not just the breath, so remember to "start where the child is at." This is far better than trying to match a child's breath rate to a respiration chart that is hard to even decipher. You can't expect someone who is running around the room to be able to do a slow yoga practice (or suddenly stop running to do slow belly breathing), and you can't expect a child who is depressed and feeling sluggish to do an energetic practice. Start where they are, and gradually move them in the direction of where you want them to be. Also bear in mind that the teacher's natural breath rate will likely be too slow for the child. According to the Cleveland Clinic (Chourpiliadis and Bhardwaj 2022) the average *adult* respiratory rate is between 12 and 20 breaths per minute, so keep in mind that there can also be a wide variation in respiratory rates, even between instructors!

It is often possible to hear and/or observe the breath rate of the child when working 1:1. In a group setting, a *general* understanding of breath rates by age can be a useful guide to help the teacher pace the breathing practice for children. The instructor should ideally encourage the children to breathe at their own pace rather than cue each breath, although if the pacing is well matched to the child, counting can help a child with anticipatory anxiety know what to expect. When breath is coordinated with movement, children should be encouraged to pace their movement to their own breath.

To help children bring their breath rate into balance, a helpful technique is to teach them that the *in-breath* is the gas pedal and the *out-breath* is the brake. Meg teaches this approach in conjunction with having students label their emotions. If the student is bored, tired, or sluggish, the teacher can encourage the student to take five deep breaths, with longer inhales (or "in-breaths") and shorter exhales (or "out-breaths") to pep them up a bit. Conversely, if the student is frustrated, worried, excited, or even mad, terrified, yelling, or out of control, the teacher can encourage the student to take five deep breaths with shorter inhales and longer exhales to aid in calming them down. This can be taught within the context of using the Pause Button or one of the other diaphragmatic breathing practices described at the end of this chapter. We recommend using the ***Zones of Regulation*** (Kuypers 2023) program to provide visual supports. This depicts emotional states in a simple self-regulation chart that is used in school settings around the country.

BREATH BIOMECHANICS

The biomechanics of the breath is the most important consideration when presenting breathing practices to children and will influence the rate of respiration. It is widely acknowledged that nasal breathing in combination with the diaphragmatic breath is the ideal natural breathing pattern (American Lung Association 2020; Cleveland Clinic 2021). We will explain the diaphragmatic breath in a minute, but first let's discuss the idea of breathing through the nose.

Nasal vs. mouth breathing

There are many benefits to breathing through the nostrils vs. through the mouth. The nose, lined with nasal hair, is especially designed to warm and filter the air that we breathe (American Lung Association 2020). It filters out dust, pollen, allergens, bacteria, and other contaminants, preventing them from entering the lungs (Allergy & Asthma Network n.d.). Think of the nasal hairs as a curtain or screen vs. germs going right through the front door of your mouth! However, many children breathe through their mouth, most commonly due to enlarged adenoids and/or tonsils. Mouth breathing in turn is associated with obstructive sleep apnea syndrome, which may lead to decreased attention, hyperactivity, impaired learning, and/or behavioral problems (Mayo Clinic 2023).

If instructors notice that a child is breathing through their mouth, it is a good idea to suggest a referral to a doctor to determine the cause, and whether nasal breathing should be encouraged or not. Try giving minor prompts to encourage nasal breathing, but don't over-correct students as some can't. Always encourage and praise their efforts, no matter what. In the greater scheme of things, it's better that they practice breath control to the best of their ability vs. none at all. The last thing we would want is for students to think they can't do something and discourage them from participating.

Developing awareness of the breath

Rolf Sovik (2013), President and Spiritual Director of the Himalayan Institute, suggested that the most important breath technique is simply to watch the breath flow in and out of the body since it takes some time to become familiar with the flow of your breath. However, children often need external props to notice their breath, as their proprioceptive and interoceptive senses are not fully developed. A weighted stuffed animal (a "breathing buddy") might be placed on the belly so that the child can use their visual and tactile senses to enhance awareness of the belly rising and falling. Mental visualizations can also be helpful, such as imagining sniffing a flower or blowing bubbles.

Helping children become aware of their natural breath has important neurological benefits. Spontaneous quiet breathing is associated with coordinated neural activity and oscillations within the brainstem, amygdala, anterior cingulate cortex, and anterior insula (Evans *et al.* 2009; Zelano *et al.* 2016). Thus, there is actually a lot going on up in the brain when lying on the yoga mat "doing nothing" but sensing the breath flow in and out. A great way to introduce this to students is by starting SMYLE™ classes with some breathwork. We have included a child-friendly breath awareness script in the ***SMYLE™ Body Scan***.

The diaphragmatic breath

The ***slower*** and ***deeper*** the breath, the more the PNS will be activated, thus inhibiting the SNS (fight–flight) response. Slow, rhythmic, diaphragmatic breathing is one of the most effective techniques to activate the PNS and produce a calmer and more relaxed state of mind. The diaphragmatic breath involves inhaling all the way down into the lower lungs, causing the diaphragm to expand into the abdominal cavity and the belly to rise due to displacement of the abdominal organs. On the exhalation, the diaphragm moves back up under the bottom of the ribcage, causing the belly to sink back toward the spine.

According to Stephen Elliott (2006), founder of Coherence, LLC, and developer of the Coherent Breathing Method, ***breathing frequency*** and ***breathing depth*** influence the SNS and PNS (see Figure 8.1): "The analysis assumes an underlying sympathetic bias, this bias resulting from the physical and emotional stress and strain of life" (Stephen Elliott, personal communication, May 2013). Findings show that when there is a combination of high breathing depth and low breath frequency it yields weak SNS stimulation and strong PNS stimulation.

		PARASYMPATHETIC STIMULATION			
		LO	HI		
BREATHING FREQUENCY	HI	Strong SNS stimulation Weak PNS stimulation Autonomic imbalance	NIL	HI	SYMPATHETIC STIMULATION
	LO	Weak SNS stimulation Weak PNS stimulation Autonomic imbalance	Weak SNS stimulation Strong PNS stimulation Autonomic balance	LO	
		LO	HI		
		BREATHING DEPTH			

FIGURE 8.1: RELATIONSHIP BETWEEN RESPIRATION AND THE ANS
Stoller (2019), adapted with permission from Elliott (2006)

Interestingly, newborns are naturally diaphragmatic breathers; however, by ten years of age most children use a predominantly thoracic breathing pattern, with more abdominal breathing noted while in a supine position (Kajander and Peper 2010). Thus, it is advised to first introduce the diaphragmatic breathing pattern to children while lying in supine. Again, it is a good idea to help children access this skill by incorporating sensory input to facilitate attention to the movement of breath in and out of the body, such as by placing a weighted stuffed animal or weighted yoga bag on the belly.

CONTROLLING THE BREATH IN DYNAMIC AND STATIC YOGA FORMS

One especially effective strategy to help students become fully present in their bodies is to help them learn to coordinate movement with the breath. As T.K.V. Desikachar (1999), the son of the "father of modern yoga," Śrī T. Krishnamacharya, wrote in *The Heart of Yoga*,

> The first step of our yoga practice is to consciously link breath and body. We do this by allowing every movement to be led by the breath as we practice the asanas. The correct linking of breath and movement is the basis for the whole asana practice. The simple exercise of raising the arms on an inhale and lowering them on an exhale helps us find the rhythm of combined breath and movement. (Desikachar 1999, p.19)

What follows are some general principles for how to incorporate the breath during static and dynamic yoga forms. While these principles are very similar to those taught in our adult-focused program, there are slight differences to take into account based on the developmental level (cognitive and language processing abilities) of children. Be sure to tell your students that if a breath pattern isn't working for them, they are free to reverse the inhalation and exhalation or let go of any control of the breath and "breathe at your own pace" or "breathe normally."

Principle 1: When teaching children how to coordinate movement with the breath, cue the inhalation and exhalation based on the natural tendency of the body. For example, the natural tendency is to exhale on a forward fold because the breath is literally being squeezed out of the lower abdomen, whereas backbends open up the front of the body, inviting air to be drawn in due to the reduced air pressure in the lungs. Thus, in yoga we generally:

- ***Inhale*** → when moving upward, expanding the chest, or moving toward center.
- ***Exhale*** → when moving downward, folding, twisting, or moving away from the center.

With children, body-sensing activities can be helpful for learning to grasp these concepts. For example, when preparing for ***Robin's Breath*** (see the "Breath Prep" activities later in this chapter), the teacher could first have the children experience each of the two postures separately (wings open, wings closed), taking several breaths in each, before flowing with their breath between them. During this exploration the teacher could ask them to sense how much space they have in their lungs in each position, and whether it feels easier to inhale or exhale. The other "Breath Prep" stretches presented at the end of this chapter—***Rainbow Breath***, ***Half Moon Breath***, ***Waterfall Breath***, and ***Ball Breath***—are also conducive for this exercise.

Principle 2: Encourage students to pace their movement to their breath, not vice versa:

- Model a pace of movement that is equal or just slightly less than the average respiratory rate for the age of the child, if the child's own respiratory rate is unknown.
- Watch for the tendency to speed up the breath in an attempt to keep up with the pace of movement, which only serves to reinforce hyperarousal.

Principle 3: Encourage students to use the ***diaphragmatic breath*** during yoga practice, starting with just a minute or two, and gradually increase the duration as they become skilled in using this breathing technique (to activate the PNS and inhibit the SNS "fight-flight" system):

- To establish this takes time and, as mentioned earlier, is usually easier initially when practiced in supine rather than sitting. Props may be needed when teaching younger children, such as placing a weighted bag, stuffed animal, or other toy on the belly, and watching it rise and fall with the breath.
- You can also have the students stand up and clasp their fingers behind their head, which blocks movement of the chest and forces movement of the diaphragm.

Principle 4: When students are holding a yoga form statically, encourage them to direct the breath into the areas being stretched. If the children are developmentally too young to follow cues to breathe into certain areas, simply ask if they can feel the movement of their [back, chest, ribcage, etc.] during the stretch. Alternatively, you might ask the child to imagine that their breath is blowing air into those areas of the body like a balloon:

- When in a *forward fold* → "breathe into the back to accentuate its expansion" (or ask if they can feel their back stretch wider as they breathe).

- When in a *backbend* → "direct the breath into the front of the chest and the heart center" (or ask if they can feel their chest stretch wider as they breathe).
- During a *lateral bend* → "breathe into the ribcage that is being stretched, feeling it expand on each in-breath" (or ask if they can feel the side of their body stretch as they breathe).
- When in a *twist* → "allow the body to grow taller as you breathe in, and maybe move just a little more into the twist as you breathe out, if you feel some space to do so."
- Even encourage your students to use their imagination to send their *breath into areas where the lungs don't stretch or reach*! For example, you might suggest that students imagine their whole body expanding like a balloon when they inhale, and deflate as they exhale. Or they might imagine breathing into any areas of tension or discomfort. Doing so invites the muscles in these areas to soften and release. The insula plays a large role in processing breath, proprioceptive, and visceral sensations and may be responsible for this effect.

An example of the breath principles in action

Meg has found that guiding students through four to five rounds of breathwork can be very helpful in preparing them for guided meditation. She also presents a breathing practice at the start of every class period. She typically chooses five Pause Button Breaths, five Waterfall Breaths, or five Rainbow Breaths. When students perform group work she has them spend 15–20 minutes at each station, and then, right before they transition to the next station, she presents a brief 1- to 3-minute breath practice. She might say, "I understand that this activity could have been challenging for you. It is finished. We are moving on to a new activity. Before we do that, let's take five deep breaths together. Breathe in to recharge your batteries...and as you breathe out, blow out any worries. Repeat five times and when complete say 'Okay, let's go to our next station and rock this next activity! We are going to erase and reset.'" Her students will often remind her if she forgets, saying "We didn't take five deep breaths" or "We didn't press our pause button." Her students have learned that they perform better and are much more attentive after they "recharge" with the breathwork. These exercises help to bring everyone back toward the center, back into their window of tolerance, back into the state that is most conducive for learning.

RECOMMENDED BREATHING TECHNIQUES

What follows are the breathing techniques most recommended for children by the SMYLE™ program to promote healing from trauma, anxiety, or related conditions. They are presented in a developmental progression, from basic breath control activities, "Breath Prep" stretches, awareness of natural breathing, and techniques to promote diaphragmatic breathing. Of all the breathing practices listed, ***the diaphragmatic breath is the most important and is worth spending a good deal of time on with your students before moving to other practices.*** Also, it is very important to instruct your students in advance to stop practicing the breathing technique if it becomes uncomfortable for them.

Body positioning during breathwork

Some of the breath practices are best performed in a supine position while others are best performed either seated or standing, depending on the exercise. For supine breathwork, invite your students to lie comfortably on their yoga mats and to make any adjustments so they feel completely comfortable. Offer a folded blanket (or light pillow or foam knee pad) to place under their head and a bolster or rolled blanket to place under their thighs so their knees are bent, with the heels of their feet resting on the mat. Some students may prefer to have a blanket (folded in half) placed on top of their mats for extra comfort and/or have a blanket placed over their body. Observe your students carefully to determine whether they may benefit from extra props, looking out for the following conditions:

- ***Kyphosis:*** Build up the folded blankets under the head, neck, and upper shoulders so the weight of the student's upper body is fully supported.
- ***Scoliosis:*** Use folded or rolled blankets or towels to comfortably support the torso.
- ***Cerebral palsy or other neuromuscular conditions:*** Some children who use wheelchairs feel more comfortable remaining in their chairs during a breathing and/or yoga practice, while others prefer to come out of their wheelchairs and be positioned in any number of positions on a mat, table mat, an extra large floor pillow, wedge, etc. If reclined on a mat, consider whether bending the knees might help to reduce overall muscle tone in the body. If so, you might position the legs on a large bolster or roll. Observe the positioning of the arms: if they are hanging in the air, provide supports (e.g., wedge, folded blankets) to ensure that they are completely supported, which will facilitate relaxation of the rest of the body.

It is best to consult with the student's physical or occupational therapist if they have one in the school setting to determine the most appropriate positioning and props to best facilitate the student's ability to access the breathing practices.

BASIC BREATH CONTROL ACTIVITIES

A. Inhale practices

1. Sniffing candles, flowers, essential oils (using the actual object).
2. Imagine sniffing your favorite ____ [flower, food, dessert, scented candle].

B. Exhale practices

1. Blow bubbles using a bubble wand, or imagine blowing bubbles.
2. Blow a pinwheel.
3. Roll up paper into a ball and try to blow it off your desk. *[If the students find it hard to purse the lips, have them use a straw.]*
4. Blow out an actual candle (if allowed in the school setting!).
5. Blow a ping-pong ball off of your fist, hand, or desk.
6. Blow paper party favors or other whistles. *[Encourage the students to not remove them from the mouth to teach them to breathe in through their nose.]*
7. Blow up a balloon. *[Encourage the students to not remove the balloon from the mouth to teach them to breathe in through their nose.]*
8. Take up a musical instrument, such as a harmonica or recorder.
9. Practice blowing bubbles in a swimming pool.

BREATH PREP STRETCHES

A. Rainbow Breath

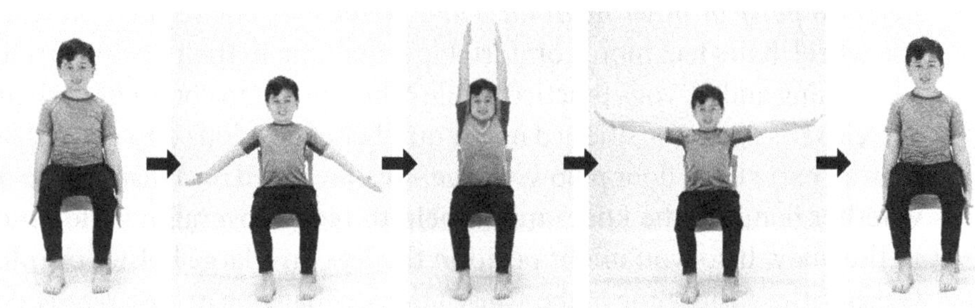

1. Cue Standing or Seated Mountain; or say "stand/sit nice and tall."
2. Start with your arms by your sides.
3. As you breathe in, lift your arms up toward the sky, as though you are tracing a rainbow with your hands.
4. As you breathe out, lower your arms back down to your sides. *[Or say: "Blow your arms back down to your side."]*

B. Waterfall Breath

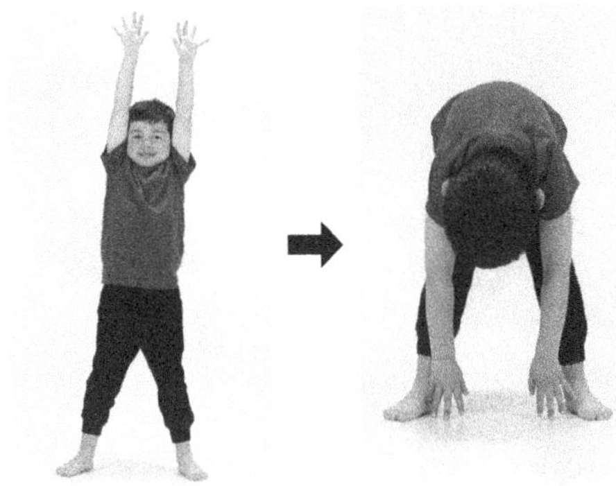

1. Breathe in as you reach your arms out and up to the sky. *[Demonstrate raising the arms out in front of them and up overhead.]*
2. Breathe out as you flow like a waterfall to the floor. *[Encourage folding at the hips and bending the knees a bit.]*

C. Seated Half Moon Breath

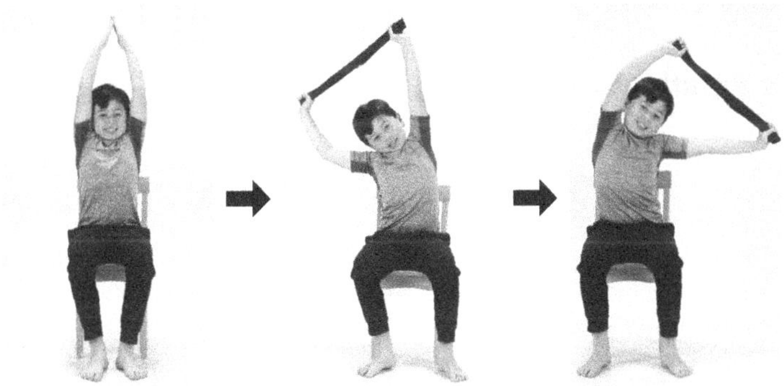

1. I invite you to join me in a Half Moon stretch. Do you want straight or bent arms for this one? Choose which one feels right for you! *[See Seated Half Moon Stretch in Chapter 15 for photographs of bent arms.]*
2. For straight arms: Reach arms up straight and press your palms together.
3. For bent arms: Clasp your hands behind your head with elbows bent.
4. Take a slow breath in through your nose.
5. Breathe out as you lean over to the right.
6. Breathe in as you come back to center.
7. Breathe out as you lean to the left.
8. Continue to move like this as you breathe in and out.

D. Reclined or Seated Ball Breath

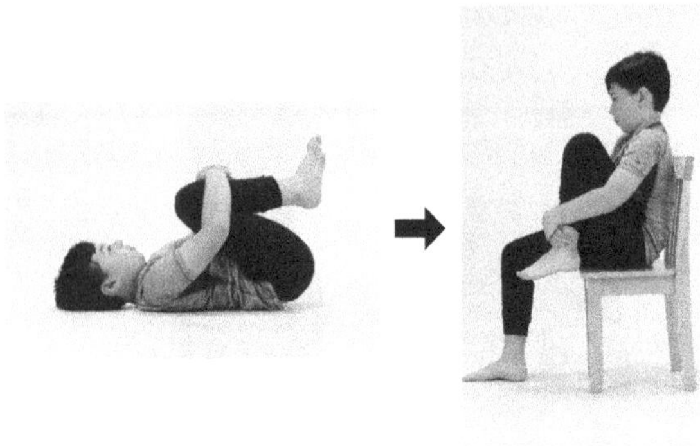

1. Take a breath in through your nose.
2. As you breathe out, bring your knees (or one knee, if seated) into your body, to fold yourself into a ball.
3. Now stay here and breathe with me for five breaths: breathe in...feel your stomach blow up like a balloon, pushing against your leg...breathe out...let all of the air flow out of the balloon as you feel your stomach sink back down.

E. Robin's Breath

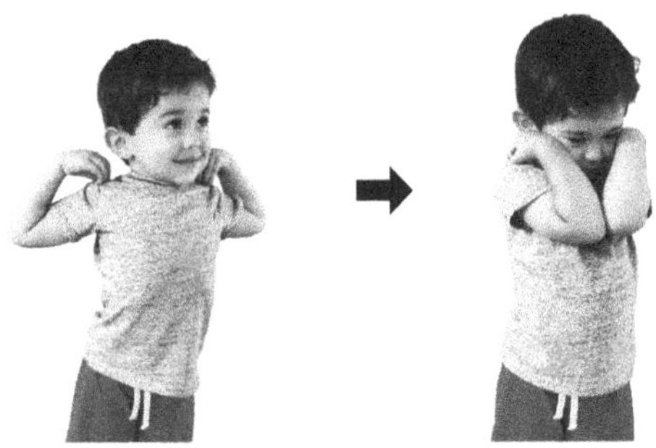

1. Sit up (or stand) nice and tall, and place your fingers on your shoulders.
2. Now lift your elbows up to the sides so your arms look like the bird wings of a robin.
3. Take a breath in through your nose as you lift up your chest and draw your wings back (hands still on shoulders).
4. As you breathe out, look down at your belly as you bring your wings (elbows) together in front of you, and curl your body forward, tucking your wings against your body.

5. As you breathe in, raise your chest back up as you spread your wings wide (fingers still on shoulders).
6. Breathe out as you close your wings...
7. Breathe in as you open your wings...

[If you find that your students don't know what a robin is, preface this exercise with a brief description. This breath is also great to help teach children the concept of Principle #1, that is, how to breathe according to the natural tendency of the body. When the wings are open, you can have them stay there while they take a few breaths and notice how much space there is in the lungs for the air to fill. Then have them take a few breaths with the wings closed, noticing the difference in the lung space now.]

AWARENESS OF NATURAL BREATHING

Speak slowly and space out the phrases to give students time to practice and really connect with what you are saying to what they are feeling...

1. I invite you to join me in a breath awareness exercise.
2. First, lie down on your yoga mat and uncross your arms and legs. Get as comfortable as you can. Would anyone like a pillow or folded blanket under their head? A rolled blanket under their knees? An eye mask over their eyes?

   [Observe your students carefully to determine whether they may benefit from extra props, as discussed earlier. Even if these students do not raise their hand when you ask the full class the above questions, go over to them subtly, and ask them the questions 1:1 to give them another opportunity to benefit from their incorporation in the practice.]
3. Begin to notice your breath... If you can, keep your mouth closed and feel the air move in and out of your nose...[pause]...
4. You may notice that the air feels cool as you breathe into your nose... [pause]...and maybe the air feels warmer when you breathe out of your nose.
5. Bring your attention to the rest of your body. Do you feel any parts moving as you breathe?
6. Now try putting one hand on your belly and your other hand on your chest. Do you feel your belly move as you breathe?...[pause]... Do you feel your chest move as you breathe?...[pause]... Which area is moving more, your belly or your chest?

   [Continue to the Diaphragmatic Breath.]

ACTIVITIES TO PROMOTE DIAPHRAGMATIC BREATHING

A. Diaphragmatic Breath Lesson #1: Balloon Breathing

1. Now we will breathe into the belly. If you want, place your hands on your belly.
2. Take a long, slow breath in, through your nose if you can, and picture a balloon blowing up in your belly. The more you breathe in, the bigger the balloon gets, and the higher your belly rises.
3. Then as you breathe out through your nose, picture yourself letting the air slowly out of the balloon. Feel your belly getting smaller and smaller as the balloon loses its air.
4. Continue to blow up the balloon and let the air out again, feeling your belly rise and sink down.
5. Now, let's blow up the balloon for 1...2...3...4.
6. And let the air out for 1...2...3...4.

[Gradually reduce the count to 3 over time, eventually returning to their normal breath rate while still feeling their stomach rise and sink as they did with the higher count. By weaning them off the count, they transition their awareness to their natural breathing rhythm, creating a more natural diaphragmatic breath.]

B. Diaphragmatic Breath Lesson #2: Breathing Buddy (or Breathing Pillow)

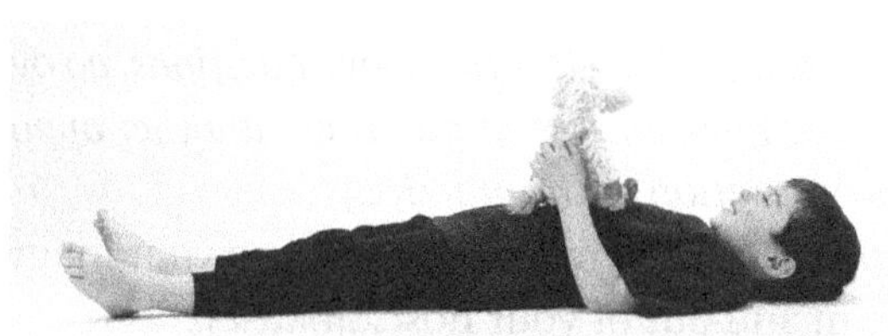

1. I invite you to join me in a breathing exercise.
2. If you would like, you may choose a "breathing buddy."
   [You might suggest that the student choose a small stuffed animal, cloth doll from a basket of "breathing buddies," or a favorite toy (that's appropriate). Alternatively, they can use a pillow or a weighted yoga bag. There are also weighted stuffed animals on the market or you can modify a stuffed animal by ripping out a seam and inserting plastic pellets or dried beans.]
3. Then lie down on your yoga mat and get as comfortable as you can. Would anyone like a pillow or folded blanket under their head? A rolled blanket under their knees?

[Observe your students carefully to determine whether they may benefit from extra props, as discussed earlier. Remember to ask those who would really benefit in a subtle 1:1 manner.]

4. Focus on your breath... What parts of your body move as you breathe?...
5. Now place your "breathing buddy" on your belly.
6. Take a nice slow breath in through your nose as you fill your belly with air.
7. As your belly rises, your breathing buddy goes up.
8. As you let the air out of your nose, your belly sinks and your breathing buddy goes down.
9. Imagine your breathing buddy surfing on the ocean... Feel it ride on the wave of your breath...watch it ride up the wave as you breathe in...and down the wave as you breathe out through your nose...in...and out...in... and out...slowly...and smoothly...

[It is okay to have children use their muscles (instead of their breath) to extend and contract their bellies when first learning the Diaphragmatic Breath. Practicing extending and contracting the belly muscles can actually facilitate learning because air naturally wants to fill up any space that is created, and will tend to expel from the body when the abdominal muscles are actively contracting.]

C. Diaphragmatic Breath Lesson #3: Breathing Ball (Hoberman sphere)

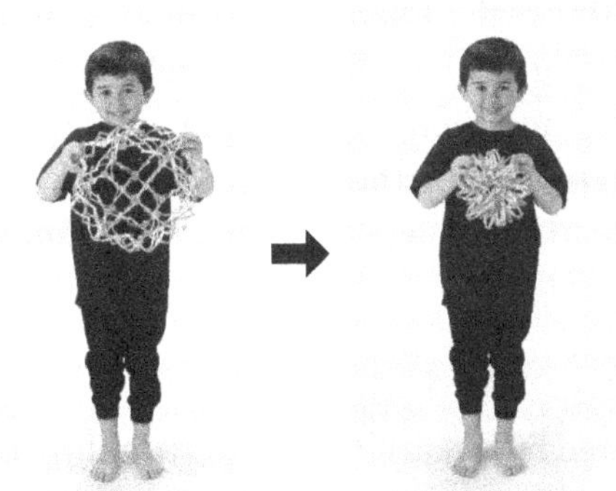

1. I invite you to join me in a breathing exercise using a Breathing Ball (Hoberman sphere).
2. Place the ball in front of your belly.
3. Breathe in as the ball and your belly get larger.
4. Breathe out as your belly and the ball get small again.[2]

2 For a video on how this works, see www.youtube.com/watch?v=YnNATiWYyxo

D. Pause Button

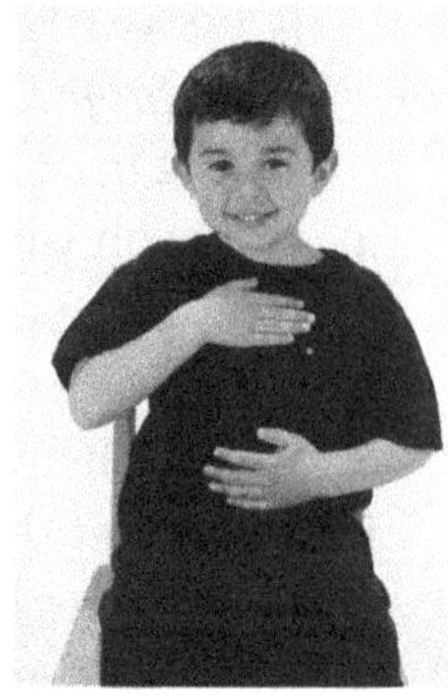

When a student appears dysregulated, suggesting pressing the "pause" button can help bring them back into their body and draw awareness to their current state of being. No matter where they are in the body and mind, it helps to pause, recharge their batteries, and bring them back to the present moment.

1. When you are watching a movie, listening to music, or watching YouTube, what happens when you press the "pause" button? *Students: "The device/ screen stops."*
2. Just as your devices stop when you press the "pause" button, your body and mind stop when you press *your* "pause" button.
3. I like to press my pause button to remind myself that I am in control of my body and breath.
4. It's also a great way to recharge your battery. Just like your devices run out of battery power if you don't plug them in, people can also run out of power if they keep running without taking a break to recharge.
5. Whenever you press your "pause" button you are telling your mind and body to stop.
6. This is how you press the pause button: Put one hand on your chest and one hand on your belly. Then close your eyes or let your eyes relax, and think of something you would like to smell. Breathe in through your nose with a big "sniff," and then breathe out through your mouth, like you are blowing out all of your birthday candles.
7. Breathe in...breathe out...(5–7 times) *[Or say: Smell the flowers...blow out your birthday candles...]*

E. Tongue Press

This breath was inspired by Sitkari Pranayama (Cooling Breath), which involves pressing the tongue to the top of the mouth while inhaling through the mouth, with the teeth lightly touching and lips slightly apart. The version below is unique to SMYLE™ and only utilizes the tongue-pressing component of Sitkari Pranayama, modified to reduce the motor coordination required, to make this a more child-friendly breath:

1. Press the tip of the tongue against the top of the mouth, a little bit behind the front teeth.
2. Close your lips, and slowly breathe in and out through the nose.
3. Focus on the calming sensation of pressure on the top of your mouth.
4. Take 10 slow, deep breaths like this, breathing in...out...in...out.

F. Hug Breath

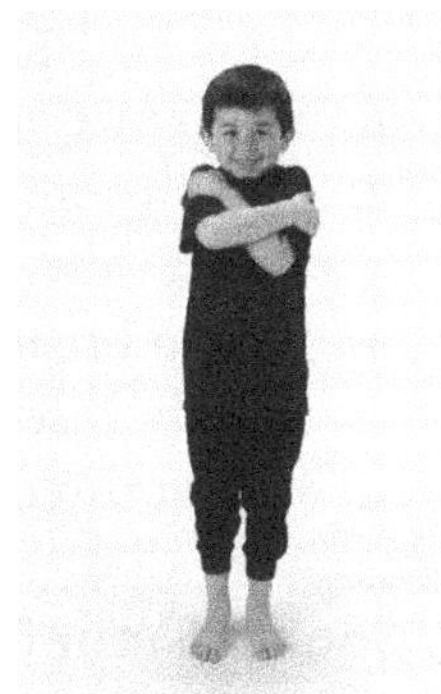

1. Breathe in as you spread your arms out to the sides.
2. Breathe out as you give yourself a big hug.
3. Repeat as many times as you want...breathing in when you open your arms wide...breathing out when you give yourself a hug...in...out...in...out.

G. Lion's Breath

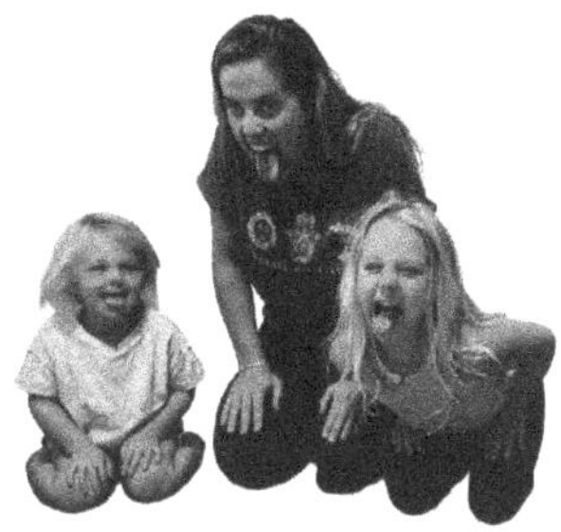

1. Sit up nice and tall (or kneel).
2. Let your shoulders hang down away from your ears.
3. Take a nice deep breath in through your nose.
4. Then open your mouth wide, stick out your tongue *[optional]*, and let out a loud roar as you breathe the air out.

   Repeat as many times as you want...breathing in through your nose...breathing out with a ROARRRR...in...out...in...out.

H. Snake Breath

1. Sit up nice and tall (or kneel).
2. Let your shoulders hang down away from your ears.
3. Take a nice deep breath in through your nose.
4. Then make the hissing sound of "sssss" through your teeth as you breathe out *[demonstrate]*.
5. Repeat as many times as you want...breathing in through your nose...breathing out with a hisssssss...in...and hiss...in...and hiss...

[This is especially fun to do when in Cobra. Breathe in through the nose when coming up into Cobra and exhale with a snake hiss when coming down to resting Cobra (lying on belly) to complete the animal play.]

I. Bees Breath

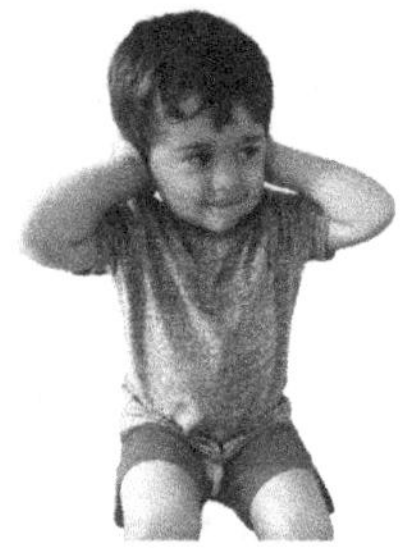

1. Sit up nice and tall.
2. Cover your ears with the palms of your hands.
3. Take a slow deep breath in through your nose.
4. As you breathe out through your nose, keep your mouth closed and hum.
5. Repeat three more times...

J. Cool Off Your Pizza Breath

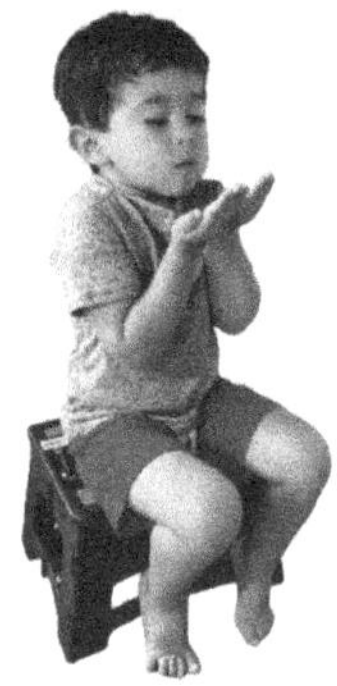

1. Hold your hands with your palms up, little fingers touching, just like you are holding a slice of pizza.
2. Pretend the pizza is too hot to eat but good to smell!
3. Take a long slow sniff with your nose to smell the pizza.
4. Then blow on the pizza to cool it down.
5. Do this a few times until your pizza is cooled down... breathe in to smell the yummy pizza...breathe out to cool it down...in...out *[demonstrate blowing out]*...in... out...

[Avoid these techniques with individuals prone to negative emotional reactions, such as children facing food scarcity or those with anorexia nervosa, bulimia nervosa, binge eating disorder, avoidant restrictive food intake disorder, pica, rumination disorder, or Prader-Willi syndrome.]

K. Lazy 8 Breathing

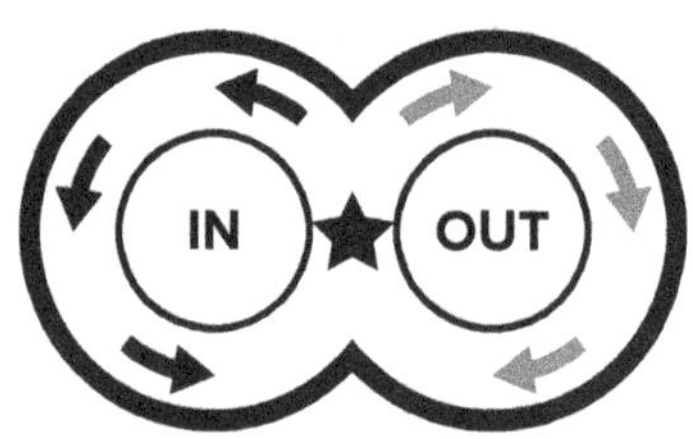

1. Put your Lazy 8 sheet[3] on your desk.
2. Place your finger on the center star.
3. As you breathe in, trace the black arrow until you reach the star.
4. As you breathe out, trace the grey arrow and come back to the star.
5. Do this 5–10 times on your own.

3 A Lazy 8 sheet is a large sideways "8" on a piece of paper with a star in the center. It is a visual and tactile resource to facilitate awareness and slowing of the breath.

PRECAUTIONS FOR BREATHING EXERCISES

- If the student has known respiratory or cardiopulmonary dysfunction or an obstruction in any part of the respiratory pathway (e.g., deviated septum, asthma), it is advised that the student's physician be consulted prior to engagement in any specific breathing practices.
- The breath must not be forced or strained.
- Avoid vigorous breathing exercises such as Kapalabhati or Mukha Bhastrika (Bellows Breath), which can activate the SNS.
- Do not teach advanced breathing practices such as unilateral or alternate nostril breathing (which are not described in this book) in a group environment or without instruction by a certified yoga therapist, as these have powerful effects on cerebral hemisphere activation, and it is important to fully understand which of these techniques are suitable for a particular person.
- Do not encourage holding of the breath, which can induce anxiety.
- Always remind your students that they may stop doing a breathing exercise at any time and return to normal breathing.

CHAPTER 9

Guideline #3: Yoga Can Promote Effective Sensory, Motor, and Cognitive Processing of Traumatic Experiences, and Thus Aid Healing

Trauma is processed at the ***sensory***, ***motor***, and ***cognitive*** levels, which together drive the ***emotional*** processing of the event. As Alan Fogel wrote, "Trauma memory is as much in the sensory receptors of the skin and in the muscles as it is in the brain" (2009, p.259). Dr. van der Kolk went even further, emphasizing how trauma affects ***every cell*** of the body and ***must be released from the body for full healing to occur*** (van der Kolk 2008, 2014). Not only does trauma affect the ANS, which controls every cell, organ, and system of our body, but it can also affect the very expression of our genes, that is, our DNA (Yehuda *et al.* 2015). Although the DNA sequence itself does not change, there are over 3,000,000 epigenetic "switches" that control how it is read and expressed in the body (Brendtro 2015, p.43).

While ANS changes are typically fluid and reversible, the ***genetic expression*** of DNA can set the stage for stress-related diseases to take hold. This is because cortisol not only provides the energy to mobilize a person for action during a stressful event, it also ***coordinates the plasticity changes to genes*** that enable a person to adapt to stressful environments over the course of a lifetime and even across generations (Kozlowska, Scher, and Helgeland 2020). The good news is that pro-inflammatory genes and pathways become downregulated in response to yoga and other mindfulness-based interventions, according to a multi-study review (Buric *et al.* 2017). Preliminary evidence also suggests that exercise can help to remediate the changes in expression of GABA receptor genes that have been found to occur in response to early life trauma (Lu *et al.* 2017).

Epigenetic expression of stress and trauma is not only evident in nerve cells—of which GABA expression is just one example (see Yehuda *et al.* 2015)—it is also evident in the cells of many other tissues and organs, and can lead to many pathological conditions including diabetes, cancer, and immune system disorders (Johnstone and Baylin 2010; Smith *et al.* 2011; also see Chapter 2). There is even evidence to suggest that epigenetics underlies skeletal muscle memory (Seaborne *et al.* 2018; Sharples, Stewart, and Seaborne 2016). Although no studies were found that specifically linked skeletal muscle memory to psychological trauma, we know that psychological trauma can affect posture and movement (Levine 1997; Ogden *et al.* 2006; Scaer 2007), which, in turn, influence a person's emotions and attitudes (Veenstra, Schneider, and Koole 2017).

Therefore, to help traumatized individuals heal, we need to help them clear out the trauma-related memory imprints, not just from the "mind," but from the entire "bodymind," as the separation of body and mind is simply an illusion. These memory imprints present as obstacles along the path to experiencing the peaceful, clear-minded existence that every human being deserves. Thus, this guideline to practice speaks to the need to process trauma through the sensorimotor (bottom-up) and cognitive (top-down) channels that influence emotional well-being, and which, when blocked, keep an individual from the blissful experience of present moment awareness, that is, the power of ***now***.

In this chapter, we present the "bottom-up" (sensory-based) elements that are incorporated into a Sensory-Enhanced Yoga® practice, which are designed to address the neurotransmitter (and resulting brain structure and network) imbalances in the brain. By doing so, there is theoretically potential to reverse epigenetic changes caused by toxic stress. In Chapter 10, we will discuss the "top-down" techniques of the program, for example positive suggestions and guided meditations. As you will recall, Sensory-Enhanced Yoga® is the methodology behind the child-focused SMYLE™ program, so when we discuss methods throughout this chapter and those that follow, we will be using the term Sensory-Enhanced Yoga®.

Our approach was strongly inspired by the insightful work of Dr. Jean Ayres (1972), founder of sensory integration theory and treatment. However, Sensory-Enhanced Yoga® differs in a few respects from a traditional sensory integration program, an important one being that, in our program, sensory-based practices are intertwined with mindfulness (including breath control) practices, which together are particularly therapeutic for rebalancing brain networks in PTSD, anxiety, bipolar disorder, and related mental health conditions.

Since we will be talking a lot about the processing of bodily based sensation, we need to introduce the neural pathways that transmit this sensory input to the brain. These pathways converge on and influence the functioning of the thalamus and certain other structures. In turn, the thalamus "controls functional connectivity within and across cortical areas," according to Nakajima and Halassa's hypothesis (2017, p.8). Yet the cerebral cortex also strongly influences the thalamus, and even dynamically manipulates its own excitatory and inhibitory processes (Crandall, Cruikshank, and Connors 2015). So clearly, the thalamus and cerebral cortex work very closely together and more collaboratively than we had previously thought, further supporting the idea that combining top-down (mindfulness) and bottom-up (sensory-based) practices would be the most powerful approach for addressing PTSD, anxiety, or related mental health conditions.

DEVELOPING A "WITNESS" MENTALITY

One powerful way that yoga draws the mind back to present-moment awareness is through "witness consciousness," which Dr. Kabat-Zinn, founder of MBSR, defined as "paying attention in a particular way: on purpose, in the present moment, and non-judgmentally" (1994, p.4). In most yoga classes, and certainly those that follow the Sensory-Enhanced Yoga® methodology, participants are encouraged to notice sensation as they move through the yoga forms and attune to their breath, and to step back and observe them as a witness when sensations get too strong, so as not to get caught up in them. Learning to step into as well as step back from sensation, mindfully, is an important skill for healthy embodiment.

To help develop the witness mentality, you might say something like this:

> You may notice strong muscle sensations in your arms and legs. When we learn to notice and accept stronger sensations in our muscles, these muscles get stronger. We strengthen our emotions in the same way, by learning to notice and accept difficult situations without getting worked up by those strong feelings. But when the sensations get *too* strong, we need to move out of the yoga form. Learning to notice, as well as move away from, strong sensations in the body is an important skill so we don't get hurt. We call that "befriending" our body, which means to "be" a "friend" to our body and treat it with kindness.

INCORPORATING THERAPEUTIC SENSORY INPUT INTO YOGA

Sensory-Enhanced Yoga® provides additional therapeutic sensation to attend to, which can be especially powerful in drawing the mind to the present moment, especially for those who suffer from intrusive thoughts or for those who feel uncomfortable with the usual sensations in their bodies (which therapeutic input can cancel out through sensory gating mechanisms). A simple seated meditation can be overwhelming for many of these individuals, but a short, seated meditation immediately following a series of yoga movements can be more accessible, as the bodymind has been prepared for it—especially if the yoga series incorporates a sufficient threshold of *therapeutic* sensory input.

You will recall from Chapter 5, in our discussion of Clancy *et al.*'s (2017) Sensory Hypothesis of PTSD, how trauma can cause excessive neuronal excitation in various cortical brain structures due to impaired sensory filtering. The inhibitory techniques presented in this chapter are designed to improve sensory filtering, especially in the thalamus so it can more effectively co-engage with higher brain structures to influence the brain networks that have been altered in PTSD. Kerr *et al.* (2013) suggested that in standardized mindfulness practices this process occurs through attention-controlled modulation of sensory alpha wave activity (via attention to sensation) and then spreads throughout the entire brain, and that this process could reduce ruminative thoughts. Sensory-Enhanced Yoga® combines sensory and mindfulness based practices to enhance this process.

Based on the work of Margaret Rood (1954), Dr. Jean Ayres (1972, 1979), and many others who have followed in their footsteps, including the late Dr. Jane Koomar (Koomar and Bundy 2002), we know that certain types and applications of sensory input can inhibit the sympathetic (fight–flight) branch of the ANS, reduce sensory overresponsivity, and facilitate self-regulation. Here are the types of therapeutic sensory input we include in this program:

- **Deep touch pressure**
- **Enhanced proprioceptive input**
- **Slow rhythmical linear movement**
- **Neutral warmth.**

Many yoga styles emphasize one or two of these sensory modalities. For example, in his book *B.K.S. Iyengar Yoga: The Path to Holistic Health*, B.K.S. Iyengar (2001) emphasized both active static holds that provide strong muscle sensation (proprioceptive input) and passive static holds (often providing deep touch pressure input using props such as bolsters) to achieve a particular bodily alignment or other therapeutic goal, and combinations of the above. Thus we could say that Iyengar exploited the benefits of therapeutic deep touch pressure and enhanced proprioceptive input in his style of yoga. Iyengar directly taught many students who subsequently became famous in their own right, including Dr. Judith Hanson Lasater, author of *Relax and Renew*, a book of restorative yoga forms that incorporates the use of yoga sandbags to provide enhanced deep touch pressure (Lasater 1995, 2011).

Other styles emphasize slow, rhythmical repetitive movement, the most famous of which is the Viniyoga style popularized in the US by Gary Kraftsow, who learned it from the founder of Viniyoga, Sri T.K.V. Desikachar of Madras, India. Some of these rhythmic flows stimulate the vestibular apparatus while others do not—the ones that do incorporate movement of the head through space (along with at least some trunk movement in the same direction). Although Kraftsow (1999) does not mention the benefits of vestibular input in his most famous book, *Yoga for Wellness*, we can easily choose rhythmic yoga movements from this rich resource that will provide the inhibitory effect in the nervous system we are looking for.

While Iyengar and Desikachar seem to have evolved their styles in completely different directions, they each learned these styles from the "father of modern yoga," Śrī T. Krishnamacharya. In fact, Desikachar is the son of Krishnamacharya while Iyengar is Krishnamacharya's brother-in-law (Desikachar 1999; Iyengar 2001). Krishnamacharya individualized his approach when working with each of them, based on their health needs, which were different from one another, and these students in turn evolved their programs based on this prescription. By individualizing the practices, it could be argued that Krishnamacharya is the father of yoga *therapy* and that modern yoga was intended to be therapy in the first place.

Krishnamacharya also mentored another famous yogi, K. Pattabhi Jois, founder of the Ashtanga Vinyasa yoga style, but, as the story goes, the nature of Jois' health needs led Krishnamacharya to suggest a more active style of movement sequences, connected with the breath. While Sensory-Enhanced Yoga® does not recommend quick yoga movements for people healing from trauma, such as the jumping or bouncing of an Ashtanga yoga class, it does incorporate flows (see Part 3), and emphasizes movement with the breath (as does Viniyoga). It is interesting to consider that Sensory-Enhanced Yoga® may not be a new way of thinking after all but rather a re-synthesis of the separate elements of Krishnamacharya's yoga style back into a unified paradigm of thinking for the purpose of healing trauma. In other words, we need to consider what effect(s) we are looking for in the bodymind, and decide what combination, dosage, and qualities of sensory input will help us reach a therapeutic threshold to achieve that effect. Let us now discuss each of these modalities in turn.

DEEP TOUCH PRESSURE

Temple Grandin, an American Professor of Animal Science at Colorado State University, livestock behavior expert, and autism spokesperson, is famous for creating the "hug box" for people on the autism spectrum, based on her own experiences with autism herself. She articulates well the therapeutic benefits of deep touch pressure:

> Deep touch pressure is the type of surface pressure that is exerted in most types of firm touching, holding, stroking, petting of animals, or swaddling. In contrast, light touch pressure is a more superficial stimulation of the skin, such

> as tickling, very light touch, or moving hairs on the skin. In animals, the tickle of a fly landing on the skin may cause a cow to kick, but the firm touch of the farmer's hands quiets her. Occupational therapists have observed that a very light touch alerts the nervous system, but deep pressure is relaxing and calming. (Grandin 1992, para. 6)

There are two major sensory pathways from the spinal cord to the brain that we need to understand in order to effectively apply this modality (see Figure 9.1):

- **The lateral tracts (including the spinothalamic pathway)** transmit information about ***pain, temperature, superficial pressure, and light touch*** to brain areas critical for arousal (e.g., reticular activating system, hypothalamus) and to the thalamus. This then travels to the sensory cortex and also targets the dACC and anterior insula, facilitating the **SN**. The spinothalamic pathway has sympathetic effects on the brain and can set off the "fight–flight" response (Menon and Uddin 2010; Neuro New Me 2021).
- **The dorsal column–medial lemniscal (DCML) pathway** transmits ***proprioception, deep touch pressure input, vibration, and discriminative touch*** to the thalamus, and from the thalamus to the sensory cortex and other areas associated with somatosensory and emotional processing (Kearney and Lanius 2022). Activation of the DCML pathway is believed to:
  - *Decrease sympathetic "fight–flight" activation* by modulating neurons in the reticular formation of the brainstem that play a large role in ANS arousal (Kimball *et al.* 2007; Reynolds, Lane, and Mullen, 2015; Salibi *et al.* 1981); and
  - *Increase parasympathetic activation* via enhanced vagal tone (Reynolds *et al.* 2015, citing Field, Diego, and Hernandez-Reif 2010).

The DCML pathway is a major system we are trying to activate in Sensory-Enhanced Yoga®/SMYLE™ classes. Experts have long hypothesized that the reason deep touch pressure and proprioceptive input helps to produce calming is due to the DCML pathway overriding the spinothalamic pathway. This is based on the understanding that both of these pathways converge in the ventral posterolateral nucleus of the thalamus, where the net sum of excitatory impulses from these pathways determines whether there will be overall arousing or calming effects on the nervous system.

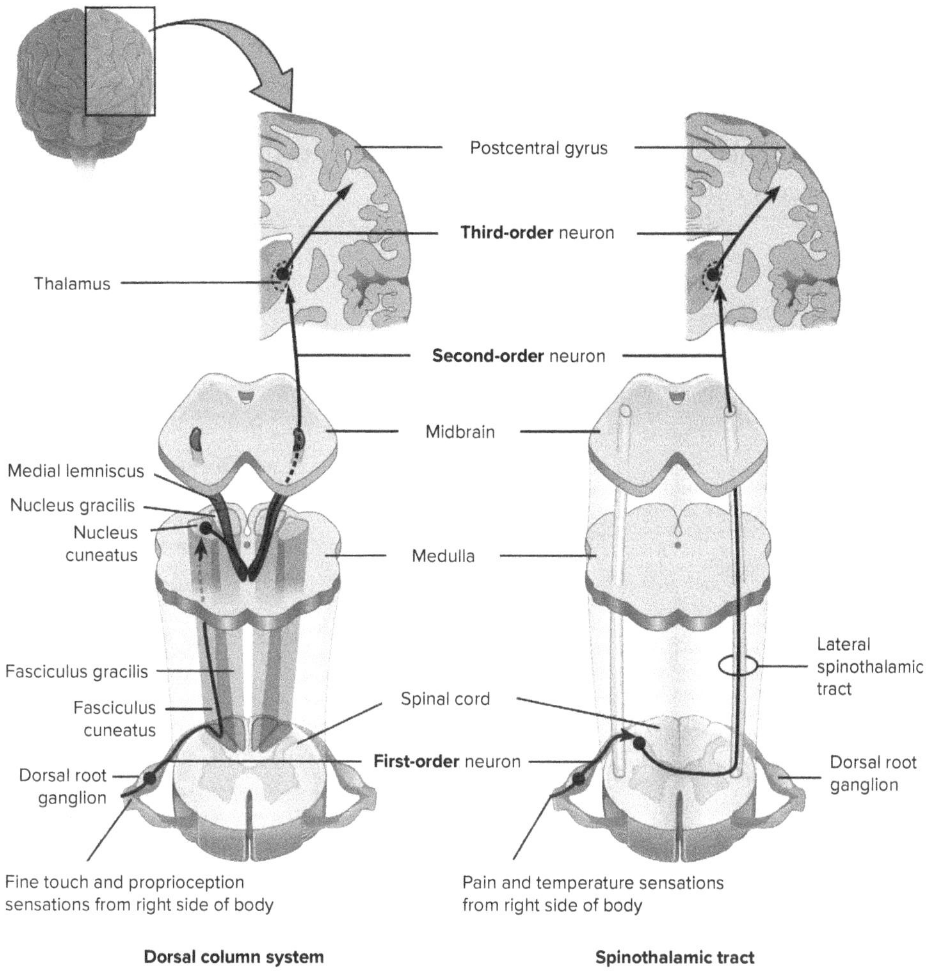

FIGURE 9.1: THE DORSAL COLUMN–MEDIAL LEMNISCAL (DCML) PATHWAY (LEFT) AND SPINOTHALAMIC PATHWAY (RIGHT). BOTH PATHWAYS CONVERGE IN THE THALAMUS.
OpenStax College, Wikimedia Commons

More recently, the triple network model has deepened our understanding of how this process works. Briefly stated, after sensory information is filtered in the thalamus (setting the "stage" for arousal or calming), it is relayed to the sensory cortex and other cortical regions, orchestrated through alpha rhythms that are influenced by this sensory input. These alpha rhythms also provide functional support for the DMN and SN (Clancy 2017). Clancy (2017) hypothesizes that by modulating these alpha oscillations it is possible to regulate these networks and thus positively impact cognition, emotion, and behavior. While he proposed using transcranial alternating current stimulation for this purpose, we propose that it can also be accomplished through the careful design of yoga and mindfulness practices that incorporate therapeutic sensory input (see Figure 5.2).

When considering how to apply therapeutic deep touch pressure to yoga practice to help achieve this goal, we need to consider how the sensory cortex is organized. The **sensory homunculus** (see Figure 9.2) depicts the relative amount of cerebral cortex surface given over to processing the different sensory inputs of the human nervous system. The image represents the sensory cortex (aka somatosensory cortex: Figure 9.3).

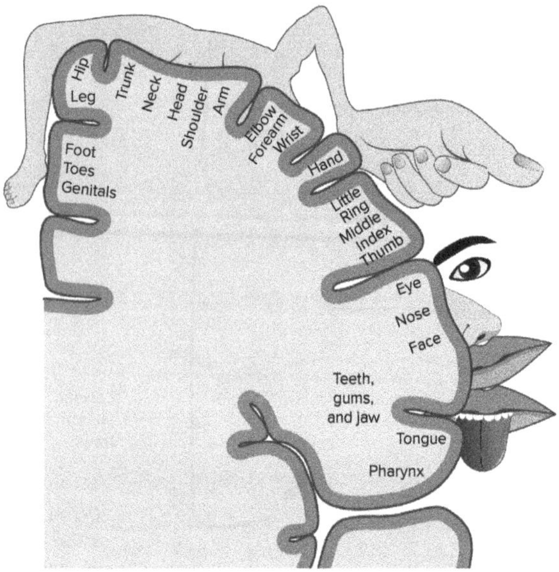

FIGURE 9.2: THE SENSORY HOMUNCULUS, FRONTAL VIEW
OpenStax College, Wikimedia Commons

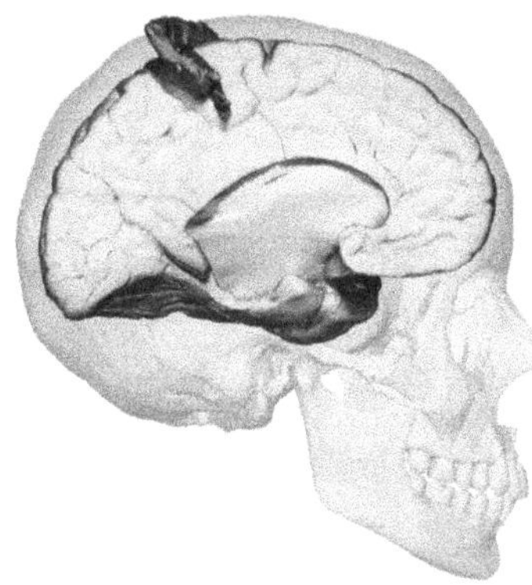

FIGURE 9.3: CORTICAL HOMUNCULUS, PRIMARY SOMATOSENSORY CORTEX
Polygon data were generated by Database Center for Life Science, Wikimedia Commons

Hands, feet, and oral areas are strongly represented in the sensory homunculus due to the much greater number of neurons and dendrites. Therefore, touch pressure to these areas can have a powerful inhibitory effect on the ANS. Pressure can be deep, such as weight-bearing through the hands and feet in Down Dog, or it can involve more subtle pressure such as pressing palms together, which is also calming and grounding.

For years, occupational therapists and other neurorehabilitation specialists have known that pressure to the hard palate is very calming to the nervous system, and they use various methods to provide deep pressure to the palate even for adults. The classic yogic Sitkari Pranayama (Cooling Breath), which is relaxing to the nerves and calming to the mind, uses the tongue to place pressure on the roof of the mouth. In SMYLE™ we use a simpler version called the Tongue Press (see Chapter 8).

Although the back and front of the torso have less density of neurons and dendrites compared to the areas discussed above, they cover wider areas of the body that can make up for it. In fact, the only study we could find on deep touch pressure that included physiological measures applied this modality to the torso. Using a convenience sample of 50 adults, Reynolds *et al.* (2015) studied the effect of deep touch pressure on arousal using an inflatable Vayu vest. The vest was inflated for a 3-minute period between two electronic game sessions. The results showed a highly significant increase in heart rate variability and decrease in skin conduction level (a measure of SNS activation) while wearing the vest, as well as a decrease in game errors during the second test that followed use of the vest. They concluded that the study "provides support for the foundational principle that deep pressure input to the thorax is capable of influencing autonomic arousal through reduction of sympathetic and enhancement of parasympathetic nervous system activity" (2015, p.4).

Ways to embed deep touch pressure into yoga

We can embed deep touch pressure into a therapeutic yoga class through the use of yoga props, such as bolsters, weighted yoga bags, and/or blocks; by offering yoga forms that naturally place pressure on various body parts (often through weight-bearing) such as the hands, feet, and various parts of the torso, for example back, shoulder blades, or belly; by presenting a breathing technique that places pressure on the belly or hard palate of the mouth (see Breathing Buddy and Tongue Press in Chapter 8); or by performing certain mudras (hand gestures) such as Adhi, which provides deep touch pressure to the thumbs (see Chapter 10).

EXAMPLES OF DEEP TOUCH PRESSURE USING PROPS

- Bolsters provide comforting deep pressure when used in restorative forms, and can be used in conjunction with other props such as blankets, blocks, bands, and weighted yoga bags. (See "Restorative yoga forms providing deep touch pressure".)
- A 5–10 pound weighted yoga bag can be placed:
  - ***On the belly*** (such as during diaphragmatic breath—see "Breathing Buddy")
  - ***Across the upper sacrum***, such as during Restorative Child or lying prone on the mat
  - ***Lengthwise over the spine or across the shoulders***, such as when lying prone on the mat, or
  - ***On the forehead*** (see the "Mental Tension Reliever" restorative form in this chapter);
  - ***Over the tops of the feet or on the lap*** while seated in a chair;
  - ***Other areas of the body*** have also been used.

Many students enjoy having two weights placed on their bodies, such as across the upper sacrum and vertically along the spine, forming an inverted "T" (see right photo in "Weighted Restorative Child"). The bags are bought from yoga supply stores (such as Yoga Accessories) and are filled with play sand from a home building supply store such as Home Depot or Lowe's.

- The wall of the room can be used to promote a sense of "grounding," such as by placing a foot (or feet) on the wall during Whole Body Stretch or during the extended leg hold at the end of Tiger Flow.
- Eye pillows can provide comforting pressure to soften and release the muscles around the eyes.

EXAMPLES OF DEEP PRESSURE TOUCH USING THE BODY (WEIGHT-BEARING)

Yoga forms can provide pressure ***through***:

- ***Back:*** Knee(s) to Chest
- ***Hands:*** Table, Down Dog, Rabbit Hop, Dolphin Flow
- ***Belly:*** Crocodile or Baby Cobra
- ***Feet:*** Warrior 1 and 2, Shining Star
- ***Upper body and/or limbs:*** Hug Breath, Clamshell Twist, Twisting Cat.

More examples are provided in the yoga form descriptions found in Part 3.

Restorative yoga forms providing deep touch pressure

Most of the restorative forms described on the following pages or variations thereof can be found in at least one of the following references:

- *B.K.S. Iyengar Yoga: The Path to Holistic Health*, by B.K.S. Iyengar (2001)
- *Rest and Renew: Restful Yoga for Stressful Times*, 2nd edition, by Judith Hanson Lasater (2011)
- *Yoga for Emotional Balance: Simple Practices to Help Relieve Anxiety and Depression*, by Bo Forbes (2011)
- *Sensory-Enhanced Yoga for Self-Regulation and Trauma Healing*, by Lynn Stoller (2019).

When adapting these restorative yoga forms for children, be sure to:

- Select form based on desired effects, e.g. ground, calm, or uplift.
- Size the props appropriately for the child.
- Position the child consistent with principles of safe body alignment.

- Fully support the child's body to invite their whole body to soften down into these supports.
- Fill in the spaces between the child's body and the surface on which it is resting using the props (e.g., bolsters, blankets, blocks).
- Fold the blankets and orient the props however they will best fit the child—there is not only one way to do it!
- Start within the person's window of tolerance and gradually move them into more expansive yoga forms as they are ready to embody them.
- Consider offering a 5–10 pound weighted yoga bag (or two) to enhance the calming effects.

Weighted Restorative Child

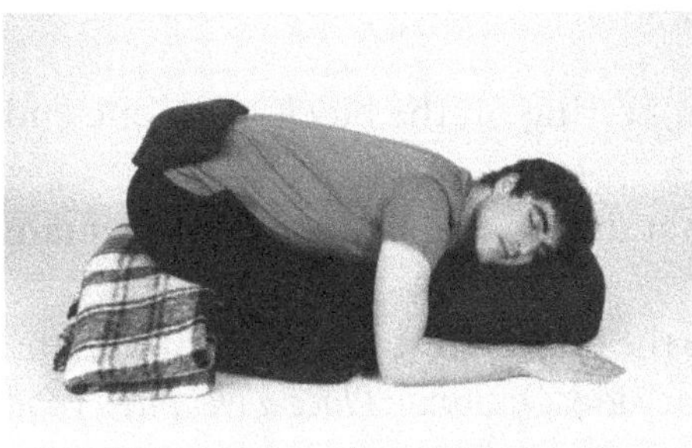

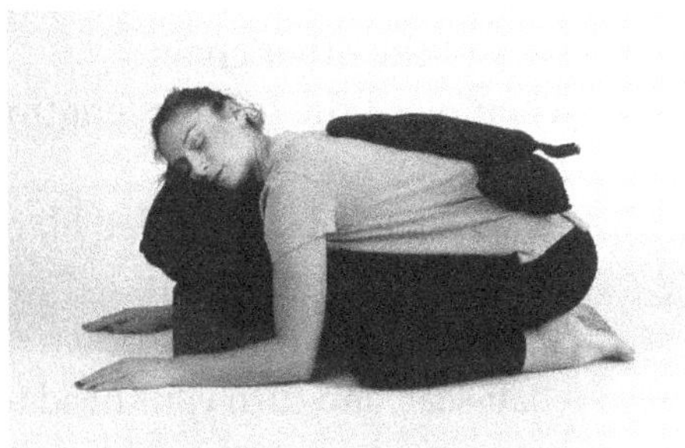

1. Place a bolster lengthwise on the mat. *Optional: During set-up, position a block (at its middle height) under the head end of the bolster to angle it.*
2. Kneel at the short end of the bolster, placing knees on each side of the bolster. *Optional: Place a firm folded blanket behind the knees to help them stay comfortable.*
3. Place your hands on the floor on each side of the bolster.
4. Slowly walk your hands away from you until you are resting on the bolster. Turn your head to one side. *Optional: Place a weighted yoga bag across the top of the sacrum to provide deep touch pressure. (Adjust the sand evenly in the bag first.) If desired, another weighted bag can be placed over the spine, overlapping the first bag to form an inverted "T."*
5. Rest for approximately 5 minutes, or however long it feels good, turning your head at the halfway point.

Restorative Child in a Chair

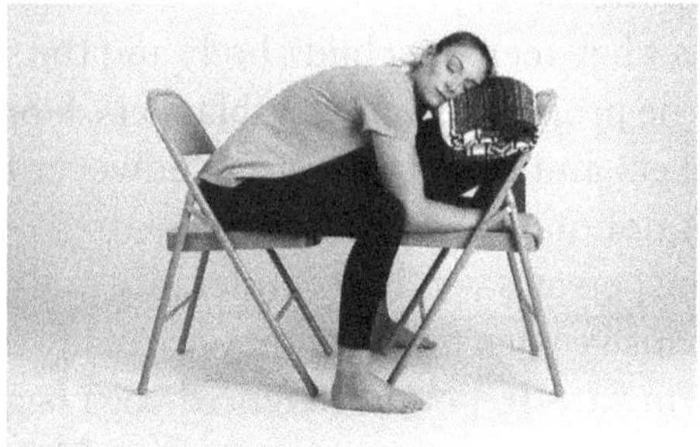

1. Position two chairs facing each other.
2. Sit in one of the chairs and position a block on its middle height at the back of the other chair.
3. Then place the bolster lengthwise, resting on the block, with one end between your legs.
4. If you'd like, place a folded blanket at the top end like a pillow (maintain neutral neck alignment).
5. Slowly lower your body down onto the bolster, rest your forearms on the chair seat, and turn your head to one side. *Optional: Place a weighted yoga bag vertically along your spine.*
6. Rest for about 5 minutes, or however long it feels good, turning your head at the halfway point.

Restorative Crocodile in a Chair

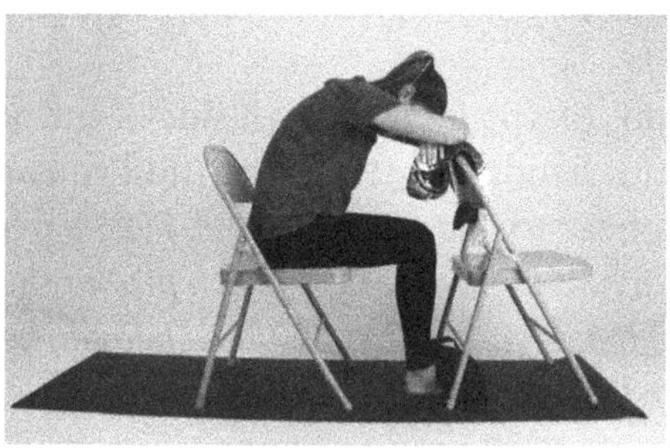

1. Position two chairs facing the same direction, one in front of the other.
2. Place a folded blanket over the back of the front chair.
3. Sit in the other chair. *Optional: Place a weighted yoga bag across the top of your feet.*
4. Place your forearms on the blanket; rest your head on your arms.
5. Stay as long as you like.

Restorative Twist over the bolster

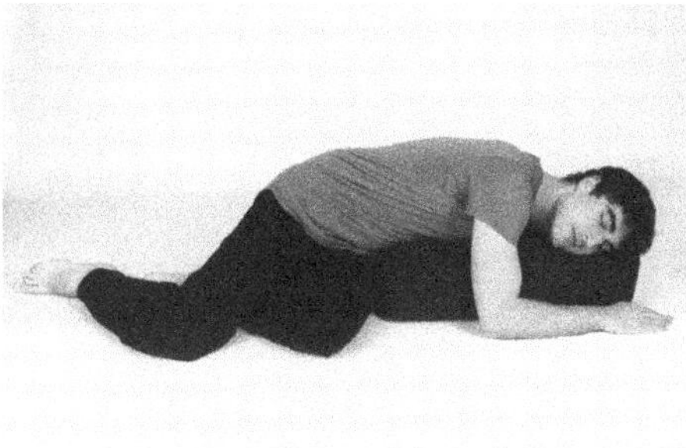

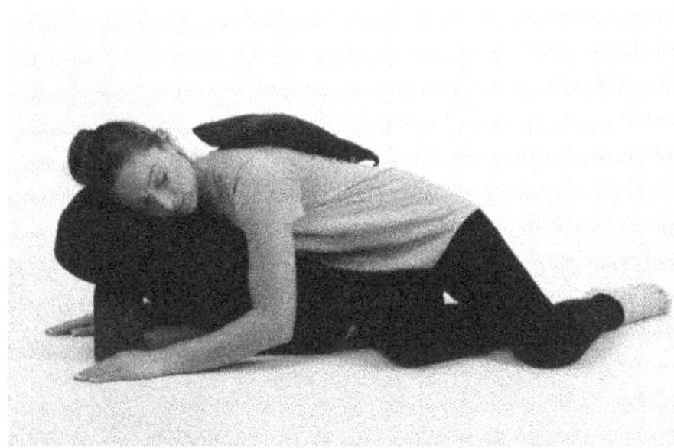

1. Lay the bolster on mat lengthwise. If desired, place a block (at its middle height) under the head end of the bolster to angle it.
2. Sit sideways so the bottom edge of the bolster is touching your top thigh.
3. Slowly walk your hands away from you until you are resting on the bolster.
4. Rest on the floor, and turn your head to face your knees.
5. If you'd like, place a folded blanket under your head (maintain neutral neck alignment). *Optional: Place a weighted bag diagonally over back (one end over the higher shoulder blade) (see right photo).*
6. Stay about 3–5 minutes or as long as comfortable; then switch sides.

Restorative Backbend

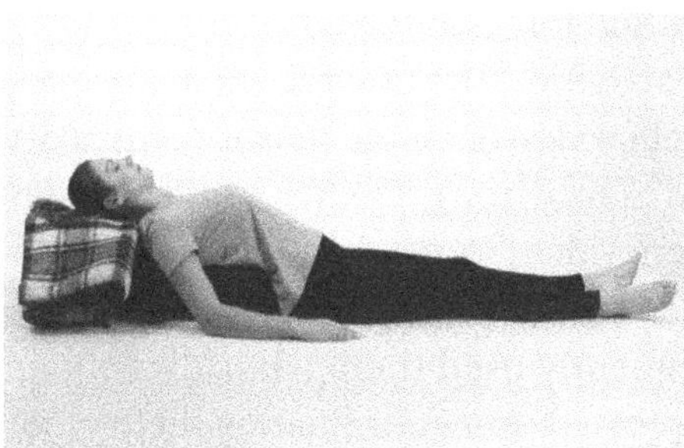

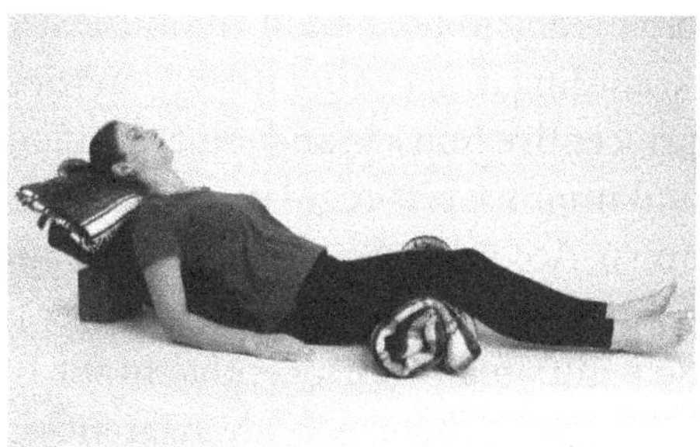

1. Sit with your back facing the bolster, and then slowly lay over it (see left photo). If this is uncomfortable for your back, move your bottom further away from the bolster or angle the bolster as described previously (see right photo).
2. Rest your head on a folded blanket.
3. Rest your forearms on the floor (or folded blankets). *Optional: Place a rolled blanket under the thighs for comfort.*

Mental Tension Reliever

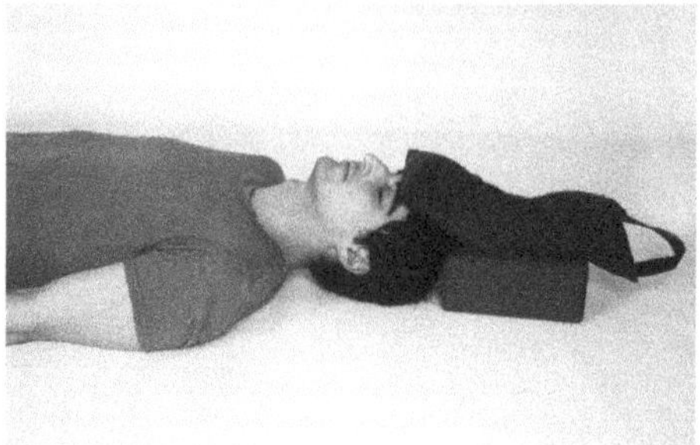

1. Lie on your back on a hard surface.
2. Position a block (4 inches thick) behind the head at its shortest height, with the short end touching the top of the head.
3. Lay a 5–10 pound weighted yoga bag over the block and forehead. (First adjust the sand inside the bag so the amount of weight on the forehead matches the student's wishes.)
4. Rest for about 5 minutes.

ENHANCED PROPRIOCEPTIVE INPUT

Proprioceptive sensation is produced by receptors in muscles and joints. The muscle spindle is the major stretch receptor within muscles. Golgi tendon organs and joint afferents monitor stresses and forces at the tendons and joints. According to sensory integration theory, activities that provide enhanced proprioceptive (muscle and joint) input are believed to decrease sensory sensitivity and improve self-regulation (Blanche and Schaaf 2001; Pfeiffer and Kinnealey 2003). According to Mollo, Schaaf, and Benevides (2008), this is hypothetically achieved by inhibiting SNS activity and by increasing activation of the PNS. Self-initiated proprioceptive input is frequently used therapeutically to help individuals "increase body awareness, improve motor coordination, help modulate arousal level, and aid in the processing of sensation through other sensory systems" (Blanche and Schaaf 2001, p.109, as cited in Mollo *et al.* 2008).

It is important to remain sensitive to the fact that trauma is held in the muscles (as well as all of the other tissues of the body) when presenting enhanced proprioceptive input to traumatized individuals. Although muscle and joint sensation is generally considered to be a very safe form of sensory input that is very integrating, there are some special considerations for trauma survivors. As you will recall, during the stress response, cortisol-, adrenaline-, and noradrenaline (aka norepinephrine)-infused blood is shunted to the limbs to assist in the "fight–flight" response. If the stress response is not adequately resolved, this excess energy is stored in the muscles, still ready to fight or flee, while the person remains in a frozen state of immobility. (One such muscle is the psoas; please see the special note in the text box that follows.) This creates trauma-based muscle tension that can present in a person's posture and movements, accompanied by psychological tension. This tension/pressure needs to be released slowly, so it is important to proceed thoughtfully when elongating the muscles. Never ask people to over-extend their own body parts into the full expression of a yoga form, or push their body parts into the full expression yourself. Always start where the person is at, staying within their physical and psychological range of motion.

The following text box describes two effective muscle-elongation methods that can help to release trauma-held muscular tensions when performed correctly. It should be noted that a muscle isn't elastic and can't actually stretch; instead, the myofibrils elongate when there is a force pulling them apart, such as gravity or an antagonistic muscle. Following elongation, a muscle should be used actively and functionally, either on or off the yoga mat. This is particularly important for loose-jointed individuals who actually need yoga forms and movements that emphasize joint compression rather than joint traction to help hold themselves together (Rothschild 2003). SMYLE™ provides plentiful opportunities for joint compression through weight-bearing forms and through use of a yoga band (for those individuals for whom a band is appropriate), which provides co-activation of muscles around the joints.

Muscle-elongation techniques used in the Sensory-Enhanced Yoga® program

1. ***Repetition and hold:*** This method consists of dynamically moving in and out of a yoga form in coordination with the breath. SMYLE™ presents most yoga forms using this technique, such as ***Cat***, ***Twisting Cat***, and ***Dynamic Warrior 1***. A leading pioneer in this approach is Gary Kraftsow, author of *Yoga for Wellness: Healing with the Timeless Teachings of Viniyoga* (1999). Dynamically moving in and out of a form *with awareness* provides us with feedback regarding our movement habits, including our protective holding patterns and release valves, so that by the time we hold the form, we are likely to be in much better alignment than had we simply gone straight into it on the first breath. Also, muscles elongate further after contracting, thus drawing us deeper into the form with each repetition. This is due to the mechanism of reciprocal innervation between antagonistic muscles. Finally, trauma survivors may start out with more constrained movements, and as they

slowly become more embodied through awareness of sensation, movement, and breath, they may begin to demonstrate greater range and ease of movement.

2. ***Maintained stretch:*** This method is used during static yoga forms or during the hold portion of a dynamic form when meeting up with a restriction in movement. A good example of its use is during Leg Stretches with a yoga band. To use this technique, move the body part just until you feel the stretch, and then stop there and simply breathe and relax into it. After several seconds, the muscles may soften and you may sense that you can move the leg a bit further (even if just a little). Once again, stop and breathe into the stretch. You might undergo this process three or four times before the final range is reached for that session. In the words of Yee (2002, p.130): "resistance...pause...breath...space...movement...resistance."

A note about the psoas muscle: The psoas muscle is the largest hip flexor and is wired tightly to the SNS, as it is needed in order to run away from the "tiger" during the fight-flight reaction. Due to its position in the body, when it contracts, it pulls on the diaphragm. It is this pull that causes us to make that short gasp when something frightens us. It contracts during activation of the SNS even if we are sitting down and not actively moving. Many trauma survivors have an especially tight psoas, which can affect diaphragmatic breathing, contributing to a shallow breath. Examples of yoga forms in the SMYLE™ program that stretch the psoas include Warrior 1 and Dynamic Warrior 1. You may notice a decreased stance during Warrior forms due to a tight psoas or psychological protection. Again, it is important to start where the person is. If you suspect a tight psoas, it is recommended that a certified yoga therapist or physical therapist be consulted for proper treatment.

Ways to increase proprioceptive input

Yoga naturally provides rich proprioceptive input; however, there are several ways we can enhance the proprioceptive qualities of a yoga session to boost its therapeutic effects. We can use yoga bands to increase the muscle activation (taking care to do so safely by not *over*stretching muscles); we can present yoga forms that offer heavy muscle work in static positions; and we can choose slower dynamic yoga flows that incorporate increased muscle loading, the latter of which also helps to modulate any hypersensitivity that may occur from the movement of the flow. When presenting yoga forms that include the use of a band, it is a good idea to offer an alternative option, in case anyone in class has experienced a whipping (see Chapter 7). This is usually easy enough by simply stating: "You can choose to do these movements with or without the yoga band."

Below are some recommended muscle-loading yoga forms. Some of the particularly effective ones involve bearing weight on the arms, such as in Down Dog, or activate more muscles in the legs due to the awkwardness of the position, such as in Shining Star. Please also see Chapters 14 and 15 for specific examples of how to use yoga bands. Here are the recommended forms:

- Tiger Flow (the holding part)
- Down Dog
- Dolphin Flow (Down Dog to Up Dog Flow)
- Rabbit Hop
- Baby Cobra
- Arm or Leg Stretches with a yoga band
- Windmill
- Warrior 1 and 2
- Shining Star (bent arms and legs).

SLOW RHYTHMICAL LINEAR MOVEMENT

In 1954, Margaret Rood proposed that through the careful selection and use of sensory stimuli, the ANS could be biased toward sympathetic or parasympathetic activation, which would influence muscle control accordingly (Rood 1954; see also Bordoloi and Deka 2018). In addition, Rood believed that it was the ***intensity***, ***frequency***, and ***rhythm*** (or lack thereof) of the sensory stimulus that determined whether it would have a sympathetic or parasympathetic effect, an assertion echoed by many other influential occupational therapists (e.g., Ayres 1972, p.59; Farber 1982, p.141). Among the sensory stimuli suggested to activate the PNS were slow, rhythmic, repetitive rocking and slow rolling (Bordoloi and Deka 2018), techniques that have been adapted for yoga in the Sensory-Enhanced Yoga® program. It is important to keep in mind, however, that context will also affect response to vestibular input, including a person's sense of safety and groundedness, and the expectation of a pleasurable or unpleasant experience.

Dr. Jean Ayres was strongly influenced by Rood when she developed her sensory integration theory and intervention program for children. It was Dr. Ayres' book, *Sensory Integration and Learning Disorders* (1972), that inspired Lynn Stoller to enter the occupational therapy field in the first place, and much later to suggest that slow rhythmic movements be integrated into the Iraq Yoga Study treatment protocol for active duty military personnel (Stoller *et al.* 2012). In her book, Dr. Ayres explains:

> Whether vestibular stimulation will have an excitatory or an inhibitory effect on human behavior through the brain stem is determined by the type of stimulation. It has been observed in the clinical situation that slow, rhythmical, passive motion with the child in a situation not demanding adaptive response can be inhibitory, whereas rapid motion is apt to be excitatory. (1972, p.59)

Although Dr. Ayres believed that passive rocking would inhibit the nervous system to a greater degree than active rocking, she stated that active participation could be encouraged to help modulate the vestibular effects if they were too inhibitory or excitatory, and that "organizing a response tends to balance the excitatory and inhibitory components of brain function" (1972, p.120). Given the popularity of rocking chairs for stress reduction, which involve active movements, Lynn wondered whether slow, ***active***, rhythmic movements along the same planes advocated for passive linear movements would also produce a calming effect. If so, she surmised that incorporating such movements into the Iraq Yoga Study treatment protocol for military personnel could potentially reduce symptoms of hyperarousal caused by living and working in combat conditions. We now know that there is a lot of neuroplasticity, even in the adult brain, which was unknown when Dr. Ayres developed her theory of sensory integration.

Here is some important background on the vestibular system as well as things to keep in mind when presenting slow, rhythmic movement input within the context of yoga. However, the reader is encouraged to read pages 167–179 of *Sensory-Enhanced Yoga for Self-Regulation and Trauma Healing* by Lynn Stoller (2019), for a much more in-depth discussion on the vestibular system, including relevant study findings and additional treatment implications.

The vestibular role in the grounded and embodied self

The vestibular system is part of the labyrinth of the inner ear, and detects our head movement through space as well as its position relative to gravity. Thus it contributes to balance and to spatial orientation, and is the dominant sense that provides information about our movement through the environment, almost like a GPS system. The vestibular system consists of the utricle and saccule, known as the otoliths, and the three semicircular canals (see Figure 9.4). They are attached to the hearing apparatus (cochlea), also located in the inner ear. These structures are lined with hair cells and are also filled with fluid (endolymph). When the head moves, the fluid moves, displacing the hair cells, which sets off nerve impulses. These nerve impulses travel to many parts of the brain, including the cerebellum, which coordinates the muscle actions necessary to maintain posture and balance (Ango and Dos Reis 2019).

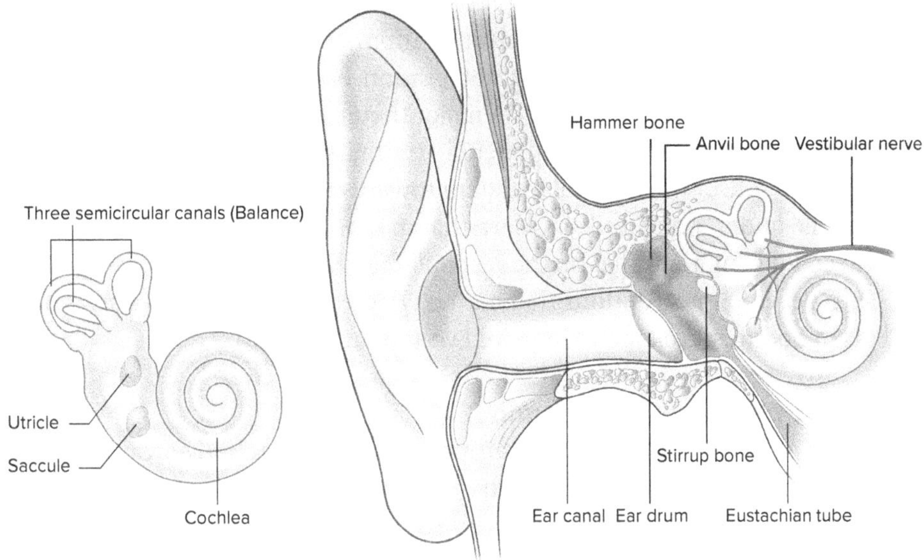

FIGURE 9.4: VESTIBULAR APPARATUS
Reproduced from Stoller (2019)

The otoliths and semicircular canals respond to different types of vestibular input:

- The **otoliths** are gravity receptors, and as such detect the position of the head in relation to gravity. They also detect linear movement through space. The otoliths consist of the ***saccule***, which detects vertical movement, and the ***utricle***, which detects forward and backward and side-to-side linear movements.
- The **semicircular canals** detect angular (or rotary) movement, such as spinning or rotating the head from side to side or doing somersaults.

The vestibular sense works closely with the proprioceptive sense to enable us to maintain balance and an upright posture. It is also closely involved with the visual system, allowing us to judge our motion in relation to the objects around us. Our sense of "grounding" is largely attributable to the vestibular sense as it detects our positional relationship to the earth/ground. When a person is feeling intense anxiety, it can be accompanied by a "floating in space" sensation due to the strong connections between the vestibular and autonomic systems. When this occurs, deep touch pressure and/or enhanced proprioceptive input will usually effectively modulate the sensations and help to psychologically "replant" the person back on the ground.

Lenggenhager and Lopez (2015) presented study findings from various fields to support their hypothesis that vestibular input contributes "to aspects of the bodily self, such as basic multisensory integration, body schema, body ownership, agency, and self-location" (abstract). A major theme of this book is on the importance of restoring a sense of embodiment in trauma survivors; therefore, studying the potential role of the vestibular system toward that goal would certainly be a worthwhile undertaking. Indeed, Harricharan *et al.* (2016) pointed to the urgent need to conduct more studies on the vestibular neural circuitry of those who have PTSD to develop interventions that address decreased interoceptive awareness and disembodiment related to impaired vestibular function.

Vestibular pathways to the brain

Vestibular pathways project to numerous areas of the cerebral cortex as well as the hippocampus, insula, and thalamus (Hitier, Besnard, and Smith 2014). Here, we will bullet just a few key points:

- The vestibular system has a strong connection with the anterior insula (Wirth *et al.* 2018), which is believed to hold a key role in switching between the CEN and DMN. This raises the question as to whether a carefully constructed vestibular program can influence the operation of these core networks.
- Activation of vestibular-related areas in the brain show a ***significant right hemisphere dominance*** (Brandt and Dieterich 1999), which is particularly interesting considering the ANS is also a right-hemisphere dominant system.
- Vestibular cortical regions activate differently to input from the semicircular canals and otoliths, which may help to explain why different types of input have different effects on arousal, mood, and other aspects of self-regulation (Kammermeier, Singh, and Bötzel 2017).
- Four main vestibular pathways have been identified that travel to the hippocampus, and furthermore, ***vestibular stimulation has been shown to activate or deactivate the hippocampus*** and related areas in humans (Hitier *et al.* 2014). This raises the question as to whether a vestibular treatment could help process traumatic memories through the hippocampus. Various study findings, in combination, lend support to this idea.
    - ***Vestibular stimulation promotes an increase in REM sleep*** (see, for example, Krystal *et al.* 2010; Woodward *et al.* 1990)
    - ***REM sleep has been hypothesized to reflect the process of memory consolidation*** (Rauchs *et al.* 2004)
    - ***Fragmented REM sleep is common in those who have PTSD*** and also

predicts the later development of PTSD symptoms (Pace-Schott, Germain, and Milad 2015)

- ***The higher the concentrations of GABA in the hippocampus, the better the mPFC can make unwanted thoughts go away*** (Schmitz *et al.* 2017)
- ***There are GABA-releasing vestibular axons throughout the whole brain in mice, which raises the question of whether this is also the case in humans*** (Shi *et al.* 2022).

- There are very strong connections between the vestibular nuclei and the thalamus (Hitier *et al.* 2014). Many vestibular nerve fibers synapse on the same thalamic nuclei that receive information from the spinothalamic and DCML pathways, where much of the integrative tactile, proprioceptive, and vestibular processing takes place (Purves *et al.* 2001).

The association between anxiety and dizziness

Many different theoretical models have been presented to explain the association of anxiety with dizziness and decreased balance control, which speaks to the fact that there are numerous vestibular connections throughout the central nervous system that could provide a plausible explanation. Balaban (2002) described vestibular-limbic neural circuits in detail, and the interested reader is referred to that resource. Here, we will just mention one of these connections. The ***parabrachial nucleus*** in the pons of the brainstem communicates information regarding whole body rotation and body position relative to gravity (linear acceleration) to neural circuits involved in anxiety responses. These neural circuits include the ***amygdala***, ***hypothalamus***, as well as a region in the ***vmPFC*** that is responsible for the inhibition of emotional responses such as fear. In Chapter 4 we identified these structures as being among the brain structures most implicated in PTSD, so it is no surprise that so many trauma survivors have vestibular symptoms (Balaban, Jacob, and Furman 2011). Balaban (2002) theorized that the processing of body motion is likely to be context-dependent since the connections between the vestibular nuclei and these higher-level structures are reciprocal. In other words, the same movement could produce a positive or negative emotional response depending on other situational factors.

Vestibulo-sympathetic reflexes and baroreceptors

There is also considerable research evidence showing that bodily movements in space adjust blood distribution throughout the body, and that these effects are controlled by the SNS. These reactions are called ***vestibulo-sympathetic reflexes*** (Yates, Bolton, and Macefield 2014). The contributions of the vestibular system to blood pressure control are higher in an upright position (Macefield and James 2016). Otherwise our blood would drain downward whenever we stand up!

The vestibulo-sympathetic reflexes are thought to interact with the baroreceptors in a complementary way to maintain homeostasis of the cardiovascular system (Yates *et al.* 2014).

Baroreceptors are mechanoreceptors located in the carotid sinus and the aortic arch that respond to changes in tension in the walls of the arteries. If the blood pressure increases suddenly (such as when doing an inversion in a yoga practice), the baroreceptors are stretched, sending impulses to certain areas of the brainstem, which inhibits sympathetic tone and increases vagal tone (on the SA node of the heart). The heart rate is then slowed to reduce the pressure. Regular dynamic exercise can increase vagal tone (Freeman 2006). Notably, slow breathing (six breaths/min.) was found to improve baroreceptor sensitivity and reduce blood pressure in people who have hypertension (Bernardi *et al.* 2001).

The link between rocking and relaxation

It has been intuitively understood across thousands of years and different world cultures that rocking movements can produce a relaxation response and even lull people of all ages to sleep, from infants in the cradle to elderly folks in rocking chairs; yet surprisingly, there remains a lack of high quality empirical evidence to establish rhythmic input as relaxing (Grabherr, Macauda, and Lenggenhager 2015; Omlin *et al.* 2016). There are also so many different variables that can be manipulated with regard to vestibular stimulation that it is impossible to make a blanket statement that "linear" or "rotary" stimulation is calming or excitatory to the nervous system. We will begin to try to tease out some of the issues here, but to do so we first need to identify the types of movement input we are talking about (see Figure 9.5):

- There are *three pure planes of linear (aka translational) movement*: ***heave*** (up and down), ***sway*** (side to side), and ***surge*** (forward and backwards), but the otoliths are also stimulated by any combination of these movements.
- There are *three pure planes of rotary movement*: **pitch** (i.e., rotating about the lateral horizontal axis, such as occurs when shaking the head "yes"), ***yaw*** (i.e., rotating about the vertical axis, such as occurs when shaking the head "no"), and ***roll*** (i.e., rotating about the longitudinal horizontal axis, such as occurs with ear down tilt). Again, there are numerous combinations of these movements that would stimulate the semicircular canals as well.

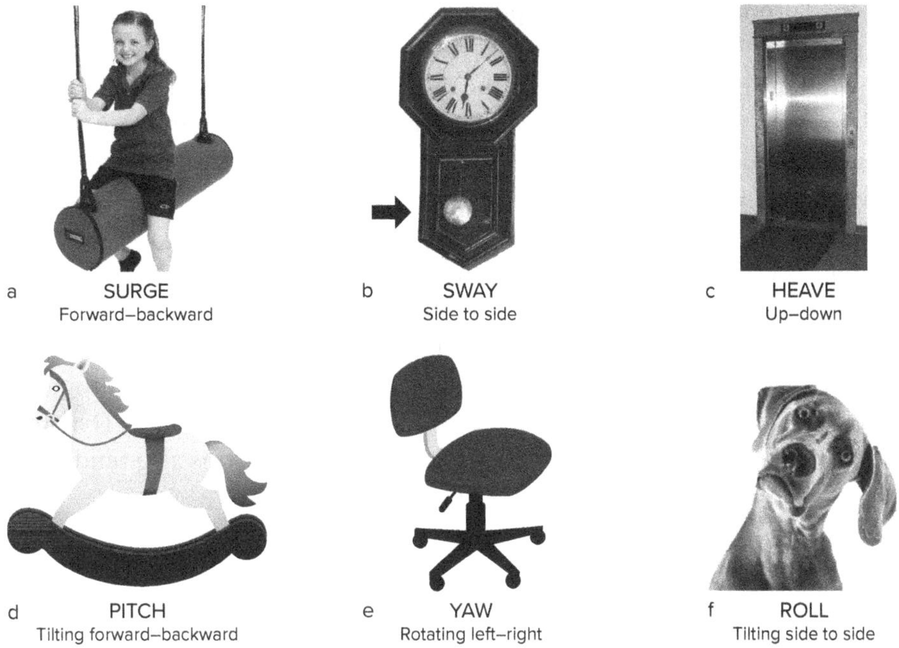

FIGURE 9.5: THE SIX DIRECTIONS OF VESTIBULAR MOVEMENT

a: Southpaw; b: Av.kumar85, Wikimedia Commons; c: Darkshark0159, Wikimedia Commons; d: gnokii at openclipart.org, Wikimedia Commons; e: anarres at openclipart.org, Wikimedia Commons; f: Shutterstock

There are many movement combinations in which the otoliths and/or semicircular canals can be activated. For example, slow rocking in a rocking chair or over a therapy ball is usually considered to be a linear form of movement (which is believed to inhibit the SNS and activate the PNS); however, they are also examples of pitch rotation, and thus provide semicircular canal stimulation as well, which has traditionally been considered stimulating as a generic category of movements. In fact, pitch movements of the head that are produced from a natural upright posture are known to stimulate both the semicircular canals and the otoliths in a coordinated fashion (Guedry *et al.* 1990). This is good to know since several of the slow, rhythmic movement patterns presented in this book involve a combination of pitch rotations with surge linear movements, such as the Dolphin and Rabbit Hop flows. Also, any rotational movement of the head stimulates all of the semicircular canals to one degree or another (Guedry *et al.* 1990). Thus, a simplified explanation of the effects of pitch, roll, yaw, heave, surge, and sway movements is likely impossible.

In occupational therapy practice, and particularly with regard to the sensory integration treatment approach (Sensory Integration International 1991), slow (mostly) linear movements emphasizing stimulation of the otoliths have been more frequently employed for the purpose of reducing hyperarousal. Common examples include slow forward/backward movement on a swing or when positioned prone over a large therapy ball. Rood's slow rolling technique (Farber 1982) is an exception, as it is designed to primarily stimulate the semicircular canals (rather than the otoliths) for the purpose of calming. This technique is simulated with the Clamshell Twist in our program (see Chapter 14). A similar rolling technique was included in a short set of vestibular exercises presented to elderly women with type 2 diabetes, which resulted in reduced anxiety, stress, and depression as study outcomes (Goothy *et al.* 2019).

Supine rocking on a therapy ball stimulates protective extension responses and is arousing to the ANS, and is to be avoided with individuals who have PTSD or anxiety. For these same reasons, backbends in yoga tend to be very alerting; this is why we only teach gentle ones with the head upright in our program. Conversely, dynamic forward folds tend to be calming, such as Seated Dynamic Warrior 1, Setting Sun, or Waterfall. Static forward inversions also tend to be calming, such as Standing Forward Fold or Down Dog.

Dizziness is less likely to be felt when the person is well-grounded, as proprioceptive and deep touch pressure input both help to modulate vestibular input. For example, Down Dog is less apt to elicit dizziness than a Standing Forward Fold due to the grounding of both hands and feet and strong muscle activation. The traditional treatment for vestibular hypersensitivity in the sensory integration field is to combine proprioceptive activities, that is, heavy muscle work, with linear (especially forward/backward) movement activities. Combining active, heavy muscle work with movement through space helps the nervous system modulate vestibular sensations, whereas passive movement (such as being swung or spun) is much more apt to cause dizziness or nausea.

Also, please be aware that when we use vestibular movement as a treatment intervention, we need to include at least some trunk movement in the same direction as the head movement. This is because the proprioceptive input generated from neck movements significantly decreases the vestibular response from such movements (Sadeghi, Mitchell, and Cullen 2009). Otherwise, we'd get dizzy every time we moved our head! Thus slow, rhythmic movements of the head in isolation from the body are not invited into the "slow, rhythmic movement" club of treatment strategies since we want the stimuli to reach the thalamus and higher brain centers, not get canceled out at the lower levels.

The effects of natural, active vestibular input on stress reduction

While a mountain of basic research has been conducted on the effects of vestibular stimulation on the nervous and cardiovascular systems, mostly with animals, there are far fewer published studies that have investigated the use of natural vestibular stimulation for stress reduction in humans, and it is very rare to find a study that investigated the effects of ***active*** vestibular stimulation on stress reduction. Many of these studies were conducted quite recently at the Little Flower Institute in India. At this Institute, Dr. K.S. Sailesh and his colleagues have performed over a dozen studies investigating the effects of natural vestibular stimulation, that is, active swinging on a standard playground-type swing, on various physiological functions and conditions, including stress and cardiovascular parameters (Archana, Sailesh, and Mukkadan 2016), insomnia (Sailesh and Mukkadan 2013a), hypothyroidism (Sailesh, Archana, and Mukkadan 2014), psychoneuroimmuno modulation (Sailesh and Mukkadan 2013b), and depression in underweight women (Sailesh *et al.* 2016).

All of these studies produced positive findings, but to highlight just one (Archana *et al.* 2016), 240 healthy college students were randomized to four groups: 60 males (stimulation group); 60 females (stimulation group); 60 males (control group); and 60 females (control group). The participants consented to swing on a swing in a back to front direction, according to their level of comfort, following standardized methods. A comparison of pre- and post-tests found that cortisol, stress score, pulse rate, and systolic, diastolic, and mean blood pressure were significantly lowered in the male and female vestibular intervention groups following vestibular stimulation, and remained within normal limits.

The researchers reported that their findings were consistent with prior study results, suggesting that the vestibular system causes the release of GABA and also activates hippocampal neurons, thereby inhibiting the HPA axis (Archana *et al.* 2016), leading to a more relaxed state of mind.

Rotary stimulation

Do not attempt to treat trauma survivors with rotary stimulation. By this we mean, do not present movements that involve consecutive 360° body rotations (e.g., spinning), or even partial body rotations that occur faster than the pace of someone's natural breath. This means even being cautious with standing rotations from side to side (e.g., "empty coat sleeves," with arms loosely swinging), which can stimulate dizziness, anxiety, and disorientation. Rotary stimulation has been shown to induce a vestibular-evoked stress response expressed by increased ACTH, noradrenaline (aka norepinephrine), and adrenaline, while caloric stimulation of the semicircular canals (which simulates rotary stimulation) has been shown to increase cortisol levels and reduce serum levels of GABA, glutamate, and glycine (Saman *et al.* 2012).

Having said this, we do present slow, rhythmical, *partial* (up to 180°) rotary movements, back and forth (A–B, A–B, A–B style), that occur at the pace of someone's natural breath or close to it. This is in line with Rood's slow rolling technique and the experience of slowly swinging in a hammock or on a swing.

Tips for learning rhythmic flows

- Focus attention on doing the movements safely and correctly before adding attention to the breath.
- Practice coordinating movement with the breath in more simpler yoga forms (e.g., Rainbow Breath, Robin's Breath) before incorporating the breath into vestibular movements (e.g., Rabbit Hop, Dolphin Flow).
- Once breath control is mastered, start at the breathing rate that comes most natural to your students when performing the movements, and very gradually reduce the rate with practice.
- Only perform these movements if it comes easily and does not cause stress or discomfort.
- To maximize the therapeutic benefits of these vestibular movements, make sure that the flow is in fact *slow* and *rhythmical*! It is important ***not*** to pause at the end ranges but instead to smoothly "swing" back and forth.

Sample slow and rhythmic flows

Here are some examples of slow, rhythmic flows that we include in our program (please see Chapters 14 and 15 for descriptions).

Performed sitting in a chair:

- Seated Cat Flow (Happy Cat/Angry Cat)
- Setting Sun
- Seated Waterfall
- Tiger Flow
- Seated Cat to Cobra
- Seated Twisting Cat
- Owl (Seated Twist)
- Dynamic Seated Warrior 1
- Warrior 2 Flow.

Performed on a mat:

- Cat Flow (Happy Cat/Angry Cat)
- Tiger Flow
- Twisting Cat
- Rabbit Hop (Hare to Knee-Down Up Dog)
- Dolphin Flow (Down Dog to Up Dog)
- Clamshell Twist
- Dynamic Warrior 1
- Warrior 2 Flow
- Waterfall.

If any students exhibit dizziness after these forms, follow with grounding yoga forms that provide heavy muscle work. Some examples include:

- Seated Forward Fold (Stage 1, leaning into elbows supported on thighs) following Seated Twisting Cat or Owl (Seated Twist)
- Down Dog following Twisting Cat or Clamshell Twist
- Shining Star following Waterfall.

NEUTRAL WARMTH

Neutral warmth is a technique that works by affecting the temperature receptors in the hypothalamus and PNS. It refers to maintaining body heat by wrapping the body (or body part to be relaxed) with a "cotton flannel or fleece blanket or a down comforter" (Sharma 2019, p.130). In therapeutic settings, it is used for 10–20 minutes. "Neutral heat" is heat no greater than body temperature so as to avoid a rebound effect in 2–3 hours (Radomski and Latham 2007). Patrick Dougherty, from the Department of Anesthesiology and Pain Medicine at the MD Anderson Cancer Center, explained the connection between warmth and the PNS: "Activation of warm-sensitive neurons results in an activation of neurons in the paraventricular nucleus (PVN) and lateral hypothalamus that result in heightened parasympathetic outflow to promote the dissipation of heat" (Dougherty n.d.).

Placing a Mexican blanket on yoga participants during Final Relaxation is an example of using neutral warmth to effect calming, but there are other times during yoga practice when draping a blanket over someone's body may be therapeutically beneficial, such as when performing seated warm-ups or reclined yoga forms. As mentioned in Chapter 8, a blanket can also help to reduce a sense of vulnerability during certain yoga forms for individuals who have experienced sexual trauma.

SOME GENERAL EFFECTS OF POSTURE FAMILIES

1. ***Forward bends:*** These tend to be calming to the nervous system and are traditionally recommended for anxiety or stress relief, but be careful how you present them to reduce the risk of eliciting dizziness in those trauma survivors who exhibit vestibular hypersensitivity. A standing ***half***-forward fold with hands on a chair seat or on the thighs and head kept above hip level is better tolerated for some people than a full forward fold. Supporting the crown of the head on a tall block during a forward fold also helps to modulate vestibular sensations.

2. ***Backward bends:*** These tend to be energizing and are often recommended to treat depression. However, they can stimulate ANS arousal and should be presented in a carefully thought-out manner with those who have PTSD. Positioning the head behind the center of gravity (such as in Camel—not presented in this book) is likely to increase hyperarousal, so it is best to choose backbends that maintain the head in a more vertical position, such as Baby Cobra or Up Dog. Also, when heart-opening (chest-expanding) yoga forms are presented, they should ideally be well grounded; thus, Baby Cobra is an ideal choice due to the increased contact with the earth/ground.
3. ***Twists:*** These are generally very calming. They help to release stress in the gut, which is considered to be the "second brain" as it is controlled by the vagus nerve. Eighty percent of the vagal nerve fibers are afferent and are considered to have a significant influence on emotional well-being. The closer to the ground and the more supportive the twist form is, the more calming the effects are. Conversely, the more balance or effort that is required in a twist, the less they will produce a calming effect; in fact, a Revolved Standing Twist will likely increase hyperarousal.
4. ***Lateral bends:*** Due to their asymmetry, lateral bends may be more difficult for those who have decreased body awareness and motor planning ability. Therefore, you may need to assist (preferably verbally, unless trust has been developed). Also, some lateral bends (such as Triangle—not shown in this book) position the head in extreme positions away from the center of gravity, which may elicit dizziness in those susceptible to this symptom. This effect can be mitigated by providing strong muscle input and/or by reducing the balance demands, for example by coming into Triangle via Extended Side Angle (when *ready* for Triangle).
5. ***Balance forms:*** These promote sensory integration on many levels and are especially powerful for helping to improve focus, bringing the mind back to the present moment. However, relatively gentle balance forms with the head upright and in midline (such as Tree or Eagle, the latter not shown in this book), or which are low to the ground and carry a minimal risk of injury (such as the extended leg/arm hold in Tiger Flow), are more therapeutic for PTSD than forms that would more strongly stimulate the sympathetic/"fight–flight" nervous system, such as Crow (not shown in this book).

Proceed with caution: Wide-legged poses, especially for individuals with a history of sexual abuse, may induce vulnerability. Standing wide-legged forms tend to be perceived as less threatening than reclined wide-legged forms. Consider participants and offer alternatives for sensitive forms.

CHAPTER 10

Guideline #4: New Beliefs and Attitudes More Easily Take Hold When We First Prepare the Body to Receive and Accept Them

We hold our emotions and traumas in our bodies, which become expressed in our posture and the ways in which we move our bodies. In children, these feelings and emotions are expressed in a more transparent way. Many adults have the cognitive awareness and ability to inhibit the expression of their true feelings in public in order to demonstrate expected or socially appropriate behaviors. In contrast, children tend to express their true feelings on their sleeves as they have not yet fully developed the capability of considering the perspectives of others around them. For example, children who are feeling depressed may slouch in their chair, walk slowly, keep their eye gaze down, put their head on their desk, reduce their speech volume, may even become mute, sleep during a group activity, and/or separate themselves from the group. In some children, behaviors can be more dramatic such as throwing themselves on the floor or hiding away from the view of others.

Children who are highly stressed or anxious may also demonstrate symptoms that are observable to those working with them, including rigid posturing, hypervigilance, fidgeting, sweating, picking, undereating, overeating, shakiness, darting eyes, distractedness, insomnia, inability to relax, and running out of the classroom or even out of the school building. Other symptoms of highly stressed or anxious students may not be so easily observed, such as stomach aches, nausea, rapid heart rate, headaches, dizziness, tingling, trouble breathing, and more (Boston Children's Hospital 2021; CDC 2021). All of these symptoms can occur at different times, settings, or contexts, depending on whether certain classes or activities are stress-inducing or positively motivating.

Thus, we easily gauge other people's emotions not only from their words and facial expressions, but also from their posture, movements, and other observable bodily indicators. We intuitively know that emotions are registered and held throughout the ***bodymind***, not just the mind. In children, the emotional transparency via physical expression provides us with a deep view into how they are feeling inside. Professionals working with children should use this to their advantage as an effective tool for gauging emotional regulation, monitoring progress, and teaching future strategies for emotional support.

Posture does not just ***reflect*** emotion; it ***induces*** emotion. Nair *et al.* (2015) found that assuming an upright sitting posture can reduce fear, increase self-esteem, and cause a person to feel more enthusiastic, excited, and/or strong, whereas a slumped posture can cause a person to feel more fearful, hostile, nervous, dull, passive, quiet, sleepy, and/or sluggish. Furthermore, a set of experiments conducted by Veenstra, Schneider, and Koole (2017) found that posture could also play an important role in helping a person recover from a negative mood that has *already been activated*. Thus, it may logically be argued that ***yoga—an activity that stretches people in all sorts of ways in which typical activities don't—is very well suited to be a natural mood lifter, which, in turn, tends to inspire more positive attitudes and beliefs***.

If linking posture to someone's personal beliefs feels like a "stretch," just imagine a teacher trying to help a child take a more optimistic or calmer perspective of a situation while their body is sending strong alarm signals that conflict with that (e.g., folded arms or head down). Dr. Ken Dychtwald (1986), author of *Bodymind*, described in detail the many ways that emotions can become blocked and expressed in the body structure, affecting someone's attitudes and beliefs. Although we personally believe he overstated the case in certain body structure presentations that have a genetic basis, there is enough deep wisdom in the book to highly recommend it for anyone doing this work, particularly yoga therapists. In *Bodymind*, Dr. Dychtwald included an elegant quote by Ida Rolf (on pp.71 and 72), which we will re-quote here since it perfectly underscores this fourth guideline of Sensory-Enhanced Yoga® (SMYLE™):

> An individual experiencing temporary fear, grief, or anger, all too often carries his body in an attitude which the world recognizes as the outward manifestation of that particular emotion. If he persists in this dramatization or consistently re-establishes it, thus forming what is ordinarily referred to as a "habit pattern", the muscular arrangement becomes set... Since it is not possible to establish a free flow through the physical flesh, the subjective emotional tone becomes progressively more limited and tends to remain in a restricted, closely defined area. Now what the individual feels is no longer an emotion, a response to an immediate situation, henceforth he lives, moves, and has his being in an attitude. (Rolf, 1963, pp.71, 72, quoted in Dychtwald 1986)

Beck's (2008) expanded ***cognitive model of depression*** describes the downward trajectory that may occur when negative attitudes and beliefs are not effectively addressed in children. The model explains that adverse developmental experiences lead to dysfunctional attitudes (schemas), which, in turn, lead to a cognitive bias toward attending to negative aspects of experiences (and interpretations) while blocking out positive aspects of experiences and memories. These cognitive schemas then become activated and reinforced by stressful events, which, over time, can lead to major depression. Beck's model has been applied to other psychological conditions beyond depression, especially anxiety (Reilly, Sokol, and Butler 1999). Unfortunately, the role of the body in the downward trajectory to psychopathology is missing from these models, despite the fact that ***the body remembers*** (Rothschild 2000) and ***keeps the score*** (van der Kolk 2014), as described in the quote by Ida Rolf above. Thus, we have taken the license to correct this omission in our own version of the model (see Figure 10.1).

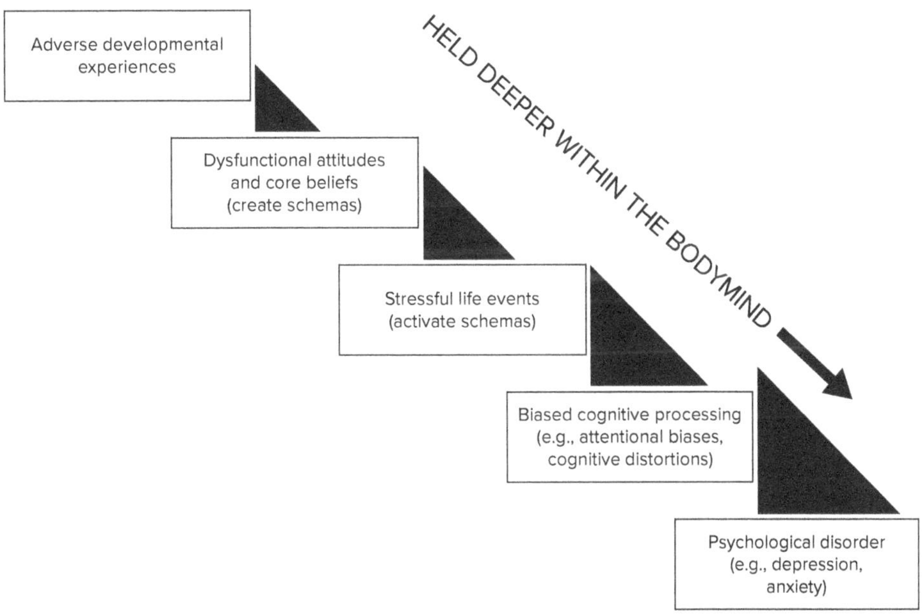

FIGURE 10.1: THE BODY AS THE MISSING LINK IN COGNITIVE MODELS OF PSYCHOPATHOLOGY

Adapted from Beck (2008) and inspired by Dychtwald (1986); Levine (1997); Ogden, Minton, and Pain (2006); Rolf (1963); Rothschild (2000); van der Kolk (2014)

THE POWER OF LANGUAGE IN THE CONTEXT OF YOGA

Through a carefully designed yoga practice delivered within the context of a "safe container," we can help highly stressed or anxious children safely release trauma- or stress-based muscular tensions and protective holding patterns. As the bodymind comes to feel safer and freer, spaces will open in the body in which new attitudes and beliefs can begin to take hold. Alan Fogel (2009) conceptualizes this beautifully from a neural standpoint in a portion of a figure in his own book *Body Sense* (formerly titled *The Psychophysiology of Self-Awareness*), which is depicted in Figure 10.2, with his permission. Of course, brain "structures" do not operate in isolation, but rather as a component of larger "systems" of neuronal activation, as discussed in Part 1; however, we will limit the discussion here to the two brain structures shown in Figure 10.2 for the sake of simplicity.

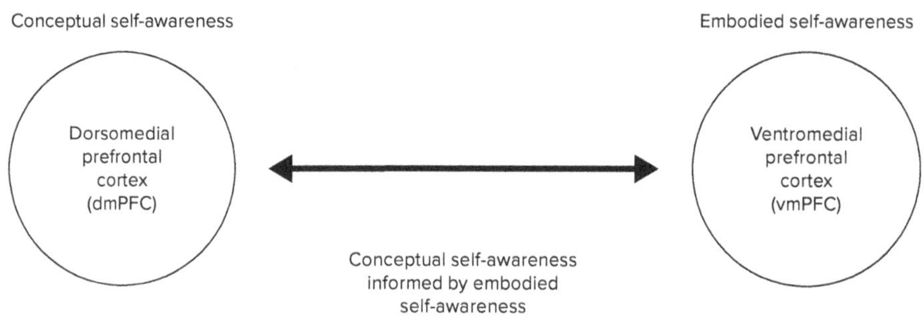

FIGURE 10.2: THE POWER OF LANGUAGE IN THE CONTEXT OF YOGA
Adapted with permission from Fogel (2009)

To summarize Fogel (2009): the dmPFC is continuously active during our waking hours and is involved in our ongoing stream of thought. Among other things, it is concerned with language-based self-judgments, that is, our ***conceptual self-awareness***: "Nobody likes me," "I am not worthy of love," "I could never do that." In contrast, the vmPFC is concerned with ***embodied self-awareness***, which Fogel (2009, p.311) describes as follows:

> the ability to pay attention to ourselves, to feel our sensations, emotions, and movements on-line, in the present moment, without the mediating influence of judgmental thoughts. It is composed of sensations like warm, tingly, soft, nauseated, dizzy; emotions such as happy, sad, threatened; and body senses like feeling the coordination (or lack of coordination) between the arms and legs while swimming, or sensing our shape and size (fat or thin), and sensing our location relative to other objects and other people.

Fogel explains that ***conceptual self-awareness is informed by embodied self-awareness*** (Figure 10.2). If we are exhibiting an anxious, tense posture or a slumped, depressed posture, the vmPFC (embodied self-awareness) will communicate that to the dmPFC (conceptual self-awareness), which then forms a thought such as "This is way too hard for me" or "Everyone is looking at me, my outfit must look weird." Conversely, if we free up the constrictions in the body and facilitate a more grounded, receptive, and confident body posture, the vmPFC will inform the dmPFC of the change, leading it to adjust its thoughts to align with this new felt experience, such as "I can do this!" or "Everyone is looking at me, they must like my new shirt!"

Interestingly, recent evidence has shown that in chronic anxiety, the amygdala becomes coupled with the dmPFC, a structure of the DMN (DeRidder *et al.* 2022), which helps to explain the negative thoughts and worry that can develop from this condition. Also, recall the **Neurocircuitry Model of PTSD**, which is based on evidence that the vmPFC plays a large role in keeping the amygdala in check. We tied all this together in Figure 10.3, which shows how the three brain structures—amygdala, dmPFC, vmPFC—relate to each other in the context of clearing out the mind of negative thoughts so new beliefs and attitudes can more easily take hold (i.e., Guideline #4).

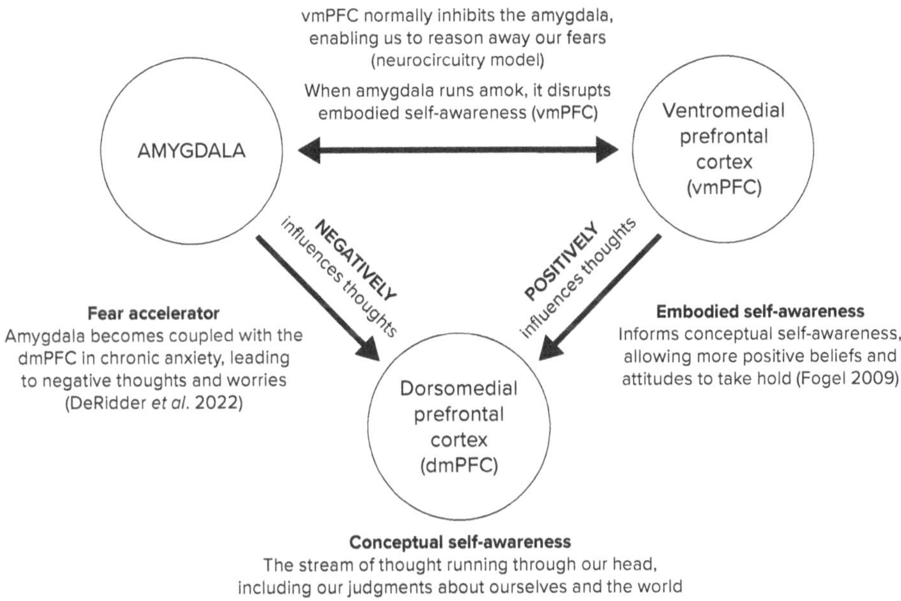

FIGURE 10.3: INFLUENCE OF SELECTED BRAIN STRUCTURES ON BELIEFS AND ATTITUDES

The concept of embodied self-awareness informing conceptual self-awareness is of very high relevance to children who have experienced maltreatment. Studies have shown that these children engage in more negative and more frequent ***self-referential processing*** (van Harmelen *et al.* 2014), which is "the cognitive process of relating information, often from the external world, to the self" (Nejad, Fossati, and Lemogne 2013, p.8). In other words, maltreated children tend to develop an exaggerated self-focus that is critical in nature (Beck 2008). This negative self-referential thinking is mediated by the dmPFC and increases vulnerability to the development of psychiatric disorders (van Harmelen *et al.* 2014).

Separate brain studies of trauma-exposed children show hyperresponsivity of the dmPFC in response to social exclusion (van Harmelen *et al.* 2014) as well as decreased thickness of the vmPFC (McLean 2016), suggesting the "double-whammy" of a negatively biased conceptual self-awareness combined with a weak sense of embodiment that hinders the ability to reframe negative thinking patterns in a more positive direction. These studies highlight the need to work with children at the body level to improve their self-esteem, and also forewarn that this process will likely be particularly difficult for traumatized children due to their weaker vmPFC. Intensive therapeutic work toward the goal of safe embodiment, such as through a carefully designed yoga program, should be the prerequisite goal for shaping attitudes and beliefs in a more positive direction.

Interestingly, Roy, Shohamy, and Wager (2012) found that the vmPFC is more associated with positive emotions while the dmPFC is more associated with negative emotions, further supporting the idea that embodied self-awareness is the better place to "be." And really, this is what Guideline #4 is speaking to: clearing out the negative ruminations, worries, and intrusive thoughts from the ***entire*** bodymind via the practices presented in Guidelines #1, #2, and #3, and then using the art of language to encourage more positive thoughts and attitudes to flourish after the body has been prepared to receive and accept them. This same exact process is embedded in the kosha model of the ancient yogis as a person progresses from feeling ***safe*** (in the annamaya kosha), ***calm*** (in the pranamaya kosha), ***clear*** (in the manomaya kosha), ***uplifted*** (our current topic, here in the vijnanamaya kosha), and ***empowered*** (in the anandamaya kosha).

CURRENT CHILD-FOCUSED APPROACHES TO SELF-REGULATION

To avoid negative outcomes from adverse developmental experiences, a concerted effort is needed to foster positive attitudes and beliefs in these children. But what happens when their bodyminds are not open to receiving them? Let's consider how this topic is currently being addressed in our society.

The emotional well-being of children and how it affects their development and overall success in life is a hot topic in education and community programming, especially after the emotional rollercoaster of the pandemic. But even prior to that, social-emotional learning (SEL) and social-emotional curriculums have become part of learning in schools throughout the USA as well as other parts of the world. Students are taught skills such as how to be a good friend, different types of feelings including their own and those of others, and strategies for managing emotions. Examples of SEL curriculums commonly in use include

Second Step (n.d.), The Incredible Years (n.d.), and MindUP (Maloney *et al.* 2016). The foundation for these SEL programs is that they are a top-down (mind affecting the body), cognitive intervention that essentially teaches strategies and skills for use in different scenarios.

Another initiative carried out by many schools, called Positive Behavioral Interventions and Supports (PBIS),[1] utilizes positive reinforcement systems at the school and classroom levels to support students in making decisions throughout the school day. PBIS is a three-tiered, evidence-based framework that has been found to improve student academic and social outcomes when carried out with fidelity. PBIS incorporates school-wide and classroom expectations for behavior and external reinforcement systems such as rewards combined with data collection and procedures for behavioral management. It taps into the drive to seek external reinforcement and a sense of reward. It provides educators with a framework to ensure that positive and expected behaviors are those that are rewarded rather than mistakenly reinforcing negative behaviors. PBIS utilizes statements such as "I can..." to frame behaviors as do-able by students, and provides specific examples of expected behaviors. For example, the core values of one elementary school include "I can be an active learner," "I can be kind," and "I can be a responsible citizen." Expected behaviors are then clearly defined for specific locations within the school setting.

Yet another layer of strategies being used within school settings are regulation strategies and skills, which are often interwoven within SEL lessons. Emotional regulation curriculums, such as the "Zones of Regulation" (Kuypers 2023) and "How Does Your Engine Run?"[2] (Williams and Shellenberger 1996), are commonly used by occupational therapists, social workers, guidance counselors, psychologists, and teachers. These programs rank feelings, emotions, and behavioral presentations into different "zones" or "speeds" depending on the program used. Feelings and emotions are divided into those that may disrupt or support a student's ability to learn and be a good friend. The "Zones of Regulation" pulls language from the "Social Thinking" curriculum (Winner 2022; Winner and Crooke 2009). In "Social Thinking," feelings, emotions, and actions that support learning and friendship are often categorized as "expected" while those that do not are categorized as "unexpected."

The "Zones of Regulation" and "How Does Your Engine Run?" programs combine bottom-up (body affects the mind) strategies, such as sensory supports, and top-down (mind affecting the body) strategies for managing difficult emotions and feelings. PBIS complements these programs by laying the foundation for what expected behaviors are within a school setting.

1 www.pbis.org
2 The Alert Program®: www.alertprogram.com

Our own program, SMYLE™, is primarily a bottom-up (body affecting the mind) approach to self-regulation with top-down components to draw the student's awareness to the effects of particular techniques on the bodymind. SMYLE™ is a framework approach that can be easily embedded within both SEL and regulation curriculums. The SMYLE™ postures and breathwork can be used as preparatory activities before engaging in SEL and regulation curriculums, and can also be taught as strategies to use for managing difficult emotions and feelings. For example, diaphragmatic breathing such as "belly breaths" is often taught as a strategy for calming the body when upset, sad, or angry. Additionally, using "I can" statements, similar to those used in PBIS, links the reinforcement of positive actions and feelings. For example, statements such as "I can be still by focusing on my breath" during meditation practices, "I can be strong by grounding my legs" during yoga posture work, or "I can try my best" during the introduction of new or difficult postures may positively influence a student's mindset.

Psychologists have found positive results in adult trauma survivors when they help them connect the muscle tension or impulse to move in certain ways back to the event that triggered that procedural memory. For example, a technique from Sensorimotor Psychotherapy involves moving back and forth between: (a) trauma-related postural holding patterns in order to explore and learn from them, and (b) practicing how it feels to assume a more relaxed posture. With children, we can't usually expect them to make a connection between a postural holding pattern or movement and a past event; however, we can help them increase their emotional self-awareness, sense of self-embodiment, and emotional flexibility by inviting them to act out "opposites" of emotions in their bodies. An example in yoga might be to alternate between Strong Warrior (e.g., a Warrior 2 with "boxing arms") and Peaceful Warrior (e.g., Warrior 1). Another is Happy Cat and Angry Cat (see Chapter 14). We recommend always following these exercises with tension-releasing yoga forms or movements and calming breathing techniques.

Having children simply imitate animals, trees, and other elements of nature provides the opportunity for them to imagine the qualities of these life forms and experience those qualities in themselves, such as the ability of a tree to go with the flow (sway) without crashing down to the ground. In fact, many of the classic yoga forms were inspired and named after animals, warriors, trees, the sun, moon, and many other things found in nature. These mindful exercises can provide a "playful break" to the students, away from the focus on high performance expectations, and give the students a time to turn "off" when most of the day they always have to be "on." Embodying these animals and nature elements helps bring their attention back to the present moment instead of hyperfocusing on what they need to do to be a "successful student" (e.g., pass the test, listen to the teacher, complete their work).

POSTURE-INSPIRED POSITIVE SUGGESTIONS AND AFFIRMATIONS

The **Sensory and Mindful-based Yoga for Learning Environments (SMYLE™)** program advocates the use of posture-inspired positive suggestions and self-chosen affirmations to enhance the healing power of yoga. These techniques help to counteract negative thought patterns that can result from traumatic experiences, and open the bodymind to more positive beliefs, attitudes, and emotions. They tend to be much more powerful when presented within the context of yoga, since, as we have just learned, how we feel in our bodies has a huge influence on how we conceptualize who we are.

Positive suggestions include statements made by the yoga instructor to draw the student's awareness to the emotional effects that tend to be naturally elicited by a particular yoga form or movement. For example, many yoga forms may naturally encourage a sense of emotional "grounding" due to the enhanced physical grounding they provide. These include forms where the energy moves downward into the earth/ground (e.g., Down Dog), the feet are encouraged to root solidly into the floor (e.g., Mountain and other standing forms), and/or there is heavy activation of the leg muscles and a lowering of the center of gravity, such as in the squatting postures (e.g., Chair, Shining Star, Warrior 1 and 2, Lunges).

Other forms tend to psychologically open the heart center, particularly those that expand the chest (e.g., Baby Cobra, Warrior 1 variations). Some forms have a self-nurturing quality, such as when hugging the knees into the chest, or a quality of feeling supported, such as lying in Child form. Yoga forms that provide a balance challenge (such as Tree or the extended leg hold in Tiger Flow) foster emotional steadiness, while forms that position the head off-kilter (such as Twisting Cat or Down Dog) change the view, quite literally inviting the person to open their mind to a different perspective on the world. The teacher or therapist can point these things out during the yoga session, as mindfulness to these qualities may accentuate these effects.

Not everyone will feel these effects, however, especially if they are experiencing mental distress. So we try to word the suggestions not by implying that they feel these qualities (which may backfire) but rather as an invitation to draw the quality into their bodymind. Alternatively, asking students to ***breathe in*** or ***inhale*** a quality is a harmless way to invite it into the bodymind, as you are not suggesting it is already present in the person but rather something outside of them being invited in, and better yet, being invited in on the power of the breath. Inviting the quality in on the thread of the breath may possibly enhance integration of sensation and emotion, since all three—sensation, emotion, and breath—are integrated in the insula.

Other language considerations

A major hallmark of any trauma-informed yoga program is the use of invitational language rather than commands in order to communicate respect and enable students to feel in control of their own bodies and experience, especially since traumatic events involve bad things happening outside of someone's control. A common way to present an invitational instruction is to preface statements with words such as "I invite you to...," "As you are ready...," "You might wish to try...," or "If you like..." Another way to help students retain control over their yoga experience is to offer them choices of yoga forms as you go along, or at least offer choices in how to vary or modify the forms.

SMYLE™ sessions are meant to be trauma-sensitive; therefore, instructors should allow children to choose whether to actively participate in the class or passively participate by observing all or portions of the class. We also strive to use invitational language and offer choices to students during SMYLE™ sessions. Having said that, for certain students, hearing language that is too "open" or "relaxed" can then lead to limited student participation. This can occur especially with neurodiverse students and/or those who are stuck in "hypoarousal" states. When using invitational language, they may see it as a choice to do the yoga form or remain still, and many would much rather just lie on the floor instead of doing something energetically taxing. Students in this population group may need that "extra positive" motivational push from their instructors to overcome their hypoarousal resistance and move into those "energetically taxing" forms that can ultimately lead to positive reactions in their bodymind (e.g., release of energetic blocks, connection to breath, breath, and body sensations) that could help them improve and/or rise above their current state.

A way to provide that "extra positive" motivational push is to praise a student's efforts, no matter how small they seem, if they are moving in the direction of the yoga form being taught. For example, the class may be doing Warrior I, but the instructor will praise a student who has been lying immobile for sitting up. Even though it is not the exact yoga form, that student showed an effort to participate in their own way at their own speed. To someone on the outside, sitting up takes minimal effort; however, for someone in a hypoarousal state, sitting up could take a concerted effort and deserves to be praised. Over time, the hope is that these small efforts continue to snowball and help encourage the person toward more engaged modes of participation.

We also found that offering choices between two specific teacher-selected actions (yoga forms) allows children to feel a sense of control while participating with the rest of the class in their own way. In addition, suggesting modifications (e.g., sitting or standing, arms bent or straight, holding on to a wall or not) helps to meet each child where they are at that given moment to allow them to feel a sense of success and achievement. All of these elements—using invitational language, offering choices, suggesting modifications, praising all efforts—can propel children to greater levels of participation and increase the overall benefits to their bodyminds.

If we are going to be offering ***invitational language*** and also encouraging ***enhanced body sensing***, we will be introducing more difficult language than some children currently know, such as "***invite*** your ***muscles*** to soften" (in Child form) vs. "***let*** your body ***rest***." The former is invitational while the latter is directive; however, the word "invite" is not typically learned until age 6 (Kelmon 2022). The former statement also mentions muscles, which are an unseen part of the body and, like the word "heart," typically takes longer for children to learn. However, we advocate teaching children the meaning of these words when developmentally appropriate (using visuals and/or videos), as the benefit of doing so far outweighs any benefit to dumbing down the language.

All of the above are important considerations when developing and implementing positive suggestions and affirmations into SMYLE™ yoga sessions. Since each student is different from one another, and each student presents differently day to day, instead of taking these considerations as rules to follow, we recommend teachers read the room, find their own voice, and provide appropriate instruction and support that best matches what their class needs.

Examples of positive suggestions

Examples of positive suggestions are listed in Table 10.1 according to the quality they are trying to elicit. Typically a few are presented per class. You will find many other examples in the yoga form descriptions in Part 3. You are also encouraged to create your own and/or modify the language according to the developmental level of your students. You will notice that some of the positive suggestions in Table 10.1 list one or more yoga forms after it, while others do not list a yoga form. We only listed forms when we had particular recommendations from our experiences.

Table 10.1: Sample positive suggestions by kosha

Category	Sample positive suggestions
Annamaya kosha (physical layer): I feel safe	
Grounding	• "Sense the strength of your legs firmly planting you on the ground." *[Shining Star]* • "Feel the strong, solid ground under your hands and feet." *[Table forms]* • "Can you feel the support of the solid earth/ground below you? How does it feel to you? It will always be there to support you wherever you go and whatever you do." *[Table forms]* • "How does it feel to be fully supported by the strength of the earth/ground?" *[Child]* • "Feel the ground through your feet and through the strength of your legs. The ground gives you power, because wherever you go, the solid ground will support you every step of the way." *[Warrior forms]*
Safe embodiment	• "Can you sense the whole length of your entire body? How does it feel to take up that much space?" *[Whole Body Stretch]* • "How does it feel to stretch your body from side to side?" *[Airplane; Half Moon Stretch]* • "How does your body feel to move and breathe like a dolphin?" *[Dolphin Flow]* • "Feel the changes in your body. No need to do anything with them, just notice and feel..." • "Listen to your body...what is it telling you? Does it want to lift higher to the sky or rest back down on the ground?" *[Baby Cobra]* • "What do you notice? How do you feel?" • "If your arms or legs start to feel tired, notice that with curiosity *['witness' mentality]*. But if you are too uncomfortable, come back down to Table or into Child to rest." *[Down Dog]* • "Learning to notice, as well as move away from, strong sensations in the body is an important skill so we don't get hurt. We call that 'befriending' our body, which means to 'be' a 'friend' to our body and treat it with kindness" *[stated while resting after an effortful yoga form]*.

<table>
<tr><th colspan="2">Pranamaya kosha (energy layer): I feel calm</th></tr>
<tr><td>Stress release/ANS balance</td><td><ul>
<li>"Just notice your breath moving in and out of your body."</li>
<li>"As you breathe out, let all your worries roll off your back." [Forward Folds]</li>
<li>"Picture yourself squeezing out all the tightness and worries in your body just like you squeeze out all the water from a wet towel." [Twists]</li>
<li>"Invite your muscles to soften with each breath in and out, feeling your body sink down into the strong support of the earth/ground." [Whole Body Stretch; Child]</li>
<li>"When we breathe into a stretch, we release tension that we are holding inside our bodies, which helps to relax us."</li>
<li>"Use this as a time of rest... There is no place to go...nothing to do... except be here now..."</li>
</ul></td></tr>
<tr><th colspan="2">Manomaya kosha (emotional/mental layer): I feel clear</th></tr>
<tr><td>Emotional awareness and regulation</td><td><ul>
<li>"Standing like a warrior brings out different feelings in different people...you may feel grounded...or strong...or balanced...confident. How does standing like a warrior make you feel?"</li>
<li>"Breathe in happy thoughts as you reach up to the sky...then breathe out your worries as you flow like a waterfall to the ground." [Waterfall]</li>
<li>"As thoughts come up, gently refocus your attention to breathing in...and out."</li>
<li>"What emotions do you feel in this yoga form? If you want to feel more .... [grounded; strong; uplifted; balanced; etc.], try .... [suggest a modification]."</li>
<li>"Feel your body sway side to side as it tries to balance itself. Welcome this swaying...as this is how we learn to find balance. Just like in life...you need to first feel off balance to learn what it means to be balanced." [Tree]</li>
</ul></td></tr>
<tr><td>Compassion for self and others</td><td><ul>
<li>"Hugging your body can be a way to show kindness towards yourself. Can you bring some caring and kindness into your yoga today?" [Knees to Chest; Hug Breath]</li>
<li>"If you like, you can draw your knee(s) into your chest and give yourself a hug, thanking your body for everything it has done for you today."[3]</li>
<li>"If you like, make a heart shape with your hands and place it on your heart. Imagine with each breath in, bringing kindness into your heart. With each breath out, share that kindness to the world around you." [Mountain]</li>
<li>"By opening your chest, you may feel more space around your heart. If it feels good to you, as you breathe in, imagine bringing kindness into that heart space, and as you breathe out, imagine you are spreading kindness in all directions." [Star; Shining Star]</li>
</ul></td></tr>
</table>

cont.

3 Thanks to Sadie Crane for this.

Vijnanamaya kosha (wisdom layer): I feel uplifted	
Mood uplifting	• "Uplifting the body helps to uplift the mind." *[Baby Cobra]* • "Sense the energy from the ground through your feet... With each breath, feel the energy rise up through your legs, to your heart, and out through your hands to the sky." *[Warrior 1]* • "Imagine your Star getting brighter and brighter with each breath in and out, shining light and joy/positive energy to the world." *[Star; Shining Star]* • "As you reach your arms to the sky, welcome good things to come your way... Open arms...open-mind..." *[Warrior 1]*
Flexible thinking	• "What happens when you don't try so hard and just go with the flow? Just let your body and breath guide your movements." *[Rabbit Hop; Dolphin Flow; Twisting Cat; Clamshell Twist; Windmill]* • "Notice how the room looks upside down and how that makes you feel. This helps us remember there is always another way to look at things!" *[Twisting Cat; Down Dog]* • "Changing our point of view helps us see things in a different light." *[Owl Twist]*
Anandamaya kosha (bliss layer): I feel empowered	
Strength and resilience	• "Is there a place in your body where you feel strong in . . . . [state yoga form you are doing]? Try sending your breath to that area. How does it make you feel? The more you notice your strength and power, the easier it is to move past challenges in our lives." • "Can you stand strong and steady like a mountain? You are deeply rooted in the ground. No wind or rain can move you. You are strong enough to handle anything that comes your way." *[Mountain]* • "You may notice strong muscle sensations in your arms and legs. When we learn to notice and accept stronger sensations in our muscles, these muscles get stronger. We strengthen our emotions in the same way, by learning to notice and accept difficult situations without getting worked up by those strong feelings." *[Down Dog; Dolphin Flow]*
Confidence	• "Breathe in balance, strength, and positive thoughts deep into your body. You've got this!" *[Tree; the extended leg/arm hold of Tiger Flow]* • "Use your deep, steady breath to help you feel strong and balanced in this yoga form." *[Tree; Warrior 1]* • "It is your mat, your practice. You make your own choices on what you can do today."
Navigating challenges	• "When you reach a tight spot, pause and breathe...soon it may open, letting you move even just a tiny bit more... Just like in life...when you get stuck, pause and breathe...try again...and you will break through those tough times. *[Leg Stretches; Twists]* • "Rooting your feet into the ground may help you to feel more stable as you change position from side to side... In the same way, when we ground ourselves, it can help us more easily handle changes and challenges in our lives." *[Airplane; Windmill]*

Other tips when developing positive suggestions

- Using TV or movie characters/animals/objects (e.g., Warriors, Superman, Elsa/Olaf, Airplane, Tree, Mountain) helps the child draw in the *psychological essence* of the yoga form, and can therefore serve as "positive suggestions" (see below).
- Although we like to use traditional labels for yoga forms, such as "Warrior 1," to prepare for participation in community yoga classes, we sometimes introduce alternative names for a yoga form to make it easier for students to connect with (e.g., animals, emotions). We also encourage drawing different qualities into yoga forms by stating things such as "Can you be a happy cat?" "...a peaceful warrior?" "...a strong, sturdy mountain?" "Can you allow your tree to blow in the wind?" or "Can you let your dolphin ride on the wave of your breath?"
- Suggesting "You might imagine you are hugging a friend" when hugging knees to chest can suggest that the child befriend *themselves*, thus drawing self-compassion into the child's heart without using that big, long word.
- ***Using motivating quotes from TV characters as mantras*** can be helpful:
  - In Rag Doll (Standing Forward Fold): "Shake away all your worries. Remember what Elsa from *Frozen* says, 'Let it go...let it go...'"[4]

Self-chosen positive affirmations are commonly used in cognitive therapy, and consist of repeating positive statements, either to yourself or out loud, to counteract negative thinking patterns and drive yourself toward more positive thoughts and experiences. Pairing affirmations with specific yoga forms that embody their essence brings the power of the thought not only into the mind but also into the body, where trauma (and often negativity) is stored. If you decide to incorporate affirmations into a therapeutic yoga practice, it is recommended that a student-directed approach be used.

Instructors should differentiate the level of support that their students will need in order to develop self-chosen affirmations, based on cognitive and language-processing abilities. For example, students who need more support could be given a range of two to four preselected choices by the teacher/therapist; students who need a little less support could be given sentence starters such as "When I focus on my breath, I feel [insert word]," while more independent students may only need basic auditory and/or visual directions to follow. One particularly effective method for using affirmations in the context of yoga is to ask the student (or group) what quality a particular yoga form suggests to

4 You can find a whole cache of child movie quotes and sayings at www.boredpanda.com/cartoon-character-life-quotes-aaa-state-play

them in their felt body sense, and invite them to create an affirmation that incorporates this quality. Several possible qualities could be suggested to help with the process, such as "Strong Tree" or "Growing Tree" or "Flexible Tree." Encourage the student(s) to focus on sensations during the yoga form so the affirmation will arise naturally from their "feeling" state rather than "thinking" mind (i.e., bottom-up approach). Inviting the person to create their own personalized affirmation based on a positive "felt experience" that a yoga form is already drawing into consciousness is quite possibly the safest and most effective way to introduce an affirmation.

In contrast, a recent study found that positive affirmations that are imposed on people may backfire for individuals who have low self-esteem, causing the person who recites them to feel worse (Wood, Perunovic, and Lee 2009). However, they only tested one affirmation, "I am a lovable person," which is a sweeping, emotionally loaded statement, and was imposed on the test subjects. To explain their findings, the study authors surmised that the subconscious mind might argue with the conscious mind, which is directing the affirmation, creating internal conflict. They also speculated that the "backfiring" would be more likely to happen with global statements such as "I am a generous person" versus moderately positive statements that are more specific, such as "I give generous gifts," to use their own example, or "When I focus on my breath, I feel calm."

Wood and her colleagues found that allowing or even encouraging the person to experience disconfirming thoughts along with the affirmative thoughts, rather than fighting the contradicting thoughts, diminished the potentially harmful effect of the positive affirmations for those with low self-esteem. This finding occurred when they suggested the participants focus on ways the statement was true for them and/or wasn't true for them, which may have communicated to them that such thoughts were to be expected. This draws to mind certain yoga nidra practices, such as iRest®, developed by Richard Miller, which work with the concept of opposite emotions and opposite beliefs as a therapeutic strategy with documented success (Stankovic 2011). However, with iRest, the student chooses the emotion or thought they wish to work with (giving them the locus of control), and the "opposites" are experienced using a body-sensing technique rather than an analytical approach, which helps to relink bodily sensation and emotion to support a healthy mind–body connection.

The SMYLE™ program is careful to avoid sweeping statements when presenting positive suggestions or affirmations. For instance, you'll notice the positive suggestion for "Knees to Chest" is presented as a gentle invitation to connect with a "feeling state" just for the present moment and within the context of a specific activity: "Hugging your body can be a way to show kindness towards yourself. Can you bring some caring and kindness into your yoga today?" This is a far cry from asking the person to globally state "I am filled with self-compassion" to which disconfirming examples may pop to mind. Similarly, emotionally loaded statements such as "I forgive myself," which have actually been used in some adult yoga classes working with individuals with PTSD, are not appropriate in any group yoga practice for adults or children. Only a qualified mental health counselor should handle such emotionally charged issues.

SMYLE™ teachers steer students away from global, emotionally charged statements that are opposite to their current felt sense. For example, if someone with depression suggests an affirmation such as "I feel happy and upbeat every moment of my life"—which is bound to backfire right out of the gate—teachers are trained to suggest one of the many excellent affirmations from the book *Mudras for Healing and Transformation*, by Joseph and Lilian LePage (2013), which are often *process-oriented* rather than statements of an achieved "end state." One affirmation they suggest for depression, for example, is "As I nourish my inner being, I experience greater enthusiasm and vitality"—which, translated for children, could be "As I take care of my bodymind, I feel more uplifted, energized, and present in my life," which includes an attainable plan to reach the stated goal. Worded in this manner, the affirmation is much more likely to resonate for someone at any stage of healing for depression, and be received as a very hopeful, self-empowering message by the bodymind.

TIPS FOR TEACHING STUDENTS HOW TO CREATE EFFECTIVE, POSITIVE AFFIRMATIONS

1. A single sentence in simple language tends to be most effective (and easy to remember!).
2. The affirmation should be stated in the first person.
3. Use positive language, e.g., "I open my heart to happiness" vs. "I am no longer depressed."
4. Structure the affirmation in the present tense, as the subconscious mind is operating in the present moment.
5. When creating affirmations for challenging or emotionally charged issues, consider choosing **process-oriented** affirmations, e.g., "Breathing brings calm," rather than global **end-state** affirmations, such as "I am calm," to avoid generating disconfirming messages from the mind.
6. When repeating the affirmation, encourage students to connect with the meaning of the affirmation with any sensations they are feeling in the yoga form (e.g., "As you say this affirmation, see if you notice any sensations in your body").

You might tell your students: If you find that your "gut" disagrees with the affirmation, allow yourself to feel the way you do without trying to judge it. You might try using the sensations that you feel in the yoga form as your "safe place" to help guide you toward a more positive viewpoint. However, if the affirmation is disturbing to you, release the affirmation and simply allow the bodily sensations of the form or movement to speak to you.

GUIDED MEDITATIONS

Guided meditations are another "top-down" approach that can be effectively used to promote healing from trauma and to promote self-regulation. They can be easily embedded into a yoga class, but need to be presented within the parameters of the instructor's training and in a manner that fosters the "safe container" for the student(s). An example of a particularly effective form of guided meditation is yoga nidra, otherwise known as "yogic sleep." Yoga nidra produces a deep state of relaxation in which the physical body is asleep while the mind is awake, yet at rest, and more readily capable of accessing the subconscious. The iRest® program in particular has been formally studied to document its effects on the symptoms of PTSD in adults and children, with positive results (Stankovic 2011). Certain components of that program are commonly integrated within yoga classes working with individuals who have PTSD. Here is a brief description of their program from their website:

> iRest enables children to gain experience in locating emotions in their body as tactile sensation, discovering various kinesthetic qualities of emotions (sharp, smooth, rough, prickly, hot, cold, etc.), describing (vocabulary development), talking about, and respectfully expressing their emotions, while discovering opposite emotions (positive and negative) and locating beliefs associated with their emotions. (https://www.irest.org/irest-kids, para. 3)

Instructors who use iRest have received formal training in these practices, particularly the Body-Sensing, Breath Awareness, Inner Resource, Heart-Felt Desire, and Intention for Practice scripts, which can be easily incorporated into a primarily asana-focused class.[5]

When working with traumatized populations, it is usually best to present meditations that help to keep the person grounded in their bodies (such as through focusing on sensation and breath) rather than take them on a "trip" somewhere, such as to a beach or some other specific type of place. Mental

5 Please refer to the iRest website (www.irest.org/irest-kids) if you would like more information about their program for children.

"trips" encourage dissociation from the body, when what we really want is to encourage reconnection with the body. An exception in our program is our use of ***yoga stories*** in which children are encouraged to "embody" particular animals, plants, or land features, such as a mountain. In these cases, it is very much a kinesthetic experience of sensing into their own body rather than a purely visual meditation in which the student is asked to summon up a scene in their head.

Zeidman and Maguire recently presented study findings to suggest that the anterior hippocampus constructs internal representations of environments based on incoming sensory information and/or prior experience, which is essential in order to "vividly re-experience past events, simulate future events and imagine fictitious scenarios, in addition to experiencing the environment we currently inhabit" (2016, p.3). As the anterior hippocampus is particularly implicated in PTSD, it is conceivable that the ability to construct internal scenes may be affected in some individuals with the condition, which should also be taken into consideration when choosing mindfulness-based strategies. That is, it is best to avoid visual meditation scripts unless they are within the person's ability to access. We do incorporate concrete visual elements (such as background scenes) into the audio-visual recordings of our yoga stories, but we do not ask the students to "imagine" these images, in order to keep their focus on the body-sensing aspects of the story.

One self-generated script that has been found to be helpful for many (though not all) traumatized individuals is the ***Inner Resource***, or "safe place," discussed in Chapter 7 (Guideline #1). In this case, the person has full control of the scene, and it is a "go-to" place in those instances where it may not feel safe in that moment to be in the body in the present setting—such as inside an MRI machine or in a dentist's chair. So it is actually a condoned form of short-term dissociation used for an adaptive purpose in a mindful way.

Gratitude meditations are another form of meditation that have been found to be helpful among traumatized populations. Vieselmeyer, Holguin, and Mezulis (2017) conducted a self-report questionnaire study of 359 students, faculty, and staff who were present during a campus shooting, and found that both "resilience and gratitude can be conceptualized as protective mechanisms, with resilience operating to prevent adverse outcomes while gratitude may promote positive outcomes following trauma" (2017, abstract). They concluded that interventions for trauma survivors should cultivate gratitude as a way to decrease post-traumatic stress and increase post-traumatic growth. Gratitude practices have also been helpful following earthquakes (Lies, Mellor, and Hong 2014) and substance misuse (Chen 2017), among other situations.

The following is a gratitude meditation for the body systems and senses. We modified the "Gratitude Meditation in Mountain," created by Sadie Crane (Stoller 2019), to be more child-friendly. You can easily adapt this script for students with different abilities by switching out/in different language and body parts. If students are able, you can also suggest they place their hands over their stomach, ribcage (lungs), and heart center as you focus on these areas.

A GRATITUDE MEDITATION

I invite you to join me in a gratitude meditation...please get into whatever position is most comfortable for you right now... Begin by noticing your body breathing in and out...say thank you to your breath for giving you life... Then notice the area around your stomach...say thank you to this area as it helps your body use the food you eat to give it energy to grow... Then, if you would like, place your hand over your heart and see if you can feel your heartbeat. This is the place where we feel joy, thankfulness, and love for ourselves and others... Say thank you to your heart for letting you feel these feelings... If you like, you may bring someone or something into that area that you are grateful for... Then move your attention to your head... Notice your mouth...say thank you to your mouth for letting you eat food and speak what you're thinking... Notice your ears...say thank you to your ears, as they let you hear what is going on around you... Notice your eyes...say thank you to your eyes, as they let us see the beauty of the world... Notice your nose...say thank you to your nose for letting you smell the flowers, trees, food you eat, and so many other wonderful smells... And finally, notice your mind...say thank you to your mind, which lets you think, make choices, and imagine new things... Now notice where in your body you feel thankful for all of these things... When you feel thankful for something, how does it make you feel?... As we end this practice, see if you can carry that feeling with you into the rest of your day...

MUDRAS

Mudras are amazing tools that can take a meditation practice to a whole new level. According to Joseph and Lilian LePage, authors of *Mudras for Healing and Transformation*, mudras are "gestures of the hands, face and body that promote physical health, psychological balance, and spiritual awakening" (2013, p.7). Who is not familiar with the image of a yogi sitting in Lotus meditating, using a hand mudra? Yet very few Americans understand what a mudra is for, or how it may impact the bodymind.

Mudras have been used in India for approximately 2000 years as well as in other countries and religious traditions, including Christianity (LePage and LePage 2013). Mudras can have a very powerful effect on a person's breath, energy level, state of alertness, level of relaxation, mood, and clarity of mind, and can facilitate higher states of meditation and well-being. It may seem surprising that the position of our hands can have such a powerful effect on the mind, especially since we move our hands all the time in our daily lives. However, we, and many of our students, have experienced many of these effects first hand, particularly with regard to how they affect our breath and the breath-related movement of energy in the body.

When we position our arms, hands, and fingers in certain ways, it produces subtle shifts in posture and muscle contractions around the ribcage and other parts of the body. For example, when the tips of the ***index fingers*** are gently pressed together in front of the solar plexus, with the remaining fingers relaxed inward toward the body, while sitting in an upright posture with shoulders relaxed and elbows held slightly away from the body, in ***Tarjani*** Mudra, the chest expands and the breath naturally rises upward into that greater expansiveness, promoting an uplifting quality. Yet when the ***little fingers*** are pressed together, with all other fingers relaxed inward, in ***Kanishtha*** Mudra, it produces a subtle postural and energetic shift that draws the breath and energy down toward the base of the body, extending the exhale and promoting a sense of grounding and calming (LePage and LePage 2013). Biomechanical postural shifts are not the only explanation or even the primary explanation for the effects of mudras, as there is a lot we still don't know about the energy systems of our bodies. The rich nerve endings of our palms and fingers, which are highly represented in the sensory homunculus of the brain, certainly play an important role (LePage and LePage 2013).

The best resource for mudras to promote self-regulation and trauma healing is *Mudras for Healing and Transformation* (2nd edn), by Joseph and Lilian LePage, published by Integrative Yoga Therapy in 2013.[6] What follows are some of the mudras from this book that have been especially beneficial for SMYLE® students and other students who have struggled with issues of anxiety and trauma (see Table 10.2). This is not an exhaustive list! Also, each of these mudras has different effects, which are explained in the book, so you will want to read the descriptions carefully and choose accordingly. Each person will experience the effects of some mudras more powerfully than others, and in slightly different ways, so allow your students to experience several of them to see which ones seem to work best for them.

Note: Students of all ages have varying language processing abilities, so we have provided examples for each mudra using simpler and more complex language.

6 https://iytyogatherapy.com/product/mudras-for-healing-and-transformation

Table 10.2: Recommended mudras for trauma and toxic stress

Kosha and goal state	Mudra(s)	Rationale	Affirmations	
			Simplified	More complex
Annamaya kosha (physical layer) I feel SAFE	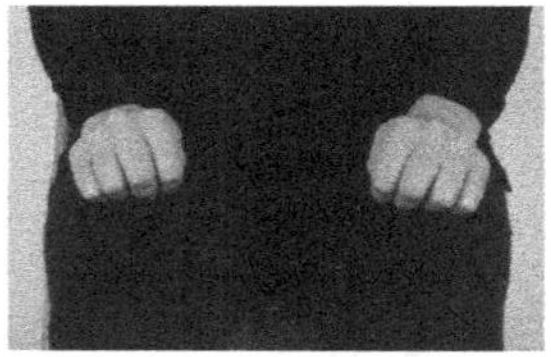 Adhi Mudra (for Stillness) Loosely hug your thumbs with your other fingers. Let your fists rest on your upper legs.	Promotes embodiment, grounding, and a sense of safety; directs breath to the pelvic floor.	"When I stop to notice how my body feels, I can better control what it does." "When I focus on my body and breath, I can slow down and be here now."	"As I become more safely present in my body, I develop greater trust in myself and the world around me." "By focusing on my breath and how my body feels, I can more easily come into stillness."
	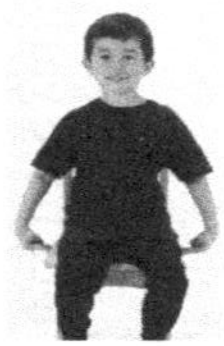 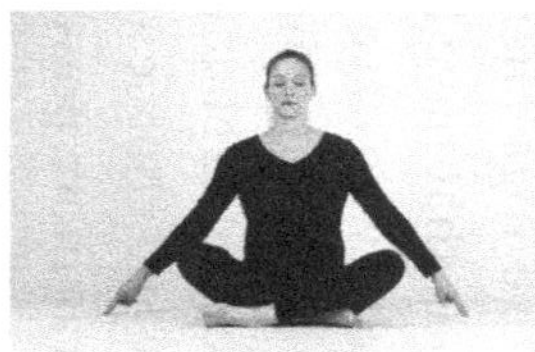 Bhu Mudra (for Grounding) Make a peace sign with your middle and pointer fingers, bend the other fingers under your thumb. Reach out to the side and touch the tips of your "peace sign" on to the ground.	Promotes embodiment, grounding, and a sense of safety; directs breath to the pelvic floor.	"When I touch the ground below me, it helps me feel more safe and more supported." "When I connect to the ground, I can feel more safe and secure."	"As I connect with the earth/ground, I develop a greater sense of safety and security." "As I become more present in my body and connected with the earth/ground, I nurture a deep sense of safety and security."

Pranayama kosha (energy layer) I feel CALM	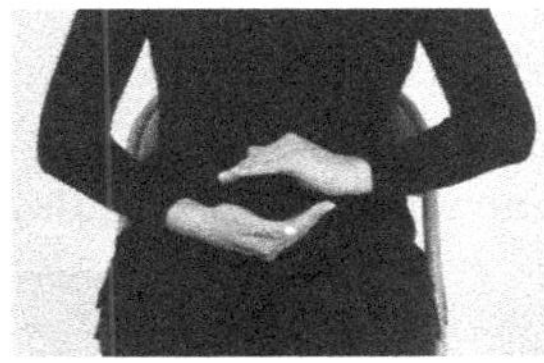 Pala Mudra (for Calming) Place one hand above your naval/belly button facing down and the other a little below, facing up. Relax your shoulders down.	Cultivates the diaphragmatic breath; relieves anxiety.	"Focusing on my breath can help bring calm." "When I slowly breathe in and out, it can help me feel more calm and peaceful."	"As I follow the rhythmic rise and fall of my breath, I experience a greater sense of calm and tranquility."
	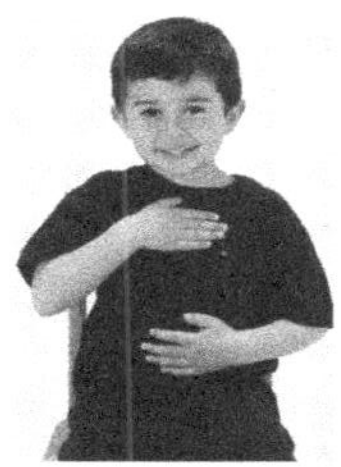 Pause Button (for Centering) Place one hand on the chest and one hand on the belly. Relax your shoulders down and feel your body move with your breath.	Cultivates the diaphragmatic breath; relieves anxiety; brings body and mind to the present moment.	"When I press my Pause Button, it helps my body and mind to slow down." "As I feel my breath moving in and out of my body, I can feel myself calm down."	"As I follow the rhythmic rise and fall of my breath, I experience a greater sense of calm and tranquility."

cont.

Kosha and goal state	Mudra(s)	Rationale	Affirmations	
			Simplified	More complex
Manomaya kosha (emotional/ mental layer) I feel CLEAR	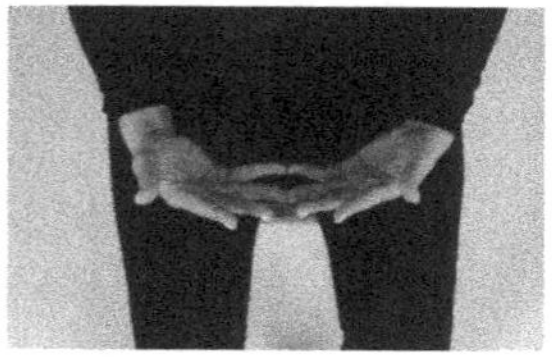 Dvimukham Mudra (for a Clear Mind) Open your hands, facing up. Touch your little fingers and ring fingers together. Place your hands just below your belly button, resting on your belly or your lap.	Draws the senses inward, instilling an inner silence; subtly digests accumulated thoughts and feelings.	"As I sense my body and breath, I quiet my mind. "By focusing on my body and breath, I clear my mind of worries and come back to what's happening now."	"By sensing my body and breath, I quiet my mind, still my body, and come into the present moment." "As my senses turn inward, my mind moves toward stillness and greater clarity."
	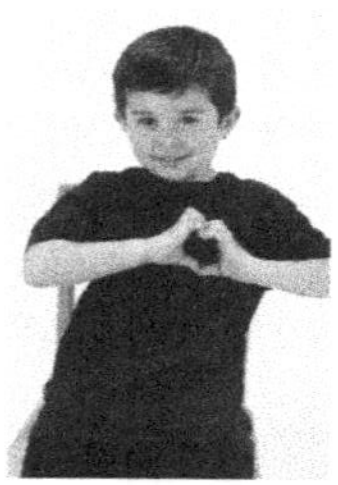 Purna Hridaya Mudra (for a Full, Uplifted Heart) Have your palms facing each other, curl the fingertips down and interlace them with each other. Stretch your thumbs down and touch them together to make a heart shape. Hold this mudra in front of your heart.	Opens and uplifts the heart; instills compassion and self-acceptance; calms the mind and creates space between thoughts.	"By listening to my thoughts and feelings, I learn to care about myself and others."	"By welcoming my thoughts and feelings, I develop compassion towards myself and others."

<table>
<tr><td>Vijnanamaya kosha
(wisdom layer)

I feel
UPLIFTED</td><td>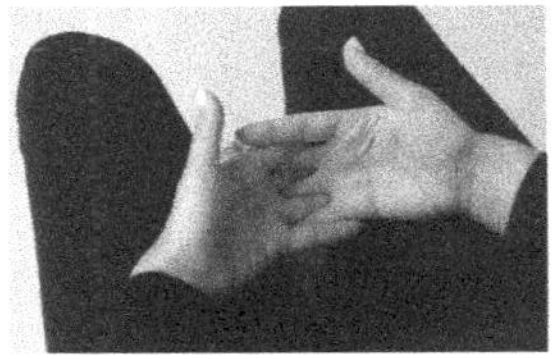
Ushas Mudra (for New Possibilities)
Interlace the fingers loosely and rest the hands on the lap, palms facing up. You can lightly touch your thumb tips together.</td><td>A subtle uplifting mudra was chosen so as not to trigger anxiety: promotes confidence, vitality, and enthusiasm; supports the treatment of depression.</td><td>"I breathe in happy thoughts and blow out my worries."
"As my mind becomes more calm and clear, it helps me see the good things in life."
"As I breathe out my worries and my problems, I make room in my body for peace and joy."</td><td>"As my mind becomes more calm and clear, I more easily recognize life's infinite possibilities."</td></tr>
<tr><td>Anandamaya kosha
(bliss layer/layer of integration)

I feel
EMPOWERED</td><td>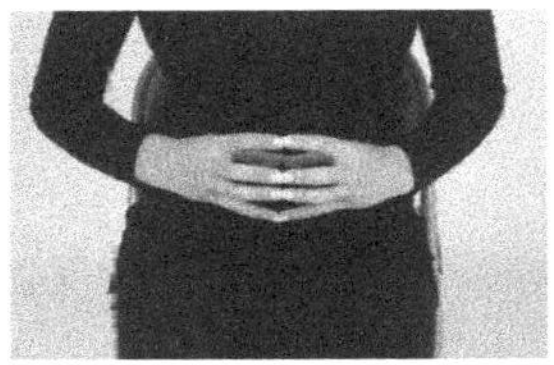
Hakini Mudra (for Focus and Empowerment)
Touch the tips of all the fingers and thumbs to the same fingers on the other hand, just above the belly button. Your hands should be open and rounded, as if holding a small ball.</td><td>Optimizes health and healing at all levels of our being; brings equilibrium to the left and right sides of the body.</td><td>"When I take care of my body and mind, I can better focus on what is important/I want to do in life."
"Having a calm, clear, and uplifted mind helps me move forward in life with more confidence."
"As my mind becomes more calm, clear, and uplifted, I develop the confidence to try new things and reach my goals."</td><td>"When I take care of my body and mind, it helps me feel safe... calm...clear...uplifted... empowered."
"As I move my body and mind into balance, I feel empowered to achieve my goals."
"As all facets of my being move into harmony, I step forward into life more confidently to manifest my life vision."</td></tr>
</table>

Note: The mudras, instructions, and rationale for all of the following, except for the "Pause Button," are taken from the second edition of *Mudras for Healing and Transformation* by Joseph and Lilian LePage (© 2014). The book also inspired the affirmations. Reprinted with permission in Stoller, L. *Sensory-Enhanced Yoga for Self-Regulation and Trauma Healing*. Pencaitland: Handspring Publishing Limited. Modified for SMYLE™ by Meg Hennessey Schofield and Lynn Stoller.

CHAPTER 11

Guideline #5: Self-Empowerment Is Born on the Wings of the Spirit Rising from the Mind–Body Connection

Oftentimes students finish a SMYLE™ session with a much calmer demeanor, clearer mind, and higher spirits. Whereas before the session they may have been acting impulsively or been hyperfocused on their phone/iPad, after class they are suddenly listening, engaging, and showing more interest in what is happening around them. Students have been noticed to act more compassionately toward themselves and others, demonstrate more emotional awareness and self-regulation, show increased flexibility, and exhibit an overall more positive mindset toward school. Suddenly, school, which could not hold their interest in the moments prior to the session, has purpose for them. And most importantly, they have more self-confidence in themselves that they can be successful in a school environment. They feel empowered!

This "yoga effect" can be particularly therapeutic for those who have been traumatized and have lost their sense of agency in the world. As explained by Ritu Sharma, former project coordinator for the JRI Trauma Center's yoga program,

> When people experience trauma, they may experience not only a sense of emotional dysregulation, but also a feeling of being physically immobilized. Body-oriented techniques such as yoga help them increase awareness of sensations in the body, stay more focused on the present moment and hopefully empower them to take effective actions. (Novotney 2009, para. 13)

David Emerson, current Director of the Trauma Center's Trauma Sensitive Yoga program, uses the term "empowerment" in the context of yoga to describe "giving our clients the space to have their own experiences without anything being imposed from the outside—namely, your experience or your ideas about what an experience within a yoga form might or should be" (Emerson 2015, p.21). So this brings us squarely back to Guideline #1, the importance of providing a sense of safety for our students by, among other considerations, giving them choices and thus a sense of control over their own process of yoga. When we place the locus of control on our students for their own experiences, they literally operate on their own "power" on the mat. For true healing transformation to occur, however, it is necessary to help the student take their "power" off the mat and into the world and their daily lives, and this is what Guideline #5 is all about.

Em-"power"-ment requires energy, and our energy levels are controlled by the ANS. When the ANS is seriously out of balance and affecting a person's emotional stability and/or ability to function, the person is said to be operating outside their window of tolerance. Ogden, Minton, and Pain (2006) speak of working at the ***edge*** of the window of tolerance rather than trying to keep the person smack in the middle of that window, totally within their safety zone and devoid of challenge. In order to "move forward in life," one must literally move forward, and that requires energy, which, in turn, requires activation of the SNS.

The thing is, to maintain health and well-being, the person must be able to rise to meet life's challenges ***and also*** calm the nervous system once a challenge has passed. As you recall from Chapter 2, this is a positive stress response. So we place our treatment emphasis at the lower koshas (i.e., the first two guidelines) at the beginning, and then carefully open Rothschild's (2009) soda bottle (see Chapter 7) just a little bit at a time, providing the "just right challenge" that will activate the nervous system in an adaptive way as well as allow it to return to a calm, resting state afterwards.

EMPOWERMENT THROUGH OCCUPATION

In one important way, we can think of Guideline #5 as somewhat of the reverse of Guideline #1. Whereas Guideline #1 is about creating a safe environment to influence the healing process, Guideline #5 is about the healing process empowering the person to influence their environment, that is, engage in the world. Working through the koshas over the course of time, a person develops clarity of mind and purpose as well as the intrinsic motivation to live in a manner consistent with their values, goals, and interests. Thus, empowerment is borne of well-"being" but is expressed in the "doing" of life, which involves living and working in the world around us, not spending the complete entirety of our lives sitting in meditation. Meditation is a means of discovering our true nature, our deepest heartfelt desires, and purpose, not the end goal.

But neither is ***achievement*** the end goal, for yoga teaches us the importance of non-attachment to the outcomes of our efforts. It is the *process* of unfolding our potential that is the important thing, which is how we conceive the term "self-actualizing" in Figure 11.2. A person's potential unfolds when their actions align with their most deeply held values and goals, and when they are fully engaged in that process in present moment awareness. In other words, "self-actualizing" is a process in which one's being and doing are in sync.

A Model of Well-Being and Well-Doing was conceptualized to better explain this relationship. The model will be explained shortly, but first, please take a moment to consider how you motivate the students you work with. ***Yoga teachers/therapists***—do you focus on perfect alignment of forms, or do you emphasize sensing the bodily experiences in the moment? ***Classroom teachers***—do you reinforce the idea that getting an "A" on a test is the reason for learning a particular lesson? Do you allow your students the time to get their creative juices flowing, or is there a time rush? ***Coaches***—do you push winning the game to be the most important thing? Do you help them connect the dots between being a "team player" on the basketball court to being a "team player" off the court? ***Therapists***—do you make efforts to show students how a strategy or exercise relates to their life, or can help them in the future?

Children across contexts are often encouraged to focus on results—the test grade, the sports "win," mastering advance yoga forms, completing a therapy session, etc. Rarely are children taught how to let go of their hyperfocus on results and just enjoy the process along the way. Worry over the end result builds, and before you know it, the child is caught up in their mind and dissociated from their body, which is likely sending signals of discomfort and stress. A focus on results raises ***fear***—fear of failure, fear of humiliation, fear of being judged, fear of rejection—which destroys concentration, any sense of creativity or flow of ideas, and any fluidity of movement.

In contrast, it is the students who let go of the results who are able to fully experience the joy of the learning process and sense the wind in their sails. If they are engaged in a motor-based activity, they become fully embodied by enjoying the pure sensation of the activity. If it is a mental task of real interest to them (with no imminent time deadline), the brain neurons start connecting in ways that further fuel their curiosity of the subject matter, or even create "brainstorms." Furthermore the information has a chance to be consolidated into long-term memory rather than quickly being forgotten due to rote memorization.

If the topic or activity does not have meaning for them, it is time to rethink how you display what is taught. Find out what makes the student "tick." Give them a wide field of choices with regard to what to research for their writing assignment or have them calculate some basic statistics on their favorite NFL football player. Also be observant to identify their interests in the first place. Do they frequently come to your sessions sporting a basketball jersey or a t-shirt from the local horse farm? What interests or hobbies do they share with you? A simple Google search is all that is needed to get ideas on how to incorporate students' interests into your activities so they can really be present and engaged.

So let's now discuss the ***Model of Well-Being and Well-Doing***. This is presented in three separate parts in order to fit in all of the information. The ***Model of Well-Being*** (Figure 11.1) is simply another way to depict the ***Transdisciplinary Model of Post-Traumatic Growth in Children*** (see Chapter 6). It is proposed that through the process depicted in the model, a person can come to feel ***safe*** (annamaya kosha), ***calm*** (pranamaya kosha), ***clear*** (manomaya kosha), ***uplifted*** (vijnanamaya kosha), and ***empowered*** (anandamaya kosha).

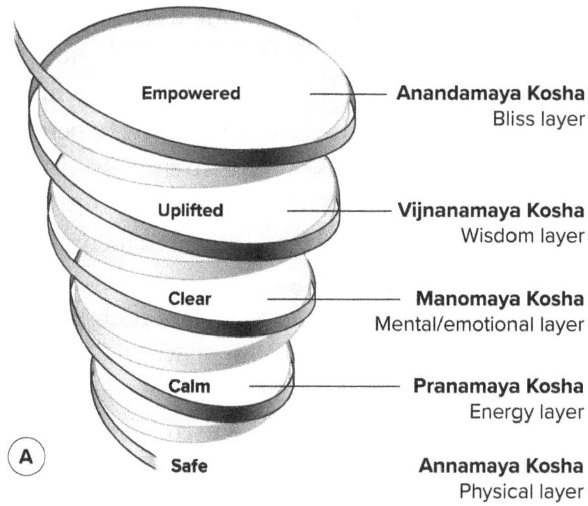

FIGURE 11.1: A MODEL OF WELL-BEING
Reproduced from Stoller (2019)

Figure 11.2 depicts a ***Model of Well-Doing***, which evolved from Lynn's Master's thesis for her occupational therapy degree (Stoller 1984). The process of "well-doing" goes as follows: when we learn to "do," we first acquire skills, and at that point we can only say we are ***capable*** of performing the skill. We then integrate these skills together into cohesive occupational behaviors as we engage with the world, at which point we can say we are showing ***competence***. We then need to learn to balance and adjust our activities and actions within the context of time and circumstances; hence, we become ***adaptable***. Over the course of time, as we engage in occupations, we connect more deeply with our felt purpose in life, which causes us to spend more time doing the things that matter most to us. This leads us to unfold our potential, and thus we become ***self-actualizing***.

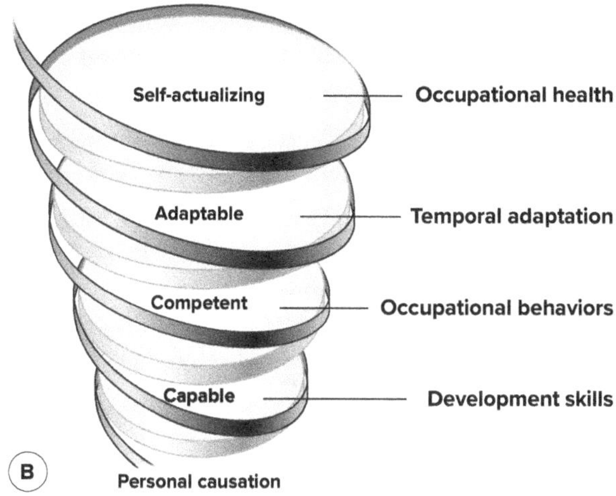

FIGURE 11.2: A MODEL OF WELL-DOING
Reproduced from Stoller (2019)

Each part of this process is continuous throughout the lifespan. As new skills are acquired, they reorganize existing occupational behaviors, and a new balance is achieved between them. For example, a child who has motor-planning difficulties may learn new skills that enable them to independently put on their clothing; that is, they become ***capable*** of performing the task. With practice, they are able to dress themselves with greater ease and efficiency and thus they become ***competent*** in dressing themselves. This shortens the amount of time spent getting dressed, allowing them more time to interact with their friends at the bus stop. Obtaining a balance that is more in step with their goals and interests allows the child to feel more in control of their life and to experience increased self-worth. Together they promote a sense of well-being.

The ***Model of Well-Being and Well-Doing*** (see Figure 11.3) depicts the relationship between, you guessed it, "being" and "doing." Each of the spirals closely influences the other; in fact, they are only separable for the purposes of explaining their togetherness. If we are not feeling safe, if we are anxious, if our head is not clear, if we have negative attitudes or beliefs floating around in our head, then we are not going to be present and fully engaged in the activities we need and want to do. Conversely, if we are particularly challenged in learning a skill, or putting skills together into occupational behaviors, or balancing or adjusting our activities to meet both our own needs and the demands of the environment, then our head will likely be filled with negative self-talk—it most certainly won't be clear; we will likely feel anxiety; and depending on the circumstances, we may even feel unsafe.

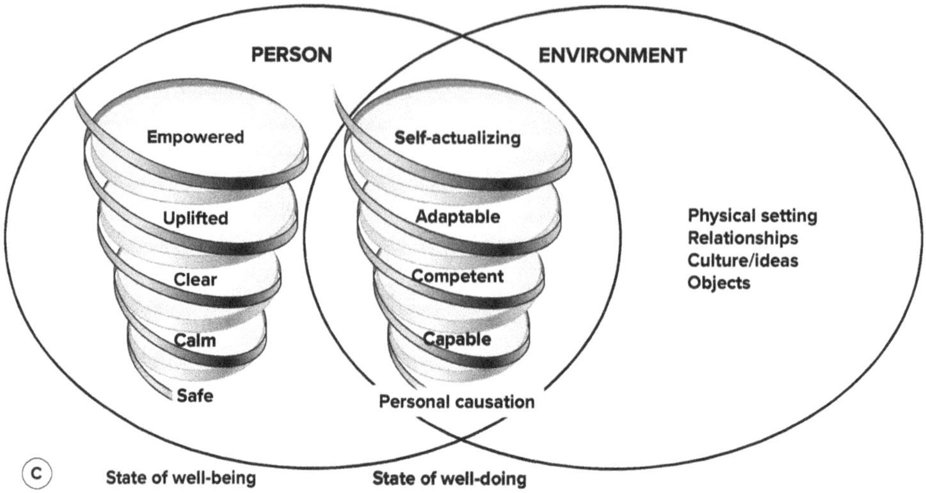

FIGURE 11.3: A MODEL OF WELL-BEING AND WELL-DOING
Reproduced from Stoller (2019)

A FEW SUGGESTIONS FOR PROMOTING SELF-EMPOWERMENT

Here are a few ideas to further promote a sense of empowerment on and off the mat:

1. We can help our students identify the state of their own valued goals and interests by using a structured approach, such as the ***Wellness Survey for Post-Traumatic Growth in Children***, to be discussed in the next section. This kosha-based survey can be administered in a 1:1 setting and also lends itself well to themed group lessons that address each layer of someone's being. In the latter context, students have opportunities to learn that other students share some of their own insecurities or concerns and can receive peer support as they problem-solve together how to address them.
2. During a yoga session, we can suggest specific ways to incorporate yoga tools into everyday life, such as chair yoga, breathwork, mudras, and/or meditations, to help the students learn how to self-regulate off the mat as well as on the mat. This is the yogic version of helping a person develop a "sensory diet," a term coined by occupational therapists. The more we can stay self-regulated, the more empowered we will be to set goals and meet them.
3. As emphasized earlier, it is crucial that we give our students choices, and thus a sense of control over their own experience of yoga, to allow them to operate on their own "power" on the mat.

4. Most importantly, we can listen to our students and ourselves. Joseph LePage, founder of Integrative Yoga Therapy®, points out that "listening already contains within it the answer to our questions" (2015, p.1.27). He adds: "As we learn to listen to ourselves, we also learn to listen to others. As we listen, we also teach the art of listening. Teaching the art of listening is synonymous with teaching yoga, as both help us open the door to who we really are."

In any group setting, it is important to not let any child get "lost in the crowd." Supervising adults should take frequent opportunities to personally connect with each child so they know that they are valued members of the group. It is worth considering when the best time is for you to do that. In a school setting, some teachers schedule this at the end of the day; however, at that time both the teacher and student may be tired, and the teacher may find themselves drifting off instead of truly listening to their student. Conversely, first thing in the morning may be too hectic, and the teacher may be distracted. Try to schedule time to talk to the student when you can be truly emotionally available to them versus thinking about your to-do list or how you will respond to what they are saying.

Also, remember to use good eye contact instead of scanning the room to check on everyone else (if you have to do that, at least don't be obvious about it!). Do not interrupt the student, and be comfortable with silence to allow the student time to formulate their thoughts. Finally, remember that the most powerful way to inhibit the "fight–flight" response is to activate the social engagement system (ventral vagal branch of the PNS). This can be done by smiling, which will invite a smile in return, and by using a melodic rather than a monotone or gruff voice when you do respond to what is being shared with you.

THE WELLNESS SURVEY FOR CHILDREN

We recommend using the ***Wellness Survey for Children*** for organizing the way you work with individual children (or older individuals who have intellectual impairments or language barriers) using the SMYLE™ approach. This is particularly helpful when working with children who have experienced trauma or who are experiencing toxic stress or high anxiety (see Table 11.1). This survey is the child version of the ***Wellness Survey for Post-Traumatic Growth*** that was published in *Sensory-Enhanced Yoga for Self-Regulation and Trauma Healing* (Stoller 2019). Adolescents who have good cognition and language processing may be best served using the original survey, while younger students and many students with special needs will benefit from the easy "thumbs up/down" choice-making format and simplified language of the child-focused version.

Many of the items on the original form were inspired by or found on materials developed by Joseph LePage and were chosen (with Joseph's permission) based on their relevance for trauma healing. They were also reorganized into the kosha model format to align with the ***Transdisciplinary Model for Post-Traumatic Growth in Children***. The scoring is not standardized and is not meaningful beyond helping to grossly identify the aspects of an individual's being (physical, energetic, emotional/mental, wisdom, or bliss) that appear to be most in need of support. The overall pattern might suggest where along the healing process a child falls, as outlined by the model.

The final section was made more "bliss-sensitive" by renaming it "Integration/resources" (not the "Bliss Body"), and by focusing on resources that may facilitate the healing process. These can be further fleshed out through follow-up questioning. For example, the teacher might ask "What are some things you like to learn about?" as a follow-up question to the item "I enjoy learning new things." You can then ask how often the student engages in the activity. Table 11.2 provides examples of appropriate follow-up questions for each item listed in the "Integration/resources" section. Follow-up questions are also appropriate for some of the items in other sections as well, but just try not to overwhelm the student with questions. Pick a few that seem most important at the moment, based on the responses on the form. You can always ask other questions on a different day.

When presenting the ***Wellness Survey for Children*** to your student(s), ask them to answer the questions the best they can by circling the thumb that matches their answer. Remind them to ask a question if they have any. When scoring, please give the following points: Yes = 2, Sometimes = 1, and No = 0. There are a few questions that are asked in the negative and have alternative scoring displayed next to the answer choices. Again, the numerical scores provide general information but are not standardized. Permission is granted to use this tool with clients only as formatted here with the proper copyright notice and reference. For all other permissions, contact lynnstoller.ot@gmail.com. We would like to collect some data on this form, so if you would be interested in contributing towards that effort (by administering the forms with a cover sheet and sending the copies to the Sensory-Enhanced Yoga® Institute), please contact us.

Table 11.1: Wellness Survey for Children

Name: Date:

How true do these statements seem to you?		
Yes = Most of the time	Sometimes	No = Not really or Never

Physical body			
My body feels comfortable with no pain or muscle aches.	Yes	Sometimes	No
I like how my body feels when I move.	Yes	Sometimes	No
I like how I feel when I sit up straight.	Yes	Sometimes	No
I feel safe in my body.	Yes	Sometimes	No
I try to be careful around strangers.	Yes	Sometimes	No
I listen to what my body needs (I eat when I am hungry, I drink when I am thirsty, I sleep when I am tired).	Yes	Sometimes	No
I feel safe and supported by people in my life.	Yes	Sometimes	No
High places bother me, like being on a high balcony, going up an escalator, or looking out of a high window.	Yes (0)	Sometimes (1)	No (2)
I like going to new places.	Yes	Sometimes	No
I feel comfortable standing next to other people at school.	Yes	Sometimes	No
Total score			

How true do these statements feel to you?			
Energy body			
I can feel my breath going in and out of my body.	Yes	Sometimes	No
Breathing is easy and comfortable for me.	Yes	Sometimes	No
I usually feel calm and relaxed.	Yes	Sometimes	No
I smile when I see people.	Yes	Sometimes	No
I get scared easily.	Yes (0)	Sometimes (1)	No (2)
I get stomach aches a lot.	Yes (0)	Sometimes (1)	No (2)
I sleep well at night and usually do not get tired at school.	Yes	Sometimes	No
I stay calm when things get hard.	Yes	Sometimes	No
I am okay if my plans change.	Yes	Sometimes	No
I work hard and take breaks when I need them.	Yes	Sometimes	No
Total score			

How true do these statements feel to you?			
Emotional/mental body			
I listen to my feelings and thoughts.	Yes	Sometimes	No
I say what I think and feel to adults that I trust.	Yes	Sometimes	No
I like exploring things with my senses (e.g., seeing, hearing, touching, tasting, smelling) such as listening to music, enjoying nature, trying new foods.	Yes	Sometimes	No
I am usually aware of what is happening around me and not stuck in my thoughts.	Yes	Sometimes	No
I am kind to myself.	Yes	Sometimes	No
I can focus on my work.	Yes	Sometimes	No
I worry about things a lot.	Yes (0)	Sometimes (1)	No (2)
I am kind and friendly to others.	Yes	Sometimes	No
I stay cool and calm when faced with a problem.	Yes	Sometimes	No
I am usually in a good mood.	Yes	Sometimes	No
Total score			

How true do these statements feel to you?			
Wisdom body			
This layer requires analytical thinking which normally does not emerge until at least age 12 and some adults never develop to this psychosocial level. We are including this layer for research purposes to gain more information on the wisdom layer of children and young adults.			
I know what I am thinking and feeling.	Yes	Sometimes	No
I make good decisions.	Yes	Sometimes	No
I make choices based on what I think is good for me.	Yes	Sometimes	No
When I have a problem, I can usually think of more than one way to solve it.	Yes	Sometimes	No
I hang out with people who make me feel good, not bad.	Yes	Sometimes	No
It is okay to make mistakes. That is how I learn.	Yes	Sometimes	No
I think good things will happen in my life.	Yes	Sometimes	No
I understand other people can think differently than me.	Yes	Sometimes	No
I feel good about myself.	Yes	Sometimes	No
I am open to trying new things.	Yes	Sometimes	No
Total score			

How true do these statements feel to you?			
Integration/resources			
I have hobbies or interests that make me happy.	Yes	Sometimes	No
I can forget my worries when I am doing an activity I enjoy.	Yes	Sometimes	No
I like to get out into nature and look at the sky, trees, flowers, or animals.	Yes	Sometimes	No
I have friends and family who are important to me and help me during difficult times.	Yes	Sometimes	No
I laugh easily.	Yes	Sometimes	No
If I am feeling upset, I can think of a good memory that helps me feel better, safe, or even happy.	Yes	Sometimes	No
I like to participate in school activities.	Yes	Sometimes	No
My schoolwork is important to me.	Yes	Sometimes	No
I feel lucky to be alive even when life is hard.	Yes	Sometimes	No
I enjoy learning new things.	Yes	Sometimes	No
I like to make plans with my friends.	Yes	Sometimes	No
I find enough time to do things I enjoy.	Yes	Sometimes	No
Total score			

Adapted from Stoller (2019). Many items were inspired or originated from materials developed by Joseph LePage and are used with his permission.

Table 11.2: Wellness Survey for Children—Follow-up questions

Items from Integration/ resources	Suggested follow-up questions	Frequency of engagement in activity (if applicable)
I have hobbies or interests that make me happy.	What are some of your hobbies and interests? When is the last time you ....?	
I can forget my worries when I am doing an activity I enjoy.	Can you name an activity that helps you to forget your worries? Any others?	
I like to get out into nature and look at the sky, trees, flowers, or animals.	Is there a favorite place you like to go to enjoy nature? Can you describe that place for me?	
I have friends and family who are important to me and help me during difficult times.	Who are the people you can rely on to help you during hard times? Who are the most important people in your life? (It's possible that the answers to these two questions may differ.)	
I laugh easily.	What types of things make you laugh? (e.g., certain TV shows, jokes) Are there certain people who make you laugh?	
If I am feeling upset, I can think of a good memory that helps me feel better, safe, or even happy.	Would you like to share that memory with me or keep that private?	
I like to participate in school activities.	What do you like to do at school?	
My schoolwork is important to me.	What are your favorite subjects?	
I feel lucky to be alive even when life is hard.	Is life hard for you now? How is it hard? Can you tell me more about how you are feeling?	
I enjoy learning new things.	What are some things you like to learn about?	
I like to make plans with my friends.	Who are some people you like to hang out with? When have you last gotten together with X?	
I find enough time to do the things I enjoy.	What would you like to do more often?	

References for Part 2

CHAPTER 6

Bremner, J.D. (1999) "Acute and chronic responses to psychological trauma: Where do we go from here?" *American Journal of Psychiatry 156*, 3, 349–351. doi: 10.1176/ajp.156.3.349.

Chaplo, S.D., Kerig, P.K., and Wainryb, C.J. (2019) "Development and validation of the moral injury scales for youth." *Journal of Traumatic Stress 32*, 3, 448–458. doi: 10.1002/jts.22408.

Fogel, A. (2009) *Body Sense*. New York: W.W. Norton & Company.

Kielhofner G. and Burke J.P. (1980) "A model of human occupation, part 1. Conceptual framework and content." *American Journal Occupational Therapy 34*, 9, 572–581. doi: 10.5014/ajot.34.9.572.

Kielhofner, G. (2008). *Model of human occupation:* theory and application. 4th Edition. Baltimore, MD: Lippincott Williams & Wilkins.

Lanius, R.A., Frewen, P.A., Tursich, M., Jetly, R., and McKinnon, M.C. (2015) "Restoring large-scale brain networks in PTSD: A proposal for neuroscientifically-informed treatment interventions." *European Journal of Psychotraumatology 6*, 27313. doi: 10.3402/ejpt.v6.27313.

Lanius, R.A., Vermetten, E., Loewenstein, R.J., Brand, B., *et al.* (2010) "Emotion modulation in PTSD: Clinical and neurobiological evidence for a dissociative subtype." *American Journal of Psychiatry 167*, 6, 640–647. doi: 10.1176/appi.ajp.2009.09081168.

Maguen, S. and Litz, B.T. (2012) "Moral injury in veterans of war." *PTSD Research Quarterly 23*, 1. https://vva1071.org/uploads/3/4/4/6/34460116/moral_injury_in_veterans_of_war.pdf

Maslow, A. (1962) *Toward a Psychology of Being*. Princeton, NJ: D. Van Nostrand. http://dx.doi.org/10.1037/10793-000

Porges, S.W. and Furman, S.A. (2011) "The early development of the autonomic nervous system provides a neural platform for social behavior: A polyvagal perspective." *Infant and Child Development 20*, 1, 106–118. doi: 10.1002/icd.688.

Rea, S. (2007) "You are here." *Yoga Journal*, August 28. www.yogajournal.com/yoga-101/philosophy/you-are-here

Riggins, T., Blankenship, S.L., Mulligan, E., Rice, K., and Redcay, E. (2015) "Developmental differences in relations between episodic memory and hippocampal subregion volume during early childhood." *Child Development 86*, 6, 1710–1718. https://doi.org/10.1111/cdev.12445

Sathiyaseelan, A. and Balasundaram, S. (2016) "A comparison of Maslow's theory of hierarchy of needs with the Pancha Kosha theory of Upanishads." *Journal of Social Sciences 15*, 1. doi: 10.12724/ajss.36.4.

Sharvananda, S. (1921) *Isha-Upanishad* (2nd edn). The Ramakrishna Math.

Siegel, D.J. (1999) *The Developing Mind: Toward a Neurobiology of Interpersonal Experience*. New York: Guilford Press.

Stoller, L. (2019) *Sensory-Enhanced Yoga for Self-Regulation and Trauma Healing*. Pencaitland: Handspring Publishing Limited.

van der Kolk, B.A. (2008) "Affect Regulation." Lecture, Pre-Conference Institute of the 19th Annual International Trauma Conference, June 25, Boston, MA.

Vermetten, E. and Bremner, J.D. (2003) "Olfaction as a traumatic reminder in posttraumatic stress disorder: Case reports and review." *The Journal of Clinical Psychiatry 64*, 2, 202–207. doi: 10.4088/JCP.v64n0214.

Wilbarger, P. and Wilbarger, J. (1990) "Sensory defensiveness and related social/emotional and neurological problems." Conference, October 13–14, Hartford, CT.

Wilbarger, P. and Wilbarger, J. (1997) *Sensory Defensiveness and Related Social/Emotional and Neurological Problems* [Self-published].

CHAPTER 7

Brown, D.K., Barton, J.L., and Gladwell, V.F. (2013) "Viewing nature scenes positively affects recovery of autonomic function following acute-mental stress." *Environmental Science & Technology 47*, 11, 5562–5569. https://doi.org/10.1021/es305019p

Burks, S.L. (1994) *Managing Your Migraine*. Totowa, NJ: Humana Press.

Burstow, B. (2003) "Toward a radical understanding of trauma and trauma work." *Violence Against Women 9*, 11, 1293–1317. doi: 10.1177/1077801203255555.

Center for Suicide Prevention (2017) "Trauma and suicide in children." March 20. www.suicideinfo.ca/local_resource/trauma-suicide-children

Emerson, D. and Hopper, E. (2011) *Overcoming Trauma Through Yoga: Reclaiming Your Body.* Berkeley, CA: North Atlantic Books.

Erikson, E. (1950, 1963) *Childhood and Society.* New York: W.W. Norton & Company.

Herman, J.L. (1997) *Trauma and Recovery: The Aftermath of Violence—From Domestic Abuse to Political Terror.* New York: Basic Books.

Herman, J.L. (1998) "Recovery from psychological trauma." *Psychiatry and Clinical Neurosciences 52*, S1, S98–S103. https://doi.org/10.1046/j.1440-1819.1998.0520s5S145.x

Hirsch, C.R. and Holmes, E.A. (2007) "Mental imagery in anxiety disorders." *Psychiatry 6*, 4, 161–165. www.sciencedirect.com/science/article/abs/pii/S1476179307000195

Khorshid, R.F., Almadani, S.H., Al Shehri, A.M., Abduljawad, L.M., and Alsaleh, A.M. (2021) "The effect of fluorescent light on anxiety patients." *Cureus 13*, 2, e13436. https://doi.org/10.7759/cureus.13436

Lanius, R.A., Frewen, P.A., Tursich, M., Jetly, R., and McKinnon, M.C. (2015) "Restoring large-scale brain networks in PTSD and related disorders: A proposal for neuroscientifically-informed treatment interventions." *European Journal of Psychotraumatology 6*, 1, 27313. https://doi.org/10.3402/ejpt.v6.27313

Lieberman, M.D., Eisenberger, N.I., Crockett, M.J., Tom, S.M., Pfeifer, J.H., and Way, B.M. (2007) "Putting feelings into words: Affect labeling disrupts amygdala activity in response to affective stimuli." *Psychological Science 18*, 5, 421–428. doi: 10.1111/j.1467-9280.2007.01916.x.

Mayo Clinic (2022) "Suicide: What to do when someone is suicidal." July. www.mayoclinic.org/diseases-conditions/suicide/in-depth/suicide/art-20044707

Mouly, A.M. and Sullivan, R. (2010) "Memory and Plasticity in the Olfactory System: From Infancy to Adulthood." In A. Menini (ed.) *The Neurobiology of Olfaction* (Chapter 15). Boca Raton, FL: CRC Press/Taylor & Francis. www.ncbi.nlm.nih.gov/books/NBK55967

Nummenmaa, L., Hari, R., Hietanen, J.K., and Glerean, E. (2018) "Maps of subjective feelings." *Proceedings of the National Academy of Sciences 115*, 37, 9198–9203. doi: 10.1073/pnas.1807390115.

Ogden, P., Minton, K., and Pain, C. (2006) *Trauma and the Body: A Sensorimotor Approach to Psychotherapy.* New York: W.W. Norton & Company.

Porges, S.W. (2011) *The Polyvagal Theory: Neurophysiological Foundations of Emotions, Attachment, Communication, and Self-Regulation.* New York: W.W. Norton & Company.

Rothschild, B. (2000) *The Body Remembers: The Psychophysiology of Trauma and Trauma Treatment.* New York: W.W. Norton & Company.

Rothschild, B. (2009) "Safe trauma recovery: 'Putting on the brakes'" [Video]. www.youtube.com/watch?v=LhuzpUlaX_k [Also available at www.somatictraumatherapy.com/videos]

Schiraldi, G. (2000) *The Post-Traumatic Stress Disorder Sourcebook: A Guide to Healing, Recovery, and Growth.* New York: McGraw-Hill.

Schneider, M. (2002) *Do School Facilities Affect Academic Outcomes?* (ED470979). ERIC. https://files.eric.ed.gov/fulltext/ED470979.pdf

Schwartz, A. (2017) "Embodiment in somatic psychology" [Web log post]. Center for Resilience Informed Therapy, March 25. https://drarielleschwartz.com/embodiment-in-somatic-psychology-dr-arielle-schwartz/#.YPbbRxNKgdU

Shabha, G. and Gaines, K. (2013) "Evidence-based classroom design for individuals with autism." *The International Journal of the Constructed Environment 2*, 4, 1–18. doi: 10.18848/2154-8587/CGP/v02i04/37359.

Singh, P. (2013) "Indoor environmental quality & student health and performance: A conceptual review." *International Journal of Physical and Social Sciences 3*, 7, 96–107.

Smolders, K.C.H.J. and de Kort, Y.A.W. (2014) "Bright light effects on mental fatigue." *Journal of Environmental Psychology 39*, 77–91.

Telles, S., Bhardwaj, A.K., Kumar, S., Kumar, N., and Balkrishna, A. (2012) "Performance in a substitution task and state anxiety following yoga in army recruits." *Psychological Reports 110*, 3, 963–976. https://doi.org/10.2466/13.02.16.20.PR0.110.3.963-976

Townsend, C. and Rheingold, A.A. (2013) *Estimating a Child Sexual Abuse Prevalence Rate for Practitioners: A Review of Child Abuse Prevalence Studies.* Charleston, SC: Darkness to Light. www.d2l.org/wp-content/uploads/2017/02/PREVALENCE-RATE-WHITE-PAPER-D2L.pdf

van der Kolk, B.A. (2008) "Affect regulation." Lecture, Pre-Conference Institute of the 19th Annual International Trauma Conference, June 25. Boston, MA.

van der Kolk, B.A. (2014) *The Body Keeps the Score: Brain, Mind, and Body in the Healing of Trauma.* New York: Viking (Penguin Random House).

van der Kolk, B.A., McFarlane, A.C., and Weisaeth, L. (eds) (1996) *Traumatic Stress: The Effects of Overwhelming Experience on Mind, Body, and Society.* New York: Guilford Press.

Vermetten, E. and Bremner, J.D. (2003) "Olfaction as a traumatic reminder in posttraumatic stress disorder: Case reports and review." *The Journal of Clinical Psychiatry 64*, 2, 202–207. doi: 10.4088/JCP.v64n0214.

CHAPTER 8

Allergy & Asthma Network (no date) "Your nose: The ultimate air cleaner." News. https://allergyasthmanetwork.org/news/your-nose-the-ultimate-air-cleaner

American Lung Association (2020) "Five ways you might be breathing wrong." Each Breath Blog, June 20. www.lung.org/blog/you-might-be-breathing-wrong

Amon, K.L. and Campbell, A. (2008) "Can children with AD/HD learn relaxation and breathing techniques through biofeedback video games?" *Australian Journal of Educational & Developmental Psychology 8*, 72–84. www.newcastle.edu.au/__data/assets/pdf_file/0014/100337/v8-amon-campbell.pdf

Bagheriyan, S., Borhani, F., Abbaszadeh, A., and Ranjbar, H. (2011) "The effects of regular breathing exercise and making bubbles on the pain of catheter insertion in school age children." *Iranian Journal of Nursing and Midwifery Research 16*, 2, 174–180.

Bhavanani, A.B. and Madanmohan, K.U. (2003) "Acute effect of Mukh bhastrika (a yogic bellows type breathing) on reaction time." *Indian Journal of Physiology and Pharmacology 47*, 3, 297–300.

Bhavanani, A.B., Ramanathan, M., and Harichandrakumar, K.T. (2012) "Immediate effect of muka bhastrika (a bellows type pranayama) on reaction time in mentally challenged adolescents." *Indian Journal of Physiology and Pharmacology 56*, 2, 174–180.

Bowlby, J. (1969) *Attachment and Loss, Vol. 1: Attachment*. New York: Basic Books.

Butler, J.E. (2007) "Drive to the human respiratory muscles." *Respiratory Physiology and Neurobiology 159*, 2, 115–126. doi: 10.1016/j.resp.2007.06.006.

Cavanaugh, J., Carp, S.B., Rock, C.M., and French, J.A. (2016) "Oxytocin modulates behavioral and physiological responses to a stressor in marmoset monkeys." *Psychoneuroendocrinology 66*, 22–30. https://doi.org/10.1016/j.psyneuen.2015.12.027

Chourpiliadis, C. and Bhardwaj, A. (2022) "Physiology, respiratory rate." StatPearls [Internet]. www.ncbi.nlm.nih.gov/books/NBK537306

Cleveland Clinic (2021) "Diaphragmatic breathing." https://my.clevelandclinic.org/health/articles/9445-diaphragmatic-breathing

Desikachar, T.K.V. (1999) *The Heart of Yoga: Developing a Personal Practice.* Rochester, VT: Inner Traditions-Bear & Co.

Eldridge, L. (2021) "Normal respiratory rate for adults and children." Verywellhealth, October 9. www.verywellhealth.com/what-is-a-normal-respiratory-rate-2248932

Elliott, S. (2006) *The New Science of Breath: Coherent Breathing for Autonomic Nervous System Balance, Health and Well-being* (2nd edn). Allex, TX: Coherence Press.

Evans, K.C., Dougherty, D.D., Schmid, A.M., Scannell, E., *et al.* (2009) "Modulation of spontaneous breathing via limbic/paralimbic-bulbar circuitry: An event-related fMRI study." *NeuroImage 47*, 3, 961–971. https://doi.org/10.1016/j.neuroimage.2009.05.025

Kajander, R. and Peper, E. (2010) "Teaching diaphragmatic breathing to children." *Biofeedback 26*, 3, 14–17. https://biofeedbackhealth.files.wordpress.com/2011/01/1998-kajander-and-peper.pdf

Khng, K.H. (2017) "A better state-of-mind: Deep breathing reduces state anxiety and enhances test performance through regulating test cognitions in children." *Cognition and Emotion 31*, 7, 1502–1510. doi: 10.1080/02699931.2016.1233095.

Kovalchick, L.V. (2015) "Use of Oxytocin as a Preventative Treatment for PTSD." Master's Thesis. Virginia Commonwealth University.

Kuypers, L. (2023) *The Zones of Regulation: Research and Scholarly Articles.* https://zonesofregulation.com/wp-content/uploads/2023/06/TheZonesofRegulation_ResearchandScholarlyArticles-MAIN2.pdf

Mayo Clinic (2023) "Pediatric obstructive sleep apnea." www.mayoclinic.org/diseases-conditions/pediatric-sleep-apnea/symptoms-causes/syc-20376196

Mersch, J. (2020) "Pediatric vital signs ranges and charts." eMedicine Health. www.emedicinehealth.com/pediatric_vital_signs/article_em.htm

Pourmovahed, Z., Dehghani, K., and Sherafat, A. (2013) "Effectiveness of regular breathing technique (hey-hu) on reduction of intrathecal injection pain in leukemic children: A randomized clinical trial." *Iranian Journal of Pediatrics 23*, 5, 564–568.

Russo, M.A., Santarelli, D.M., and O'Rourke, D. (2017) "The physiological effects of slow breathing in the healthy human." *Breathe (Sheffield) 13*, 4, 298–309. doi: 10.1183/20734735.009817.
Saoji, A.A., Raghavendra, B.R., and Manjunath, N.K. (2019) "Effects of yogic breath regulation: A narrative review of scientific evidence." *Journal of Ayurveda Integrative Medicine 10*, 1, 50–58. doi: 10.1016/j.jaim.2017.07.008.
Saunders, H., Kraus, A., Barone, L., and Biringen, Z. (2015) "Emotional availability: Theory, research, and intervention." *Frontiers in Psychology 6*, 1069. www.frontiersin.org/article/10.3389/fpsyg.2015.01069
Semple, R.J., Reid, E.F.G., and Miller, L. (2005) "Treating anxiety with mindfulness: An open trial of mindfulness training for anxious children." *Journal of Cognitive Psychotherapy 19*, 4. doi: 10.1891/jcop.2005.19.4.379.
Sonne, T. and Jensen, M.M. (2016) "Evaluating the ChillFish Biofeedback Game with Children with ADHD." The 15th International Conference. www.researchgate.net/publication/305727043_Evaluating_the_ChillFish_Biofeedback_Game_with_Children_with_ADHD
Sovik, R. (2013) "Learn diaphragmatic breathing for deep relaxation" [Video]. July 18. www.youtube.com/watch?v=Q82YnmLoKr8
Stoller, L. (2019) *Sensory-Enhanced Yoga for Self-Regulation and Trauma Healing*. Pencaitland: Handspring Publishing Limited.
Su, Y.H., Luh, J.J., Chen, H.I., Lin, C.C., Liao, M.J., and Chen, H.S. (2010) "Effects of using relaxation breathing training to reduce music performance anxiety in 3rd to 6th graders." *Medical Problems of Performing Artists 2*, 82–86.
Veerman, T.J. (2017) "A Deep Breathing Intervention for Stress Reduction in 5-Year-Old Children." Doctoral dissertation. Knoxville, TN: University of Tennessee, TRACE (Tennessee Research and Creative Exchange). https://trace.tennessee.edu/cgi/viewcontent.cgi?article=6345&context=utk_graddiss
Zaccaro, A., Piarulli, A., Laurino, M., Garbella, E., *et al.* (2018) "How breath-control can change your life: A systematic review on psycho-physiological correlates of slow breathing." *Frontiers in Human Neuroscience 12.* doi: 10.3389/fnhum.2018.00353.
Zelano, C., Jiang, H., Zhou, G., Arora, N., *et al.* (2016) "Nasal respiration entrains human limbic oscillations and modulates cognitive function." *Journal of Neuroscience 36*, 12448–12467. https://doi.org/10.1523/JNEUROSCI.2586-16.2016

CHAPTER 9

Ango, F. and Dos Reis, R. (2019) "Cerebellum: Sensing how to balance." *eLife 8*, e46973. https://doi.org/10.7554/eLife.46973
Archana, R., Sailesh, K.S., and Mukkadan, J.K. (2016) "Effect of vestibular stimulation on stress and cardiovascular parameters in healthy college students." *Biomedical Research 27*, 3, 985–990.
Ayres, A.J. (1972) *Sensory Integration and Learning Disorders*. Los Angeles, CA: Western Psychological Services.
Ayres, A.J. (1979) *Sensory Integration and the Child.* Los Angeles, CA: Western Psychological Services.
Balaban, C.D. (2002) "Neural substrates linking balance control and anxiety." *Physiology & Behavior 77*, 4–5, 469–475. https://doi.org/10.1016/s0031-9384(02)00935-6
Balaban, C.D., Jacob, R.G., and Furman, J.M. (2011) "Neurologic bases for comorbidity of balance disorders, anxiety disorders and migraine: Neurotherapeutic implications." *Expert Review of Neurotherapeutics 11*, 3, 379–394. doi :10.1586/ern.11.19.

Bernardi, L., Gabutti, A., Porta, C., and Spicuzza, L. (2001) "Slow breathing reduces chemoreflex response to hypoxia and hypercapnia, and increases baroreflex sensitivity." *Journal of Hypertension 19*, 12, 2221–2229. doi: 10.1097/00004872-200112000-00016.

Blanche, E.I. and Schaaf, R.C. (2001) "Proprioception: A Cornerstone of Sensory Integrative Intervention." In S. Smith Roley, R.I. Blanche, and R.C. Schaaf (eds) *Understanding the Nature of Sensory Integration with Diverse Populations* (pp.109–124). San Antonio, TX: Therapy Skill Builders.

Bordoloi, K. and Deka, R.S. (2018) "Scientific reconciliation of the concepts and principles of Rood approach." *International Journal of Health Sciences and Research 8*, 9, 225–234.

Brandt, T. and Dieterich, M. (1999) "The vestibular cortex: Its locations, functions, and disorders." *Annals of the New York Academy of Sciences 871*, 1, 293–312. doi: 10.1111/j.1749-6632.1999.tb09193.x.

Brendtro, L.K. (2015) "Our resilient brain: Nature's most complex creation." *Reclaiming Children & Youth 24*, 2, 41–49.

Buric, I., Farias, M., Jong, J., Mee, C., and Brazil, I.A. (2017) "What is the molecular signature of mind-body interventions? A systematic review of gene expression changes induced by meditation and related practices." *Frontiers in Immunology 8*, 670. https://doi.org/10.3389/fimmu.2017.00670

Clancy, K.J. (2017) "Assessing the clinical utility of non-invasive brain stimulation in the treatment of anxious arousal and sensory hypersensitivity: A targeted transcranial alternating current stimulation study." The Graduate School Theses and Dissertations. http://purl.flvc.org/fsu/fd/FSU_FALL2017_Clancy_fsu_0071N_14146

Clancy, K.J., Ding, M., Bernat, E., Schmidt, N.B., and Li, W. (2017) "Restless 'rest': Intrinsic sensory hyperactivity and disinhibition in post-traumatic stress disorder." *Brain 140*, 7, 2041–2050. https://doi.org/10.1093/brain/awx116

Crandall, S.R., Cruikshank, S.J., and Connors, B.W. (2015) "A corticothalamic switch: Controlling the thalamus with dynamic synapses." *Neuron 86*, 768–782.

Desikachar, T.K.V. (1999) *The Heart of Yoga: Developing a Personal Practice.* Rochester, VT: Inner Traditions-Bear & Co.

Dougherty, P. (no date) "Central Control of the Autonomic Nervous System and Thermoregulation." In *Neuroscience Online: An Electronic Textbook for the Neurosciences* (Chapter 3). https://nba.uth.tmc.edu/neuroscience/m/s4/chapter03.html

Farber, S. (1982) *Neurorehabilitation: A Multisensory Approach*. Philadelphia, PA: W.B. Saunders Co.

Field, T., Diego, M., and Hernandez-Reif, M. (2010) "Preterm infant massage therapy research: A review." *Infant Behavior & Development 33*, 2, 115–124. https://doi.org/10.1016/j.infbeh.2009.12.004

Fogel, A. (2009) *Body Sense*. New York: W.W. Norton & Company.

Forbes, B. (2011) *Yoga for Emotional Balance: Simple Practices to Help Relieve Anxiety and Depression*. Boston, MA: Shambhala Publications, Inc.

Freeman, R. (2006) "Assessment of cardiovascular autonomic function." *Clinical Neurophysiology 117*, 4, 716–730. doi: 10.1016/j.clinph.2005.09.027.

Goothy, S.S.K., Padmanabha, B.V., Goothy, S., and Mukkadan, J.K. (2019) "Effect of selected vestibular exercises on depression, anxiety and stress in elderly women with type 2 diabetes." *International Journal of Biochemistry and Physiology 4*, 4, 000169.

Grabherr, L., Macauda, G., and Lenggenhager, B. (2015) "The moving history of vestibular stimulation as a therapeutic intervention." *Multisensory Research 28*, 5–6, 653–687. doi: 10.1163/22134808-00002495.

Grandin, T. (1992) "Calming effects of deep touch pressure in patients with autistic disorder, college students, and animals." *Journal of Child and Adolescent Psychopharmacology 2*, 1,

63–72. doi: 10.1089/cap.1992.2.63. www.grandin.com/inc/squeeze.html#:~:text=Deep%20touch%20pressure%20is%20the,moving%20hairs%20on%20the%20skin

Guedry, F.E., Norman, J., Turnipseed, G., and Rupert, A. (1990) *Vestibular Responses and Motion Sickness During Pitch, Roll, and Yaw Sinusoidal Whole-Body Oscillation.* Interim Report, March 1. Pensacola, FL: Naval Aerospace Medical Research Lab.

Harricharan, S., Rabellino, D., Frewen, P.A., Densmore, M., *et al.* (2016) "fMRI functional connectivity of the periaqueductal gray in PTSD and its dissociative subtype." *Brain and Behavior 6*, 12, e00579. http://doi.org/10.1002/brb3.579

Hitier, M., Besnard, S., and Smith, P.F. (2014) "Vestibular pathways involved in cognition." *Frontiers in Integrative Neuroscience 8*, 59. doi: 10.3389/fnint.2014.00059.

Iyengar, B.K.S. (2001) *B.K.S. Iyengar Yoga: The Path to Holistic Health.* London: Dorling Kindersley Ltd.

Johnstone, S.E. and Baylin, S.B. (2010) "Stress and the epigenetic landscape: A link to the pathobiology of human diseases?" *Nature Reviews. Genetics 11*, 11, 806–812. https://doi.org/10.1038/nrg2881

Kabat-Zinn, J. (1994) *Wherever You Go, There You Are: Mindfulness Meditation in Everyday Life.* New York: Hachette Book Publishing.

Kammermeier, S., Singh, A., and Bötzel, K. (2017) "Intermediate latency-evoked potentials of multimodal cortical vestibular areas: Galvanic stimulation." *Frontiers in Neurology 8*, 587. http://doi.org/10.3389/fneur.2017.00587

Kearney, B.E. and Lanius, R.A. (2022) "The brain–body disconnect: A somatic sensory basis for trauma-related disorders." *Frontiers in Neuroscience 16*, 1015749. https://doi.org/10.3389/fnins.2022.1015749

Kerr, C.E., Sacchet, M.D., Lazar, S.W., Moore, C.I., and Jones, S.R. (2013) "Mindfulness starts with the body: Somatosensory attention and top-down modulation of cortical alpha rhythms in mindfulness meditation." *Frontiers in Human Neuroscience 7*, 12. http://doi.org/10.3389/fnhum.2013.00012

Kimball, J.G., Lynch, K.M., Stewart, K.C., Williams, N.E., Thomas, M.A., and Atwood, K.D. (2007) "Using salivary cortisol to measure the effects of a Wilbarger protocol-based procedure on sympathetic arousal: A pilot study." *American Journal of Occupational Therapy 61*, 406–413. http://dx.doi.org/10.5014/ajot.61.4.406

Koomar, J.A. and Bundy, A.C. (2002) "Creating Direct Intervention from Theory." In A.C. Bundy, S.J. Lane, and E.A. Murray (eds) *Sensory Integration Theory and Practice* (pp.261–308). Philadelphia, PA: F.A. Davis Company.

Kozlowska, K., Scher, S., and Helgeland, H. (2020, October 1) "The HPA Axis and Functional Somatic Symptoms." In K. Kozlowska, S. Scher, and H. Helgeland (eds) *Functional Somatic Symptoms in Children and Adolescents* (pp.161–173). Basingstoke: Palgrave Macmillan.

Kraftsow, G. (1999) *Yoga for Wellness: Healing with the Timeless Teachings of Viniyoga.* New York: Penguin Putnam Inc.

Krystal, A.D., Zammit, G.K., Wyatt, J.K., Quan, S.F., *et al.* (2010) "The effect of vestibular stimulation in a four-hour sleep phase advance model of transient insomnia." *Journal of Clinical Sleep Medicine (JCSM): Official Publication of the American Academy of Sleep Medicine 6*, 4, 315–321. doi: 10.5664/jcsm.27871.

Lasater, J.H. (1995, 2011) *Relax and Renew: Restful Yoga for Stressful Times.* Brookline, MA: Shambhala Publications.

Lenggenhager, B. and Lopez, C. (2015) "Vestibular Contributions to the Sense of Body, Self, and Others." In T. Metzinger and J.M. Windt (eds) *Open MIND.* Frankfurt am Main: MIND Group. doi: 10.15502/9783958570023.

Levine, P.A. (1997) *Waking the Tiger: Healing Trauma.* Berkeley, CA: North Atlantic Books.

Lu, C.Y., Liu, X., Jiang, H., Pan, F., Ho, C.S., and Ho, R.C. (2017) "Effects of traumatic stress induced in the juvenile period on the expression of gamma-aminobutyric acid receptor type A subunits in adult rat brain." *Neural Plasticity 2017*, 5715816. https://doi.org/10.1155/2017/5715816

Macefield, V.G. and James, C. (2016) "Superentrainment of muscle sympathetic nerve activity during sinusoidal galvanic vestibular stimulation." *Journal of Neurophysiology 116*, 6, 2689–2694. doi: 10.1152/jn.00036.2016.

Menon, V. and Uddin, L.Q. (2010) "Saliency, switching, attention and control: A network model of insula function." *Brain Structure & Function 214*, 5–6, 655–667. https://doi.org/10.1007/s00429-010-0262-0

Mollo, K., Schaaf, R., and Benevides, T. (2008) "The use of kripalu yoga to decrease sensory overresponsivity: A pilot study." *Sensory Integration*, Special Interest Section Quarterly, *31*, 3.

Nakajima, M. and Halassa, M.M. (2017) "Thalamic control of functional cortical connectivity." *Current Opinion in Neurobiology 44*, 127–131. https://doi.org/10.1016/j.conb.2017.04.001

Neuro New Me (2021) "Ascending Sensory Pathways." Chapter 10. https://pdtr-global.com/upload/pdf/AscendingSensoryPathways.pdf

Ogden, P., Minton, K., and Pain, C. (2006) *Trauma and the Body: A Sensorimotor Approach to Psychotherapy*. New York: W.W. Norton & Company.

Omlin, X., Crivelli, F., Heinicke, L., Zaunseder, S., Achermann, P., and Riener, R. (2016) "Effect of rocking movements on respiration." *PLoS ONE 11*, 3, e0150581. https://doi.org/10.1371/journal.pone.0150581

Pace-Schott, E.F., Germain, A., and Milad, M.R. (2015) "Sleep and REM sleep disturbance in the pathophysiology of PTSD: The role of extinction memory." *Biology of Mood & Anxiety Disorders* 5, 3. doi: 10.1186/s13587-015-0018-9.

Pfeiffer, B. and Kinnealey, M. (2003) "Treatment of sensory defensiveness in adults." *Occupational Therapy International 10*, 3, 175–184. doi: 10.1002/oti.184.

Purves, D., Augustine, G.J., Fitzpatrick, D., Katz, L.C., *et al.* (eds) (2001) "Vestibular Pathways to the Thalamus and Cortex." In D. Purves, G.J. Augustine, D. Fitzpatrick, L.C. Katz, *et al., Neuroscience* (2nd edn) (Chapter 14). Sinauer Associates. www.ncbi.nlm.nih.gov/books/NBK10862

Radomski, M.V. and Latham, C.A.T. (2007) *Occupational Therapy for Physical Dysfunction* (6th edn). Philadelphia, PA: Lippincott Williams & Wilkins.

Rauchs, G., Bertran, F., Guillery-Girard, B., Desgranges, B., *et al.* (2004) "Consolidation of strictly episodic memories mainly requires rapid eye movement sleep." *Sleep 27*, 3, 395–401. doi: 10.1093/sleep/27.3.395.

Reynolds, S., Lane, S.J., and Mullen, B. (2015) "Effects of deep pressure stimulation on physiological arousal." *American Journal of Occupational Therapy 69*, 3, 6903350010p1–6903350010p5. https://doi.org/10.5014/ajot.2015.015560

Rood, M.S. (1954) "Neurophysiological reactions as a basis for physical therapy." *Physical Therapy Review 34*, 9, 444–449. doi: 10.1093/ptj/34.9.444.

Rothschild, B. (2003) *The Body Remembers Casebook: Unifying Methods and Models in the Treatment of Trauma and PTSD*. New York: Norton Professional Books.

Sadeghi, S.G., Mitchell, D.E., and Cullen, K.E. (2009) "Different neural strategies for multimodal integration: Comparison of two macaque monkey species." *Experimental Brain Research 195*, 1, 45–57. doi: 10.1007/s00221-009-1751-3.

Sailesh, K.S. and Mukkadan, J.K. (2013a) "Can controlled vestibular stimulation reduce stress?" *Health Sciences* 2, 3, JS001.

Sailesh, K.S. and Mukkadan, J.K. (2013b) "Psychoneuroimmuno modulation by controlled vestibular stimulation." *Journal of Clinical & Experimental Research 1*, 68–70.

Sailesh, K.S., Archana, R., and Mukkadan, J.K. (2014) "Controlled vestibular stimulation: Supplementary treatment for hypothyroidism." *Research Journal of Pharmaceutical, Biological and Chemical Sciences* 5, 1842–1845.

Sailesh, K.S., Archana, R., Sajeevan, A., and Mukkadan, J.K. (2016) "Effect of controlled vestibular stimulation on depression, spatial and verbal memory scores in underweight female students: A pilot study." *Biomedical Research 27*, 3.

Salibi, N.A., Saadé, N.E., Banna, N.R., and Jabbur, S.J. (1981) "Dorsal column input into the reticular formation." *Nature 288*, 5790, 481–483. doi: 10.1038/288481a0.

Saman, Y., Bamiou, D.E., Gleeson, M., and Dutia, M.B. (2012) "Interactions between stress and vestibular compensation—A review." *Frontiers in Neurology 3*, 116. doi: 10.3389/fneur.2012.00116.

Scaer, R.C. (2007) *The Body Bears the Burden: Trauma, Dissociation and Disease*. New York: Taylor & Francis Group (Routledge).

Schmitz, T.W., Correia, M.M., Ferreira, C.S., Prescot, A.P., and Anderson, M.C. (2017) "Hippocampal GABA enables inhibitory control over unwanted thoughts." *Nature Communications 8*, 1311. https://doi.org/10.1038/s41467-017-00956-z

Seaborne, R.A., Strauss, J., Cocks, M., Shepherd, S., *et al.* (2018) "Human skeletal muscle possesses an epigenetic memory of hypertrophy." *Scientific Reports 8*, 1898. https://doi.org/10.1038/s41598-018-20287-3

Sensory Integration International (1991) *Sensory Integration and Praxis Tests Training Manual.* Los Angeles, CA: Sensory Integration International.

Sharma, K.N. (2019) *Advanced Techniques in Physiotherapy & Occupational Therapy*. New Delhi, India: Jaypee Brothers Medical Publishers (P) Ltd.

Sharples, A.P., Stewart, C.E., and Seaborne, R.A. (2016) "Does skeletal muscle have an 'epi'-memory? The role of epigenetics in nutritional programming, metabolic disease, aging and exercise." *Aging Cell 15*, 4, 603–616. https://doi.org/10.1111/acel.12486

Shi, X.B., Wang, J., Li, F.T., Zhang, Y.B., *et al.* (2022) "Whole-brain monosynaptic outputs and presynaptic inputs of GABAergic neurons in the vestibular nuclei complex of mice." *Frontiers of Neuroscience 16*, 982596. doi: 10.3389/fnins.2022.982596.

Smith, A.K., Conneely, K.N., Kilaru, V., Mercer, K.B., *et al.* (2011) "Differential immune system DNA methylation and cytokine regulation in post-traumatic stress disorder." *American Journal of Medical Genetics. Part B, Neuropsychiatric Genetics: The Official Publication of the International Society of Psychiatric Genetics 156B*, 6, 700–708. https://doi.org/10.1002/ajmg.b.31212

Stoller, C.C., Greuel, J.H., Cimini, L.S., Fowler, M.S., and Koomar, J.A. (2012) "Effects of sensory enhanced yoga on symptoms of combat stress in deployed military personnel." *The American Journal of Occupational Therapy 66*, 59–68. doi: 10.5014/ajot.2012.001230.

Stoller, L. (2019) *Sensory-Enhanced Yoga for Self-Regulation and Trauma Healing*. Pencaitland: Handspring Publishing Limited.

van der Kolk, B.A. (2008) "Affect Regulation." Lecture, Pre-Conference Institute of the 19th Annual International Trauma Conference, June 25, Boston, MA.

van der Kolk, B.A. (2014) *The Body Keeps the Score: Brain, Mind, and Body in the Healing of Trauma.* New York: Viking (Penguin Random House).

Veenstra, L., Schneider, I.K., and Koole, S.L. (2017) "Embodied mood regulation: The impact of body posture on mood recovery, negative thoughts, and mood-congruent recall." *Cognition and Emotion 31*, 7, 1361–1376. doi: 10.1080/02699931.2016.1225003.

Wirth, A.M., Frank, S.M., Greenlee, M.W., and Beer, A.L. (2018) "White matter connectivity of the visual-vestibular cortex examined by diffusion-weighted imaging." *Brain Connections 8*, 235–244. doi: 10.1089/brain.2017.0544.

Woodward, S., Tauber, E.S., Spielmann, A.J., and Thorpy, M.J. (1990) "Effects of otolithic vestibular stimulation on sleep." *Sleep 13*, 6, 533–537. https://doi.org/10.1093/sleep/13.6.533

Yates, B.J., Bolton, P.S., and Macefield, V.G. (2014) "Vestibulo-sympathetic responses." *Comprehensive Physiology 4*, 2, 851–887. https://doi.org/10.1002/cphy.c130041

Yee, R. (2002) *Yoga: The Poetry of the Body*. New York: St Martin's Press.

Yehuda, R., Hoge, C.W., McFarlane, A.C., Vermetten, E., *et al.* (2015) "Post-traumatic stress disorder." *Nature Reviews. Disease Primers 1*, 15057, 1–22. https://doi.org/10.1038/nrdp.2015.57

Figure attributions

Figure 9.1: Anatomy & Physiology, Connexions, http://cnx.org/content/col11496/1.6, CC by 3.0, https://commons.wikimedia.org/wiki/File:1417_Ascending_Pathways_of_Spinal_Cord.jpg

Figure 9.2: This file was derived from: https://commons.wikimedia.org/wiki/File:1421_Sensory_Homunculus.jpg, CC by 3.0, https://commons.wikimedia.org/wiki/File:Sensory_Homunculus-en.svg

Figure 9.3: Polygon data are from BodyParts3D, CC by SA 2.1, https://commons.wikimedia.org/wiki/File:BA312_-_Primary_Somatosensory_Cortex_-_lateral_view_-_with_homunculus.png

Figure 9.5b: Transferred from en.wikipedia to Commons, Public Domain, https://commons.wikimedia.org/w/index.php?curid=11087888

Figure 9.5c: Transferred from en.wikipedia to Commons, Public Domain, https://commons.wikimedia.org/w/index.php?curid=2539199

Figure 9.5d: OpenClipart, CC0, https://commons.wikimedia.org/w/index.php?curid=64375759

Figure 9.5e: Openclipart, CC0, https://commons.wikimedia.org/w/index.php?curid=88868812

CHAPTER 10

Beck, A.T. (2008) "The evolution of the cognitive model of depression and its neurobiological correlates." *The American Journal of Psychiatry 165*, 8, 969–977. https://doi.org/10.1176/appi.ajp.2008.08050721

Boston Children's Hospital (2021) "Anxiety disorders." www.childrenshospital.org/conditions-and-treatments/conditions/a/anxiety-disorders

CDC (Centers for Disease Control and Prevention) (2021) "Anxiety and depression in children." www.cdc.gov/childrensmentalhealth/depression.html

Chen, G. (2017) "Does gratitude promote recovery from substance misuse?" *Addiction Research & Theory 25*, 2, 121–128. doi: 10.1080/16066359.2016.1212337.

DeRidder, D., Vanneste, S., Smith, M., and Adhia, D. (2022) "Pain and the triple network model." *Frontiers in Neurology 13*, 757241. https://doi.org/10.3389/fneur.2022.757241

Dychtwald, K. (1986) *Bodymind*. New York: Tarcher Putnam Books.

Fogel, A. (2009) *Body Sense: The Science and Practice of Embodied Self-Awareness*. New York: W.W. Norton & Company.

Incredible Years, The (no date) "Online workshops and video streaming now available!" The Incredible Years: Parents, Teachers, and Children Training Series. www.incredibleyears.com/research/library/article/the-incredible-years-parents-teachers-and-children-training-series

Kelmon, J. (2022) "Academic vocabulary words for 1st graders." GreatSchools, November 10. www.greatschools.org/gk/articles/academic-vocabulary-words-for-first-graders

Kuypers, L. (2023) *The Zones of Regulation: Research and Scholarly Articles*. https://zonesofregulation.com/wp-content/uploads/2023/06/TheZonesofRegulation_ResearchandScholarlyArticles-MAIN2.pdf

LePage, J. and LePage, L. (2013) *Mudras for Healing and Transformation.* Sebastopol, CA: Integrative Yoga Therapy.

Levine, P.A. (1997) *Waking the Tiger: Healing Trauma.* Berkeley, CA: North Atlantic Books.

Lies, J., Mellor, D., and Hong, R.Y. (2014) "Gratitude and personal functioning among earthquake survivors in Indonesia." *The Journal of Positive Psychology 9*, 4, 295–305. https://doi.org/10.1080/17439760.2014.902492

Maloney, J.E., Lawlor, M.S., Schonert-Reichl, K.A., and Whitehead, J. (2016) "A Mindfulness-Based Social and Emotional Learning Curriculum for School-Aged Children: The MindUP Program." In K.A. Schonert-Reichl and R.W. Roeser (eds) *Handbook of Mindfulness in Education: Integrating Theory and Research into Practice* (pp.3–16). New York: Springer.

McLean, S. (2016, June) *The Effect of Trauma on the Brain Development of Children: Evidence-Based Principles for Supporting the Recovery of Children in Care.* Child Family Community Australia Practice Resource. https://aifs.gov.au/resources/practice-guides/effect-trauma-brain-development-children

Nair, S., Sagar, M., Sollers, J. III, Consedine, N., and Broadbent, E. (2015) "Do slumped and upright postures affect stress responses? A randomized trial." *Health Psychology 34*, 6, 632–641. http://dx.doi.org/10.1037/hea0000146

Nejad, A., Fossati, P., and Lemogne, C. (2013) "Self-referential processing, rumination, and cortical midline structures in major depression." *Frontiers in Human Neuroscience 7*, 1–9. doi: 10.3389/fnhum.2013.00666.

Ogden, P., Minton, K., and Pain, C. (2006) *Trauma and the Body: A Sensorimotor Approach to Psychotherapy.* New York: W.W. Norton & Co.

Reilly, C.E., Sokol, L., and Butler, A.C. (1999) "A cognitive approach to understanding and treating anxiety." *Human Psychopharmacology: Clinical & Experimental 14*, S1, S16–S21. https://doi.org/10.1002/(SICI)1099-1077(199908)14:1+<S16::AID-HUP113>3.0.CO;2-N

Rolf, I. (1963) "Structural integration." *Systematics 1*, 1, 67–84.

Rothschild, B. (2000) *The Body Remembers: The Psychophysiology of Trauma and Trauma Treatment.* New York: W.W. Norton & Company.

Roy, M., Shohamy, D., and Wager, T.D. (2012) "Ventromedial prefrontal-subcortical systems and the generation of affective meaning." *Trends in Cognitive Sciences 16*, 3, 147–156. http://doi.org/10.1016/j.tics.2012.01.005

Second Step (no date) "Empowered with skills for life." www.secondstep.org

Stankovic, L. (2011) "Transforming trauma: A qualitative feasibility study of integrative restoration (iRest) yoga Nidra on combat-related post-traumatic stress disorder." *International Journal of Yoga Therapy 21*, 23–37.

Stoller, L. (2019) *Sensory-Enhanced Yoga for Self-Regulation and Trauma Healing.* Pencaitland: Handspring Publishing Limited.

van der Kolk, B.A. (2014) *The Body Keeps the Score: Brain, Mind, and Body in the Healing of Trauma.* New York: Viking (Penguin Random House).

van Harmelen, A.L., Hauber, K., Gunther Moor, B., Spinhoven, P., *et al.* (2014) "Childhood emotional maltreatment severity is associated with dorsal medial prefrontal cortex responsivity to social exclusion in young adults." *PLoS ONE 9*, 1, e85107. https://doi.org/10.1371/journal.pone.0085107

Veenstra, L., Schneider, I.K., and Koole, S.L. (2017) "Embodied mood regulation: the impact of body posture on mood recovery, negative thoughts, and mood-congruent recall." *Cognition and Emotion 31*, 7, 1361–1376. doi: 10.1080/02699931.2016.1225003.

Vieselmeyer, J., Holguin, J., and Mezulis, A. (2017) "The role of resilience and gratitude in posttraumatic stress and growth following a campus shooting." *Psychological Trauma: Theory, Research, Practice, and Policy 9*, 1, 62–69. doi: 10.1037/tra0000149.

Williams, M.S. and Shellenberger, S. (1996) *How Does Your Engine Run? Leader's Guide to the Alert Program for Self Regulation.* Albuquerque, NM: TherapyWorks, Inc.

Winner, M.G. (2022) "It's not about appropriate vs. inappropriate! Teaching expected & unexpected behaviors the right way. Social Thinking, July. www.socialthinking.com/Articles?name=why-use-expected-unexpected-social-thinking-vocabulary

Winner, M.G. and Crooke, P.J. (2009) "Social thinking: A training paradigm for professionals and treatment approach for individuals with social learning/social pragmatic challenges." *Perspectives on Language Learning and Education 16*, 2, 62–69. doi: 10.1044/lle16.2.62.

Wood, J.V., Perunovic, W.Q.E., and Lee, J.W. (2009) "Positive self-statements: power for some, peril for others." *Psychology of Science 20*, 7, 860–866. doi: 10.1111/j.1467-9280.2009.02370.x.

Zeidman, P. and Maguire, E.A. (2016) "Anterior hippocampus: The anatomy of perception, imagination and episodic memory." *Nature Reviews. Neuroscience 17*, 3, 173–182. https://doi.org/10.1038/nrn.2015.24

CHAPTER 11

Emerson, D. (2015) *Trauma-Sensitive Yoga in Therapy: Bringing the Body into Treatment.* New York: W.W. Norton & Company.

LePage, J. (2015) *Professional Yoga Therapist Internship Study Guide.* Fort Lauderdale, FL: Integrative Yoga Therapy. www.iytyogatherapy.com

Novotney, A. (2009) "Yoga as a practice tool." *Monitor on Psychology (American Psychological Association) 40*, 10, 38.

Ogden, P., Minton, K., and Pain, C. (2006) *Trauma and the Body: A Sensorimotor Approach to Psychotherapy.* New York: W.W. Norton & Company.

Rothschild, B. (2009) "Safe trauma recovery" [Video file]. www.youtube.com/watch?v=LhuzpUlaX_k [also available at www.somatictraumatherapy.com/videos].

Stoller, C.C. (1984) "Toward a Unifying Theory of Occupational Therapy: A Comparison and Synthesis of Developmental and Systems Theories." Thesis. San Jose State University, San Jose, CA.

Stoller, L. (2019) *Sensory-Enhanced Yoga for Self-Regulation and Trauma Healing.* Pencaitland: Handspring Publishing Limited.

PART 3

The Practice

CHAPTER 12

Student Factors to Consider

In this chapter we will discuss factors to consider when planning a SMYLE™ session for students who are trauma survivors or who are dealing with toxic stress, anxiety, sensory modulation disorder, ADHD, mixed anxiety/depression, or other mental health challenges. Many of the ideas presented in this chapter were inspired by the experiences of SMYLE™ co-creators Meg Hennessey Schofield as a lead teacher and Lynn Stoller as occupational therapist working with a wide range of students experiencing a variety of developmental, intellectual, physical, and mental health challenges. The structure of the SMYLE™ program was particularly inspired by Meg's experiences integrating yoga and mindfulness within a classroom setting, which meshed perfectly with the guidelines to the practice of Sensory Enhanced Yoga®. Although informed by our work in school settings, most of these recommendations apply just as easily to other settings, such as summer camps, group residential homes, yoga studios, and typical home settings.

HOW TO STRUCTURE A SMYLE™ SESSION

Designing a SMYLE™ session requires thoughtful selection and sequencing of the yoga forms and flows, breathing practices, and the meditative components including the Body Scan, Final Relaxation, and Mudra meditation segments. Various environmental and student factors should be considered when planning these elements. Many environmental considerations were discussed in detail in Chapter 7, including the location and sensory elements of the setting. We encourage you to present yoga and other mindfulness practices in various locations to spread the calm energy across contexts, although they will obviously be most effective in a quiet space.

In a school environment, these practices can be conducted any time of the day that best fits the classroom schedule; however, ideal times include on arrival at school, transitions between classes and activities, after lunch to prepare for the afternoon activities, and whenever students need a quick calming or energizing sequence to return to balance. In addition, there may be opportunities to present a longer session, such as during a group occupational therapy session, physical education class, or after-school club.

The next chapter will present sample practices. But first, in this chapter, we will focus on student-specific needs that we have encountered in our work over the years, which have informed the structure of our yoga and mindfulness sessions. We will discuss the lessons we have learned and the strategies we developed to enable all students to be successful with our program. Keep in mind that this is not an exhaustive list of student-specific needs to consider, but ones that we have had the most experience addressing in our work settings.

Student considerations when planning a SMYLE™ session include:

- Emotional regulation needs
- Receptive language levels
- Arousal regulation needs
- Attention span
- Familiarity with sequences/routines
- Mobility challenges.

Considering these components ahead of time is crucial for a successful SMYLE™ session. Since the focus of this book is to provide professionals with tools to help children, adolescents, and individuals with special challenges recover from trauma, toxic stress, high anxiety, and/or related conditions, it is important to find frequent opportunities to help them move out of their minds and safely back into their bodies. "Body-sensing" language, movements, and scans are very helpful towards this end. These elements are incorporated into all components of the SMYLE™ program including the meditative scripts for the Body Scan, Tension and Release Exercise, and Savasana (the final rest portion of class). They are also included in all of the SMYLE™ sequences discussed in the next chapter.

EMOTIONAL REGULATION NEEDS

Every student each day could be dealing with a different emotional need, so make sure to always begin SMYLE™ sessions with an open, non-judgmental, and unbiased mindset. Also remember that students can be dealing with multiple emotions at the same time. For example, some students may struggle with mixed anxiety and depression, which can make planning a therapeutic sequence a challenge. The typical yogic protocol for treating anxiety involves moving the energy downward to help ground the individual. In contrast, people in depressed states need to be uplifted. When these two emotions are present at the same time, try to find a balance between grounding and uplifting.

One usually effective way to do this is to present some chest-expanding (heart-opening) yoga forms, which move the energy upward, while being careful to only choose ones that keep the student well grounded in the process (e.g., Warrior 1, Rainbow Breath, Shining Star). Otherwise, you could potentially exacerbate the student's anxiety. If you still notice some hesitancy moving into one of these forms, you might try offering a yoga band. Yoga bands are a great yogic tool because they help students more easily move into more expansive yoga forms while also providing significant proprioceptive input that can keep the student feeling grounded. But don't push it: if the student is not feeling ready to open their heart center, we need to honor that to keep this a safe practice for the student.

In order to be prepared for emotions of all sizes that may arise, instructors should always start a SMYLE™ session stating: "If at any point during class you feel you need a break, please choose any yoga form that feels good for you and helps you rest. Join back in when you are ready." Child is the standard yoga form that yoga instructors offer for rest, but remember that Child is not accessible or "restful" for everyone. Some yoga forms we recommend using for rest during SMYLE™ sessions include Seated Forward Fold, Lying Down Rest Form (Savasana), Crocodile, Seated Crocodile, or any restorative yoga form that the student can get into (or have another staff member who can help).

Also consider that you may be suggesting positions for students to move into that they have never gotten into before, or maybe not for a long while, which can release a lot of emotional energy that has been stagnant for long periods of time. When students get into these forms, they may experience feelings, thoughts, or emotions that they are unfamiliar with or may recognize but haven't fully processed. This was discussed in Chapter 7 (Guideline #1). Students' daily routines can be very busy as they move from one thing to the other throughout their entire day. SMYLE™ sessions are a planned time for students to return back to the present moment and truly be with themselves in a safe way. Yet keep in mind that some people cannot handle too much silence because they will get wrapped up in their concerns, thoughts, and emotions. Therefore, it is important to carefully pace the breath, movements, guided meditation, and silence in an effort to provide the "just right" amount of each to be effective in their healing.

RECEPTIVE LANGUAGE LEVELS

Clear and *concise* language, with significant *modeling*, are key elements to success in a SMYLE™ session. The language level of the practice should be planned in advance to best connect with the majority of the class. Remember—we are trying to encourage students to disconnect from their thoughts and reconnect their mind with their bodies. SMYLE™ session instructions should help the students easily and safely get into the yoga forms, but should then focus the students' attention on the breath and bodymind connection while in the forms. There is an "art" to ***balancing language with silence***. We want to guide students into their minds and bodies, to return them to the present moment, and then allow them to experience the bodymind connection at a deep level, without teacher intrusion.

When giving verbal instructions, it is important to know your students' receptive language levels, especially the level of vocabulary, pacing, and amount of verbiage they can process, before teaching a SMYLE™ session. Be sure that the verbal instructions you are giving are understood by everyone in the session. If the language is too high for the group, it will negate the intended effect of the practices. In these situations, students could feel confused, lost, and not able to keep up, and turn their attention to negative self-deprecating thoughts (e.g., "I can't do this," "This is too hard for me," "I never want to do this again," "I am not good at anything").

On the other hand, if the language level is too low for students in your session, negative reactions could also arise. In these circumstances, the students could feel like the instructor is downgrading their ability or treating them like a child. This tends to happen more often in higher elementary levels (5th grade), middle school, and high school years when students start to mature and want to be treated more like a young adult. In these situations, it is best to avoid the "child-like" yoga forms and descriptions and include more age-appropriate vocabulary. For example:

- **The classic names for yoga forms**, e.g., Cat/Cow vs. "Happy Cat/Angry Cat;" Down Dog to Up Dog vs. "Dolphin Flow."
- **More mature names for body parts**, e.g., stomach (belly is okay, too!) vs. tummy; buttocks vs. bottom; torso vs. body; ribcage vs. chest.
- **More specific rather than general body parts**, e.g., forearm vs. arm; thigh vs. leg.
- **More advanced directional and positional words**, e.g., right side vs. other side; above vs. up; below vs. down.
- **More advanced body-related action verbs**, e.g., extend vs. raise; flex vs. bend; expand vs. get bigger (as in belly).
- **More precise points of attentional focus during Body Scans**, e.g., center of the forehead vs. forehead; center of the palm vs. hand.

In every group setting there will be outliers with respect to language levels. Visuals such as those in Figures 12.1–12.4 are a great tool to provide that extra level of support to students who may need it. In some groups, ***all*** students may benefit from the use of visual aids. It is suggested that these visuals include the title of the yoga form along with a picture of a person doing each step of the form. Simplified visual instructions for breath directions could also be included. Also having the repetition number (e.g., "Do five times") listed at the bottom helps to decrease anxiety for some students.

How to incorporate visuals into your SMYLE™ sessions

A. To remember the routine sequences:

- It can be very helpful to present a visual overview of the entire yoga/mindfulness routine at the beginning of the yoga session (see Figure 12.1), as well as visuals of the specific practices (see Figures 12.3 and 12.4).
- If a projection or interactive whiteboard (such as a SmartBoard) is available, the visuals can be displayed for the whole group to see.
- The visuals can also be printed and put into page protectors, and can then be connected with rings to make a book. These books can be displayed on mats, desks, or inclined surfaces (such as a slant board) for easy reference. This is also a great resource for home practice.
- For those who benefit from knowing what is coming next and how much longer they need to participate, a "**To Do/Finished**" board could be displayed (see Figure 12.2). Instructors should reference this board after every yoga form is complete and move it to the "Finished" column.

Mindfulness routine

1. Deep breathing
2. Yoga forms
3. Relax and listen to meditation
4. Say positive thoughts out loud
5. Check in with our emotions
6. Clean up and have an AMAZING day

FIGURE 12.1: SAMPLE MINDFULNESS ROUTINE

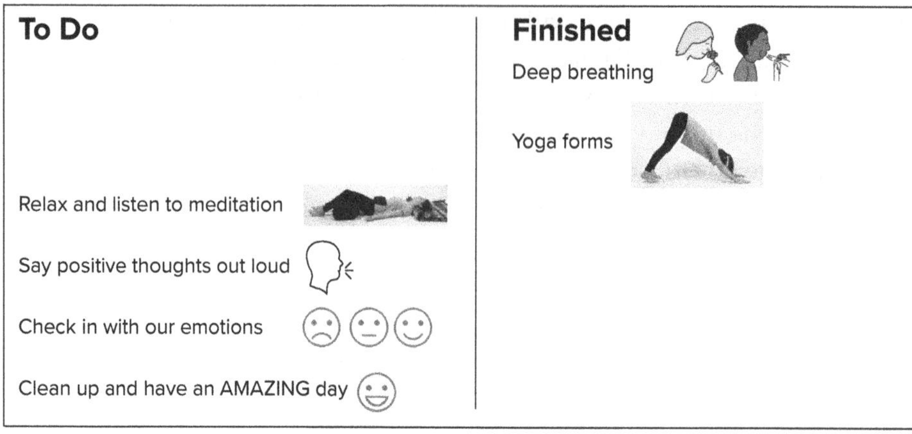

FIGURE 12.2: SAMPLE "TO DO/FINISHED" BOARD

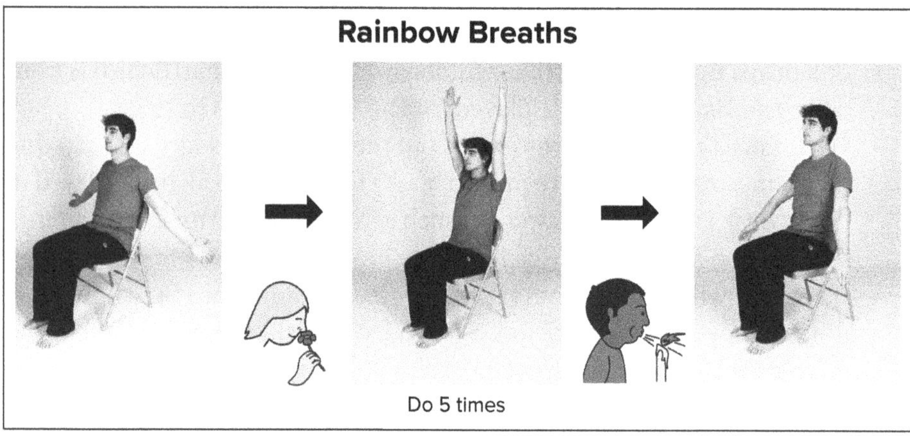

FIGURE 12.3: YOGA FORM VISUAL—RAINBOW BREATH

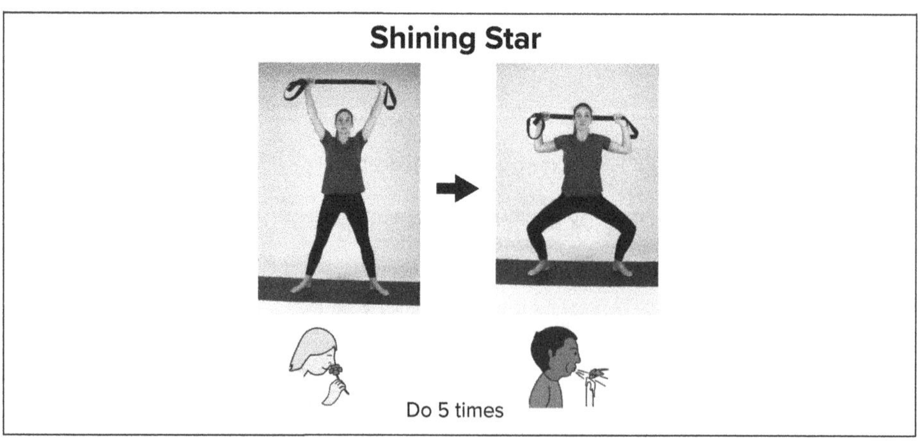

FIGURE 12.4: YOGA FORM VISUAL—SHINING STAR

B. For body positioning:

- Hand and feet markers (made of yoga mat material or Dycem) can be very helpful for some students to know where to plant their feet and/or hands on the mat.
- Bracelets can be made by the students to assist with learning right vs. left. Some instructors place colored floor tape along the edges of the mat; however, when the student changes body position to face a different direction, the "green" edge may no longer be on the "left" side (for example), which may be confusing for the student. Placing the visual cue directly on the body will always represent the left–right directional cues accurately, and is recommended.
- You might also consider giving each student a different-color yoga sock or glove for each hand/foot to help them discriminate left vs. right. These yoga socks and gloves have special rubber bumps on the bottom to help prevent slippage.

AROUSAL REGULATION NEEDS

Students fluctuate throughout the day between various levels of alertness. They may be feeling hyperaroused and anxious, or low, slow, and hypoaroused, or maybe they feel good, calm, and ready to learn. As mentioned in Chapter 2, "window of tolerance" is a term used to describe the zone of arousal in which a person can function most effectively (see Figure 2.7). When planning a SMYLE™ session it is important to keep these levels of alertness in mind. Some students may operate at one of these levels for the majority of their time at school. If this is the case, then SMYLE™ instructors should plan accordingly for those specific students in the sessions. It is also common for students who are usually quite stable in their arousal levels to have an "off day" or "tough moment" due to a variety of factors (such as test anxiety, lack of sleep, sickness, family troubles, social anxiety, and/or other causes). Thus, it is important for SMYLE™ instructors to be prepared to adapt their sessions in order to best meet the needs of each student.

Working with students who are hyperaroused

As you will recall from Chapter 3, students who are feeling ***hyperaroused*** can present as quite fidgety, irritable, easily startled, and have difficulty focusing or concentrating on one thing. Even though the threat or stressful situation may no longer be present, students' bodies could still be in a state as if it were. Examples observed in the classroom include an inability to sit in one place for extended or even short amounts of time, constant fidgeting with physical items, excessive wandering around the room, repetitive movements (e.g., rocking, picking, stimming), ruminating thoughts (observed as the student is lost in thought or exhibiting self-talk), asking anxiety-related questions over and over, and constantly looking at the door/window/clock. Some of these behaviors could be viewed as ADHD, obsessive-compulsive disorder, or other anxiety disorders. However, in all of these circumstances, unresolved trauma or toxic stress could be an additional underlying factor or even the real culprit.

To best support students in hyperaroused states, we have found it is best to match the pace of yoga to the student's level of arousal, so they can harness their attention and work toward gradually slowing themselves down over the course of the yoga session. The idea is to give the student a movement to focus on at all times, in coordination with the breath (if that is accessible to them). If the practice moves too slowly, they will find other, extraneous, ways to move, and if the verbal instruction is not appropriately paced, their anxious thoughts will fill the silence. It is also helpful to incorporate a lot of yoga forms and tools that could improve sensory filtering. Intense proprioceptive feedback through weight-bearing forms, especially while using a yoga band, can help draw the student's attention back into their body. Instructors can also cue students to focus their attention on specific body parts, movements, sensations, or breath exercises in an effort to increase grounding elements. What follows are some recommended grounding yoga forms and modification cues for addressing hyperarousal symptoms in students.

Grounding yoga forms:

- Lying Down Twist
- Standing Forward Fold
- Table
- Child
- Down Dog—grounding the hands and feet
- Crocodile
- Mountain
- Seated with hands in Adhi Mudra
- Pause Button (seated/standing/lying down)
- Seated or Standing in Pala Mudra
- Warrior 1 and 2
- Seated with hands in Bhu Mudra
- Shining Star.

When students demonstrate hyperarousal symptoms, it would be beneficial for instructors to give cues to the whole class to draw their attention to the grounding aspects of the yoga forms. This way, students will not feel singled out or embarrassed.

Some ways to increase the sense of grounding include:

- Drawing students' attention to the points of contact between their body and the surface(s) on which it rests.
- Focusing attention on energy (e.g., breath) in the body moving downward on the exhalation.
- Breathing out with slow breaths that come from deep in the belly or diaphragm (see Chapter 8).
- Using a yoga band to increase proprioceptive awareness (see Chapter 9).
- Holding weight-loading yoga forms to tolerance level, to accentuate the connection to ground and sensation in their bodies.
- Suggesting props to ensure the student is fully supported.

Here are some examples of verbal cues to encourage a sense of groundedness:

- In supine forms:
  - Feel the firm support of the earth/ground below your body.
  - Bring your attention to the parts of your body that are connected to the ground...your .... [list specific body parts, e.g., back, back of your legs/head].
- In Table forms:
  - Spread your fingers and press down with your whole hand—feel your connection to the solid ground.
- In standing yoga forms:
  - Press down through your feet, as though you have tree roots growing into the earth/ground.
  - Push your feet down and away from each other, as though you are trying to stretch your mat longer (in Warrior yoga forms and Star).

Here are some equipment suggestions for students who have limited mobility, to facilitate grounding:

- Use a blanket, block, or chair to help a student gain a sense of connection to the ground if they have limited flexibility. For example:
  - If *sitting cross-legged*: You might want to place a block under each knee if they don't come all the way to the floor, in order to help you feel more grounded.
  - If in a *reclined twist*: To help you relax all of your muscles, you may

wish to place a folded or rolled blanket or block under the parts of your body that don't reach the floor.
- If in a *standing yoga form*: You can lean against a wall or hold onto a chair if you would like extra support.

Working with students who are hypoaroused

On the other end of the arousal spectrum, some students in your SMYLE™ sessions may fall into the ***hypoaroused*** category. They may present as exhausted, overwhelmed, lost in their thoughts, depressed, and/or shutdown. Hypoarousal can be a bit trickier to work with than hyperarousal, as it can be the outcome of an unresolved freeze response, in which case, as Levine (1997) has noted, there is still an increase in adrenaline that needs to be discharged from the body. Therefore, it is important to keep an extra eye on those students who could potentially veer too far in the opposite arousal direction into unsafe or explosive states due to activation of their fight–flight response.

To best support students in hypoaroused states, we again match the pace of yoga to the student's current level of arousal. So, in this case, we start slowly to avoid overwhelming them with demands that are out of sync with their own bodymind state, and then we gradually work toward increasing the pace and energy demands over the course of the yoga session. We emphasize more uplifting yoga forms to move the energy upward. However, judging where to start can depend on the individual student. Some may be more motivated to attend the yoga session if they anticipate starting in a reclined position; however, a portion of these same students may tend to fall asleep if they do! In the latter case, it may be best to begin in a seated position. It can also be helpful to adjust your voice level, background music, and lighting just a half note higher than where your students are at, to gently nudge them along. However, if you increase the pace too fast, the students may start to withdraw from the session mentally and physically. So be sure to continually read the room to gauge students' responses and adjust the session accordingly. If students are still responding low and slow as the session progresses, respect their current state and teach a slower, restorative session.

Here are some recommended yoga forms and accommodations for addressing hyporarousal symptoms in students:

Uplifting yoga forms:

- Robin's Breath
- Seated Cat to Cobra
- Extended Mountain
- Standing Half Moon (Flow)

- Standing Waterfall (Flow)
- Clamshell Twist
- Rainbow Breath
- Star
- Static Warrior 1
- Dynamic Warrior 1
- Airplane
- Baby Cobra
- Hands in Ushas Mudra (seated or standing)
- Hands in Hakini Mudra (seated or standing)
- Hands in Full Heart Mudra (seated or standing).

Uplifting accommodations for students who are hypoaroused include:

- Encouraging students to soften their facial muscles, and even put a smile on their face.
- Spending more time on instructions to encourage extra expansion in chest (heart) opening forms.
- Adding in uplifting affirmations or comments when in certain yoga forms.
- Providing alternative positions (e.g., chair, mat, standing) to promote a more uplifting posture.
- Performing modified moves that are easier in exertion and flexibility.
- Offering students to take breaks when needed.
- Asking staff to help assist students who need more physical and/or emotional support.

ATTENTION SPAN

According to Helen Neville, whose research was spotlighted on PBS, a reasonable attention span to expect for a student is 2–3 minutes per year of their age (Brain Balance 2021). It is worth keeping these ranges in mind for planning purposes:

- 4 years old: 8–12 minutes
- 6 years old: 12–18 minutes
- 8 years old: 16–24 minutes
- 10 years old: 20–30 minutes
- 12 years old: 24–36 minutes
- 14 years old: 28–42 minutes
- 16 years old: 32–48 minutes.

These are only estimations. Each student's attention span will vary depending on a variety of ***environmental*** (e.g., distractions, sensory stimuli), ***interpersonal*** (e.g., comfort level with staff and peers, language processing), and ***individual*** (e.g., interest, hunger, fatigue, emotions, stress, disability) factors. Current research also is showing a decrease in attention span due to the digitized world we now live in (Paul, Baker, and Cochran, 2012). Students do not have to learn to wait for things they want to see or do; in most cases they click a link and it is instantaneous. SMYLE™ practices allow students a break from the fast-moving, tech-focused world, and provide them a scheduled time to turn their attention inward and focus on their body–mind connection.

In school settings, learning academic content is the primary focus. As a result, very few classroom schedules have enough wiggle room to allow for 15–20 consecutive minutes per day for mindfulness practices. This is why it is so important for teachers to plan ahead and make their allotted mindfulness time the most meaningful for the students. The duration of a yoga or mindfulness session should depend on the needs of the students at that moment and the purpose of the session, such as to prepare for the day, improve focus on a difficult lesson, or transition more easily to a new activity. Even a minute or two can be very helpful during transition times, to get up and do a few stretches in coordination with the breath. Done in this manner, the yoga techniques are used as "sensory diet" tools to help students stay self-regulated during the school day. In addition, some schools can afford to schedule longer yoga or mindfulness sessions often as part of a physical education class, occupational therapy/physical therapy session, or after-school club. These sessions are generally the same length as a typical school class period (45–60 minutes), and can allow for more content. But for a classroom of students with short attention spans or low endurance, it is often helpful to break up the session into two activities or yoga and a break time.

In the next chapter you will find SMYLE™ sessions of different lengths to meet the varying needs of students in the classroom or other group settings throughout a typical day. We suggest teaching the sequences that match the length of the attention spans of the students you are working with. For younger students, incorporate a sense of play, or stimulate their imagination using yoga stories (see Chapter 10) to make it fun and engaging. For older students, match your directions, pace, and breathwork to their own abilities in an effort to maintain their attention.

FAMILIARITY WITH SEQUENCES/ROUTINES

When planning a SMYLE™ class, we recommend teaching the same sequence or repeating large chunks of it from week to week. Consider the energy level and abilities of the students in your class, and continue the repetition period until they seem comfortable and confident with the given yoga forms. Then add in one or two new forms into that basic sequence. Repeat the updated sequence as long as necessary until the students demonstrate the confidence and openness to try new yoga forms. Students of all ages and abilities tend to like repetition and can relax more into a class when it is somewhat predictable and they can anticipate what is coming next. For students with special needs, this is crucial, while typically developing students—especially older ones—may need the routine updated on a more frequent basis to keep the class fresh. Themed classes work well in the latter case, so the instructor can teach new yoga forms in each class but keep the focus around a central theme, such as breath, grounding, resiliency, and so on. We have found that Guideline #5 statements often serve as great inspiration for developing themed sessions. Across all contexts, it comes down to the instructor's ability to read the needs and interests of their students and then plan the SMYLE™ session accordingly. Unfortunately in a group class, students will likely not all have the same needs. Therefore, it is extremely important to plan *in advance* how you might modify the yoga forms and movements for certain students in your class to make the yoga experience accessible for all.

MOBILITY CHALLENGES

Students who use wheelchairs should make their own choice on how they want to participate in SMYLE™ sessions. Some may choose to participate in their chair and others out of their chair (if there is enough staff support to do so safely). If they participate out of their chair, they can be positioned with props such as pillows and bolsters on the floor or on a mat table. It is most important that the least anxiety-provoking position is chosen by the student themselves or with the help of the staff working with them. Some students who spend most of their school day in their chair and have very limited mobility may feel anxiety at the thought of getting out of their chair. These students can participate to the best of their ability in their chair, or possibly recline their chair and place a weighted bag on their lap instead. If the "rest option" is their choice, instructors can make this time a mindful moment by cuing up relaxing music or a guided meditation for them to listen to in their headphones while their classmates are doing the yoga sequence. The school day is very stressful and chaotic for many students, so a "relaxing rest time" for highly anxious students (with mobility challenges or not) could be extremely beneficial for the overall mental health of that student, if that is what their body is telling them they need. However, it is important to encourage all students to take off their headphones and join in during the Body Scan and Final Relaxation/meditation sections of class, so they can benefit from them.

When working with a group of students with mixed mobility levels, it is desirable to have an assistant, preferably an occupational therapist, physical therapist, or adaptive physical education teacher, who can assist with the demonstrations and be an extra set of eyes to ensure everyone's needs are taken care of. In school settings, we have found it most effective for the lead instructor to model the mat versions of the program while the assistant listens to the lead instructor's words and adapts for the students in the chairs. The students using chairs then copy the assistant's moves "Simon Says" style. We have found that most of the verbal cues from the lead instructor will apply for both groups of students (those practicing on the mat or in a chair). The major difference occurs in the initial set-up of the yoga form when providing grounding and alignment cues for positioning the body on the mat or chair. The cues involving movement of the spine, upper extremities, and coordinating breath with movement usually apply to everyone. If the lead instructor tried to verbally communicate every detail to both groups of students, the class would hardly be relaxing at all as there would be twice as much chatter from the instructor, and the students would not know which directions are intended for them! When there are no assistants in a class of students with mixed mobility levels, it is often easier and more effective for the instructor to present a chair class without a mat option.

CREATING YOGA AND MINDFULNESS SEQUENCES

In this book, we present a variety of sequence options for various situations, to help take the "guesswork" out of it for those instructors who do not have formal training as yoga or mindfulness teachers. However, there may be times when you feel that something a bit different is needed for a situation, so here we offer some things to consider in these circumstances. First, please remember that yoga forms were originally developed for the purpose of preparing the body for meditation. This is clearly expressed in the sequence of ***Patanjali's Eight Limbs of Yoga*** (see Chapter 6). So, in a combined yoga and meditation session, the most meditative portion of the session should follow the active practice, although typically we start with a short Body Scan to begin to draw the person out of their thoughts and into their body and the room prior to presenting the yoga forms.

Beginning: We start the active practice with warm-up stretches for the spine, which also prepare the muscles around the lungs for breathwork. These "Breath Prep"/spinal warm-ups help students create a strong breath–body connection, which is essential for grounding the student and helping them achieve a sense of safety and calm. Focusing on and integrating sensation, movement, and breath in present-moment awareness also promotes clarity of mind. This creates a strong foundation on which to include other elements of practice to help uplift and empower the students.

Warm-up stretches can be performed in the following positions:

- ***Reclined*** (e.g., Whole Body Stretch, Reclined Half Moon, Knees to Chest)
- ***Table*** (e.g., Table to Cat Flow, Tiger Flow)
- ***Seated*** (e.g., Rainbow Breath, Robin's Breath, Seated Half Moon, Cat Flow)
- ***Standing*** (e.g., Extended Mountain with yoga band, Standing Half Moon Stretch Flow).

By lengthening the spine through whole body stretches, side bends, and forward spinal bends, we help to loosen the muscles around the spine so they are better able to make subtle adjustments and also avoid injury during more challenging yoga forms, such as Down Dog or the Warrior forms.

Middle: After the students are warmed up, the middle of the session is where the bulk of the yoga forms are presented. During this position of the class we emphasize body sensing (Guideline #3) and offer positive suggestions (Guideline #4) for some of the yoga forms to help students connect to the emotional qualities often elicited by particular forms. It is important to remember that you do not need to include a positive suggestion for every yoga form you teach, because this could be too much language for students to process. However, including one or two that match the purpose or theme of your session could be very impactful for the students. When choosing the structure of your session keep in mind these questions—What is your purpose? Is it to help ground students? Is it to uplift them at that moment? Is it to calm them down from a distressing situation? Meet the students where they are at that moment, and choose which positive suggestions best match their needs.

End: We recommend ending all SMYLE™ sessions in a resting form where the students can relax and let the changes in their bodymind sink in. Depending on the attention span and level of support needed, some SMYLE™ classes rest quietly in the final yoga form in silence for 30 seconds to 3 minutes. Other students who have difficulty resting in silence could benefit from guided breathwork (e.g., breathe in...breathe out...etc.), or listening to a guided meditation. We use several different scripts for Final Relaxation, but every one of them includes some sort of body sensing and breath awareness element. As mentioned earlier, we stay away from sending people on "trips" to places in guided meditations when working with traumatized individuals unless they create the trip themselves (to access their Inner Resource/"safe place"). As with the positive suggestions, choose guided meditations based on the intended theme or message for your session (e.g., uplifting, calming, ocean, nature, etc.).

CHAPTER 13

Sample SMYLE™ Practices

This chapter presents a variety of routines that can be easily implemented at various times of the day across different settings (e.g., schools, camps, group residential programs, yoga studios, home programming, clubs, health centers) to address the self-regulation needs of the children and adolescents in the moment. These include the following:

SMYLE™ session sequence:

- SMYLE™ Master Sequence for mat and/or chair.

Body-sensing scripts:

- Child-friendly Body Scan
- Tension and Release Exercise.

Scripts for Final Relaxation (resting/integration):

- Short Script for Final Relaxation
- Longer Script for Final Relaxation
- 39-Point Meditation
- Safe Place Meditation.

Short situational routines:

- Morning Routine (10–15 minutes)
- Mindful Transitions Between Classes/Activities (1–3 minutes)
- Practices for After Lunch (5–10 minutes)
- Self-Regulation Mini-Routines:
  - Reclined Calming Sequence (5–10 minutes)
  - Reclined Energizing Sequence (5–10 minutes)

- Table Calming Sequence (5–10 minutes)
- Table Energizing Sequence (5–10 minutes)
- Seated Calming Sequence (5–10 minutes)
- Seated Energizing Sequence (5–10 minutes)
- Standing Calming Sequence (5–10 minutes)
- Standing Energizing Sequence (5–10 minutes).

Table 13.1 presents a Sensory-Enhanced Yoga® class session designed for a group of students using mats, chairs, or a mixture of both. Oftentimes, students who use chairs are also able to perform some standing yoga forms. Students with mobility challenges usually have the most difficulty transitioning up and down from the mat. Some may choose to do the majority of the session in the chair, and may then lie down on the mat for final relaxation. Some students who remain in the chair during final relaxation find it helpful to have another chair positioned in front of them, with a blanket folded over the backrest to rest their heads on.

Table 13.1: SMYLE™ Master Sequence for mat or chair

	Segments	On a mat	Using a chair
1	Segment A: Breathwork prep	Whole Body Stretch	Rainbow Breath
		Half Moon Stretch Breathe into stretched ribcage	Seated Half Moon Stretch Breathe into stretched ribcage
		Knees to Chest	Knee to Chest
2	Segment B: Centering/body sensing/breath	SMYLE™ Body Scan	SMYLE™ Body Scan
3	Segment C: Supine forms	Leg Stretches 1, 2, 3 (with yoga band)	Leg Stretch (with yoga band) Optional: *Can support leg on another chair when using yoga band*
		Clamshell Twist or Lying Down Twist	Owl (Seated Twist)
4	Segment D: Table forms	Table Cat Flow Choose a flow (*in italics*): *Tiger Flow* *Twisting Cat* *Rabbit Hop* Down Dog Dolphin Flow	Seated Cat Flow Choose a flow (*in italics*): *Seated Tiger Flow* *Seated Twisting Cat* *Setting Sun*

5	Segment E: Standing stretches (with yoga band)	Mountain Extended Mountain *(with yoga band)* Standing Half Moon *(with yoga band)* Standing Twist *(with yoga band)*	Seated Mountain Seated Extended Mountain *(with yoga band)* Seated Half Moon *(with yoga band)* Seated Twist *(with yoga band)*
6	Segment F: Standing forms	Star/Shining Star Airplane Warrior 1 and/or 2 Windmill	Seated Star/Shining Star Seated Airplane Seated Warrior 1 and/or 2 Seated Windmill
		Standing Forward Fold Waterfall	Seated Forward Fold (two-stage) Seated Waterfall
		Tree	Modified Tree using chair or wall *(if capable)* or Seated Tree
7	Segment G: Prone forms	Baby Cobra *Then Knees to Chest as counterform*	Seated Cat to Cobra
		Crocodile	Seated Crocodile
8	Segment H: Resting form	Lying Down Rest Form (Savasana)	Seated Mountain
9	Segment I: Mudra meditation	Student-centered Mudra meditation	Student-centered Mudra meditation

BODY-SENSING SCRIPTS

SMYLE™ Body Scan

Note: The headings are listed below to organize the information, but are not intended to be stated out loud.

POSITIONING

I invite you to join me for an exercise to notice different parts of your body and how they feel right now. Take a moment to get yourself into a comfortable position... You can sit in a chair or lie on the floor... Do whatever feels right for you, right now.

[If you have bolsters, blankets, or pillows, feel free to offer them to your students.] You may close your eyes or let your eyes rest open...[pause].

LISTENING TO THE BODY AND MIND

Please always listen to your body and mind during this practice. If something hurts or makes you feel uncomfortable, please stop and make a change so that you feel better. If something feels too hard or makes you too tired, you can rest and join back in when you're ready.

Remember, it is normal for thoughts, emotions, or worries to come up during practice. You might imagine that those thoughts are clouds up in the sky...and as you breathe in and out...just watch them pass by.

SENSING SURROUNDINGS

Now notice what is around you...any sounds...smells...the feeling of your clothes on your skin...and the feeling of the parts of your body touching the floor or the chair...

BODY SENSING

And now let's move our attention to different parts of the body... Just notice what you feel...starting with your feet... Do they feel warm or cool?... Relaxed or tight?... These feelings are called sensations... No sensation is right or wrong... just practice being aware of these sensations in your body.

Now notice your legs, from your feet all the way up to the top of your legs... Do your legs feel warm or cool?... Relaxed or tight?... Are they comfortable?... If not, feel free to move your legs to a better position...

As you are ready, move your attention to your back...notice the bottom of your back...and then slowly move your attention all the way up to the top of your back... Are there any areas of tightness in your back?... Any areas that feel relaxed?... Does your back feel warm or cool?... Just notice what you find... If you notice that your thoughts have wandered, just bring your attention back to my voice and your body.

Now, move your attention to the front of your body...starting with your belly... Does it feel empty or full?... Relaxed or tight?... What sensations do you feel in your belly right now?

As you're ready, move your attention up to your chest...what sensations do you feel here?... Does your chest feel calm or tight?... Does it move with your breath?... In the middle of your chest is your heart, can you feel it beating?... If you can, is it beating slow or fast?... Remember, nothing you feel is right or wrong... Noticing sensations in your body helps you understand how you are feeling... If you want, you can take a few nice slow breaths here to help the muscles in your chest soften and relax...

Now let your awareness travel down your arms all the way to your hands... Notice sensations in your hands and fingers... Are your fingers resting or moving?... Do you feel any tingling?... Now notice your arms, all the way from your hands up to your shoulders... Do they feel warm or cool?...relaxed or tight?... Are they comfortable? If not, feel free to move your arms to a better position...

When you're ready, bring your attention to your neck and throat... Do the muscles here feel tight or comfortable?... Now move up to the face...jaw...mouth... eyes...forehead...all the way to the top of your head... Do the muscles in your face feel tight, or soft and relaxed?... Now focus your attention on the thoughts inside your head... Are they racing thoughts or quiet thoughts?... If you want, try to notice your next thought that comes up...now let it travel by like a cloud up in the sky...

BREATH AWARENESS

As you're ready, notice the body breathing by itself. Without controlling it in any way, try to be aware of the air moving in...and out...in...and out... Notice what your breath is doing today...is it fast or slow?... Calm or tight?... Just notice your breath in this moment...right now.

Inner Resource: This is a natural spot to insert the Inner Resource/"safe place" (see Chapter 7).

DIAPHRAGMATIC BREATH

If you want, you can put your hand on your belly to feel your body breathing... feel your belly rise when you breathe in...and sink down when you breathe out...

Breathing in...breathing out...

Breathing in...breathing out...

Continue breathing in and out...at your own pace...

As you are ready, you may move your hand from your belly and rest it in a comfortable position...as you continue to focus on your breath...

WHOLE BODY AWARENESS

Now become aware of your whole body...the front side...and back side...inside... and outside...welcoming every sensation that you now feel...

If you like, stay with these sensations for a little while longer.

After 30 seconds to 1 minute: Now take a slow breath in...and out...

[If you are using this script as a Body Scan exercise prior to an active yoga practice, move into "Breath Prep" stretches next. Otherwise, end the Body Scan as described below.]

Bring your attention back to your body in the room.

Wiggle your toes and fingers...turn your head from side to side...move the muscles in your face. If you want, put a smile on your face because you took time to care for your body and mind. Open your eyes when you're ready.

Take a moment to smile and wave to your friends and teachers, wishing them a good day. When you're ready you can sit up and get ready for ....

SMYLE™ Tension and Release Exercise

It is quite common for traumatized individuals to dissociate from their bodies in order to numb out powerful bodily sensations arising from overwhelming emotions. In doing so, they are often unaware of how much tension they are carrying in their bodies. A primary goal of trauma-informed yoga is to help these individuals become safely re-embodied, which requires attending to bodily sensation. However, this needs to proceed in a careful manner in order to avoid becoming inundated by these sensations. Remember Rothschild's (2009) pressurized soda bottle analogy (Chapter 7): the safest way to release the pressure is to open and close the cap in a slow, cautious, and intentional manner, so that the contents don't burst out.

Although difficult emotions may arise in any mind–body exercise, the Tension and Release Exercise is considered to be a generally safe way to help traumatized individuals begin to identify what they are feeling in their bodies and learn how to release it. In general, focusing on "muscle tension" is much more innocuous than asking a person to focus on other types of bodily sensations—such as the feeling in the gut—that are more representative of strong emotions such as grief, sadness, or fear. That said, the SMYLE™ version of this exercise avoids asking students to tense the hips and buttocks, so as not to risk triggering children who may have experienced sexual abuse. The exercise can be presented alone or at the beginning of a yoga practice for the body-sensing component. Note that the headings are listed below to organize the information, but are not intended to be stated out loud.

POSITIONING

I invite you to join me in an exercise to practice squeezing and relaxing the muscles in your body. You can lie down or sit in a chair. I will ask you to squeeze a body part, hold it, and then let it go. As you squeeze, imagine you are giving that body part a big hug. As you let go, notice what you feel there... It may feel tight or loose and relaxed... These feelings are called sensations... You may notice sensations or you may not, and that's okay. Just notice what you feel... Please breathe in any way that is comfortable for you.

MOUTH AND FACE

Focus on your mouth... Open your mouth wide...then close it... Press your lips together, close your eyes tight, and squeeze all the muscles in your face toward your nose... When you are ready, relax your muscles by letting them go soft... Notice any sensations... Let's do that one more time. Breathing in, squeeze all the muscles in your face... As you breathe out...let the muscles go soft. Notice what you feel.

NECK AND SHOULDERS

Now, squeeze the muscles of your neck and shoulders by lifting your shoulders toward your ears...squeeze these muscles tight...and then turn the muscles off... Notice any sensations... If your mind starts to wander...that is okay...just bring your attention back to your breath and body. Let's try it one more time...neck and shoulder muscles tight...then let the muscles go soft... Notice what you feel.

ARMS AND HANDS

Now slowly make fists with both hands. You can straighten your arms if you want to. Tighten your fists...forearms...elbows...upper arms...squeezing the muscles in your arms... Then let the muscles go soft...letting all your arm muscles go soft... Notice any sensations... Let's try that again...squeeze your fists and arms tight...and...then let them go soft... Notice what you feel.

LEGS AND FEET

Now straighten your legs out in front of you, keeping the heels of your feet on the floor. Then, as you are ready, point your toes away from you...and slowly squeeze the muscles of your feet...ankles...lower legs...knees...and thighs... squeezing all the muscles of your legs... Then let the muscles relax, letting all your leg muscles go soft... Notice any sensations...

Let's try that again, but this time, press your heels away from you...as you squeeze the muscles of both legs, squeezing them tight...and...then let them go soft... When you are ready, you can move your feet back under your knees if you are seated in a chair... Notice what you feel.

WHOLE BODY

Now squeeze your whole body tight, from your head to your toes...including both arms and legs...making the muscles as tight as you can...and then let the all the muscles relax...letting your whole body go soft... Once again, tighten all the muscles in your body...squeeze...squeeze...then let them all relax, letting your whole body go soft... Notice what you feel.

NOTICING SENSATION WITH BODY AT REST *[SOFTER, SLOWER VOICE]*

Now let's notice the body at rest...feel all sensations in your face...jaw...tongue... inside of your mouth...lips...corners of your eyes...forehead...and top of your head.

Notice or sense your neck and shoulders...invite the muscles to go soft.

Sense your arms...all the way to your hands and fingers... Arms soft and completely at rest. Sense your belly...inside and outside...you might notice your belly move with your breath.

And then sense your legs...all the way down to your feet and toes... Legs soft and completely at rest.

Now become aware of your whole body...the front side...and back side...inside... outside...welcoming every sensation that you now feel...

If you like, just stay with these sensations for a little while.

[Allow (1–2) minutes of rest.]

As you're ready, take a slow breath in...and out...

Slowly bring your attention back to your body in the room.

Wiggle your toes and fingers...turn your head from side to side...move the muscles in your face. If you want, put a smile on your face because you took time to care for your body and mind. Open your eyes when you're ready.

Take a moment to smile and wave to your friends and teachers.

Wish them a good day.

When you're ready you can sit up and get ready for ....

SCRIPTS FOR FINAL RELAXATION

SMYLE™ Short Script for Final Relaxation (Savasana)

I invite you to join me in a short resting meditation... If you would like/when you're ready, find a comfortable position in your chair or lying down on your mat... If you are lying down on your mat, you may wish to place a small pillow under your head and a larger pillow under your knees, and then rest your arms by your sides. You may close your eyes or let your eyes rest open.

Now think about relaxing all the muscles of your arms and legs to let them completely soften and rest... Let the weight of your body sink lower and lower into the support of the floor or your chair... Notice and feel the firm support of the earth/ground under you. The earth is solid and strong... See if you can feel the strength of the earth rise up through your own body, giving you strength... The earth is always there to support you.

As you are ready, notice your breath moving through your whole body as you breathe in...and breathe out...in...and out...

As you breathe out, sense your body sinking down deeper into the ground, every muscle softening even more into the support of the earth/ground... Invite your whole body to completely rest into this support...

As you rest here, welcome all parts of this experience...every feeling...every sensation...every breath... There is no place to go...nothing to do...except be here now.

[Pause for 30–90 seconds, and then invite the students back to a state of alertness, with the script below.]

Slowly bring your attention back to your body in the room.

Wiggle your toes and fingers; turn your head from side to side, move the muscles in your face.

If you want, put a smile on your face because you took time to care for your body and mind.

Open your eyes when you're ready.

Take a moment to smile and wave to your friends and teachers... Wish them a good day.

When you're ready you can sit up and get ready for ....

SMYLE™ Longer Script for Final Relaxation (Savasana)[1]

Roll your head from side to side, and then let it rest in a comfortable position back in the center. Let your mouth open if it wants. Soften the eyes—you can keep them open or let them close.

And notice any sensations or feelings in your ears...cheeks...nose...eyes...forehead... Next we will focus our attention on other parts of our body...no need to do anything, just notice and feel...the back of the head and neck...shoulders...and follow any sensations or feelings down through the shoulders and into the arms.

Just feel your right arm...starting with your right shoulder...upper arm...lower arm...all the way down to your hand...noticing how your whole right arm feels.

Let's move our attention to your left arm...starting with your left shoulder... left upper arm...lower arm...all the way down to your left hand...noticing how your whole left arm feels.

And bring your attention into your throat and let the muscles go soft in your throat.

Draw your awareness from the throat down to the chest and heart center... into your ribcage and around to your upper back...down to your lower back... and around to your belly...noticing sensation inside and around the belly area...

Draw attention to the right hip...upper right leg...lower right leg...right foot... entire leg from the hip to the foot.

1 This meditation uses more complex language. It is best used with older students who have good receptive language skills.

Then shift your awareness over to the left leg...left hip...left upper leg...left lower leg...left foot...entire left leg...

Feel both feet and legs simultaneously...simply noticing sensation...

Allow all of the sensations throughout the entire body to blend together...so the entire body is perceived simultaneously...front side and back side...right side and left side...inside and outside...feeling the entire physical body as pure sensation...and welcoming every experience that is now present in awareness...

[Pause for several minutes.]

You may begin to wiggle your fingers and toes, taking your time as you now transition into your waking life...stretching however you wish... You may wish to lie on one side for a few additional moments before coming up to a sitting position...and when you are ready, slowly open your eyes and come fully back to your wide-awake and alert state of being.

Slowly bring your attention back to your body in the room.

Wiggle your toes and fingers, turn your head from side to side, move the muscles in your face.

If you want, put a smile on your face because you took time to care for your body and mind.

Open your eyes when you're ready.

Take a moment to smile and wave to your friends and teachers.

Wish them a good day.

When you're ready you can sit up and get ready for ....

SMYLE™ 39-Point Meditation

(Adapted from the traditional 61-Point Meditation.)

Roll your head from side to side, and then let it rest in a comfortable spot... Allow your jaw to hang open if it wants, and your tongue to fall to the back of your throat. Soften your eyes, and the muscles in your forehead...

Sense the parts of your body that touch the ground below you, and invite your body to soften and rest down on the ground.

Rest the muscles of your throat...rest the muscles of your belly...and start to notice your breath, the way it moves on its own...in...and out...of your body with no need to change it...

And now we will focus your attention on different parts of your body.

Picture a butterfly flying over you and landing for a split second on each point before flying off to the next spot. There is no need to do anything but simply notice:

1. Your forehead
2. Your throat
3. Your right shoulder
4. Your right elbow
5. Your right wrist
6. Your right hand
7. Your right wrist
8. Your right elbow
9. Your right shoulder
10. Your throat
11. Your left shoulder
12. Your left elbow
13. Your left wrist
14. Your left hand
15. Your left wrist
16. Your left elbow
17. Your left shoulder
18. Your throat
19. Your heart
20. Your belly
21. Your right hip
22. Your right knee
23. Your right ankle
24. Your right foot
25. Your right ankle
26. Your right knee
27. Your right hip
28. Your belly

29. Your left hip
30. Your left knee
31. Your left ankle
32. Your left foot
33. Your left ankle
34. Your left knee
35. Your left hip
36. Your belly
37. Your heart
38. Your throat
39. Your forehead (repeat this last one three times).

[Stay just long enough on each point for the students to register it, but not long enough for the mind to wander, i.e., about 6 seconds, including the time it takes to state the body part.]

Slowly bring your attention back to your body in the room.

Wiggle your toes and fingers, turn your head from side to side, move the muscles in your face.

If you want, put a smile on your face because you took time to care for your body and mind.

Open your eyes when you're ready.

Take a moment to smile and wave to your friends and teachers.

Wish them a good day.

When you're ready you can sit up and get ready for ....

SMYLE™ Safe Place Meditation

As a reminder, the Safe Place Meditation in Chapter 7 is another script that works very well at the end (or at any point) of a SMYLE™ session.

SHORT SITUATIONAL ROUTINES

SMYLE™ Morning Mindfulness Routine (10–15 minutes)

How students feel when they enter your classroom sets the tone for the rest of the day. As mentioned in Chapter 7, Meg prepares her classroom to try to relax every sense (i.e., relaxing music playing in background, dimmed lights, nature scene displayed on screen, consistent four-step arrival routine displayed on screen). The combination of a consistent, calm environment along with visually displaying clear expectations for their arrival routine significantly decreases students' anxiety. Students start their day off with a sense of greater independence and accomplishment, which sets a positive tone for the rest of the school day ahead. Once everyone has gotten settled, Meg rings the bells three times, signaling it is time for the Morning Mindfulness Routine to begin. Since she does this every day, all the students know to make their way to their yoga spaces. Here is the routine that Meg found to be highly successful for the students in her classroom.

Morning Mindfulness Routine (see Figure 13.1):

- Pause Button (deep breathing)
- Rainbow Breath
- Owl (Seated Twist)
- Standing Half Moon Stretch
- Standing Waterfall
- Standing Shining Star
- Relax and listen to a meditation
- Say positive thoughts out loud (see Figure 13.2)
- Check in with our emotions (see Figure 13.3)
- Clean up and have an AMAZING day! (see Figure 13.4).

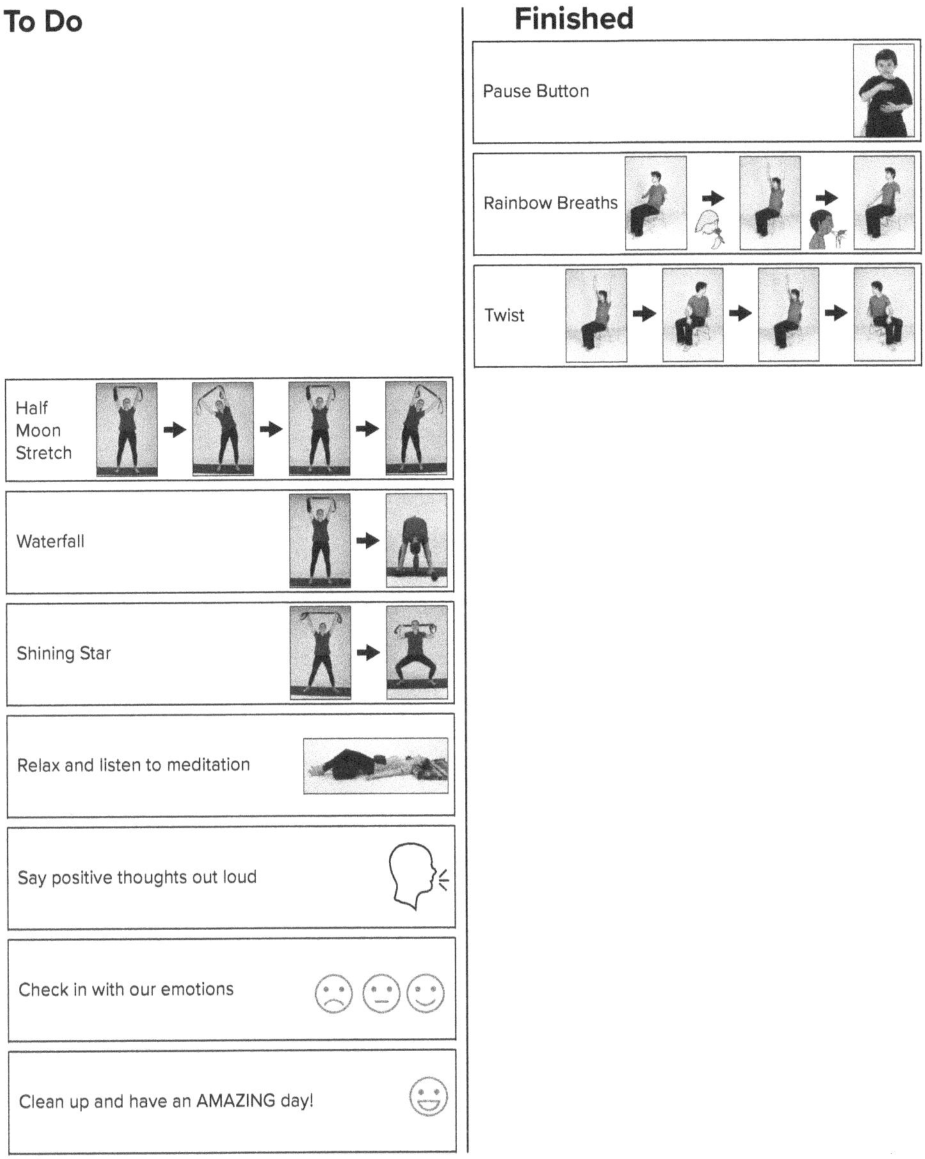

FIGURE 13.1: MORNING MINDFULNESS ROUTINE SLIDE (PROJECTED ONTO FRONT BOARD)

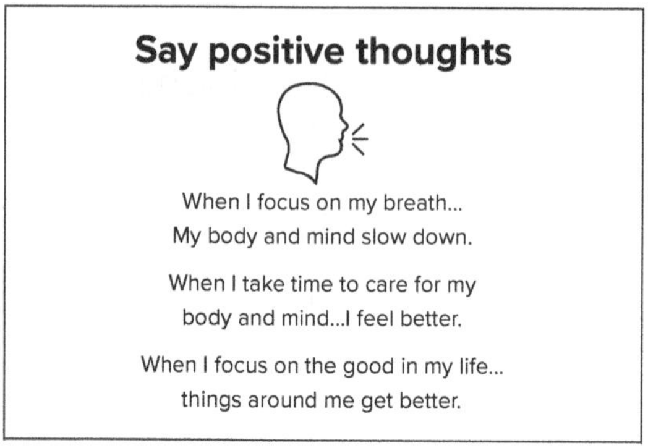

FIGURE 13.2: POSITIVE THOUGHTS SLIDE (PROJECTED ONTO FRONT BOARD)

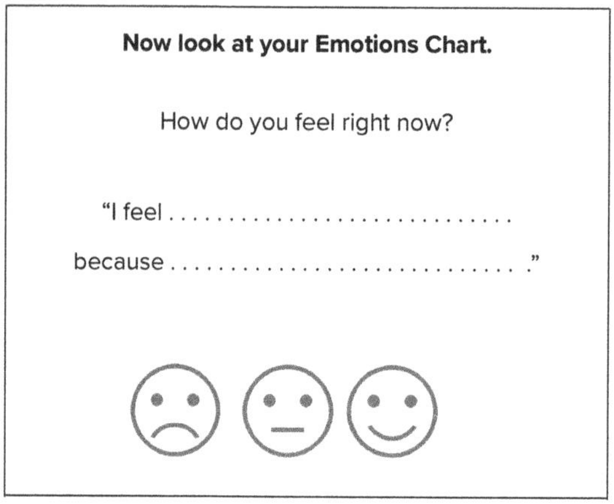

FIGURE 13.3: EMOTIONAL CHECK IN SLIDE (PROJECTED ONTO FRONT BOARD)

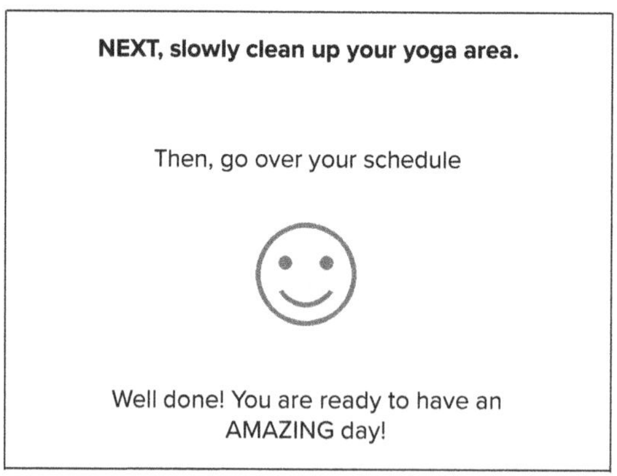

FIGURE 13.4: END OF MORNING MINDFULNESS ROUTINE SLIDE (PROJECTED ONTO FRONT BOARD)

SMYLE™ Mindful Transitions Between Classes/Activities (1–3 minutes)

As discussed in Chapter 8 (Guideline #2), breathing practices lend themselves well to helping students transition from one activity to the next, as they are the most powerful way to self-regulate, and can be performed within just a couple of minutes. The following practices have been found to be especially effective for this purpose (see Chapter 8 for directions):

- Five Pause Button Breaths
- Five Waterfall Breaths
- Five Rainbow Breaths
- Five Robin's Breaths
- Mindful moment 3–2–1 (see Figure 7.2)
- Five Snake Breaths.

These practices also help students release any frustration and tension that may have developed from a challenging task, so they can start fresh on the next task.

SMYLE™ Practices for After Lunch (10–15 minutes)

After lunch, it is important to allow time for students to digest their food, and so we do not recommend having students participate in active yoga forms at this time. However, after lunch is a perfect time to schedule a guided meditation or restorative yoga practice. We recommend any of the following, which are presented later in this chapter, except as noted:

- Safe Place Meditation (see Chapter 7)
- Child-friendly Body Scan
- Short Script for Final Relaxation
- Tension and Release Exercise
- 39-Point Meditation
- Restorative Yoga Session (see Chapter 9).

SMYLE™ Mini Routines for Self-Regulation

Table 13.2 shows a variety of mini-routines designed to help students who are either hyperaroused or hypoaroused rebalance their autonomic nervous systems to prepare for their next activity. Before beginning a short SMYLE™ session, first read the energy level of your students to determine what they would most benefit from in that moment. Are they moving low and slow, or are they amped up and in need of some calming practices? Maybe you have a combination of both! If you have a group with students with ranging energy levels, we recommend doing the "Energizing in a grounding way" sequences in Table 13.2 because all of the forms are heart-opening in a grounding and calming way, which could benefit all.

Next, decide which body position you want your students to work from. Make this decision based on time of day, best use of the space you are located in, and which positioning would be most conducive for the next activity on their schedule. In a school setting, if math work is next, we recommend doing work from the seated or standing position to increase ease of transitions for students to academic work. However, if it is the end of the day and students need to calm down or recharge from the day's many activities, a Table or reclined practice might work better.

Table 13.2: Mini Routines for Self-Regulation

The most important suggestion is to start where the student is at...in...that...very... moment, and then gradually move them into balance through more calming or energizing practices. This will improve the student's ability to function, learn new information, and handle unanticipated changes.

Starting position	Calming	Energizing in a grounding way
Reclined	1. Whole Body Stretch 2. Reclined Half Moon 3. Knees to Chest 4. Clamshell Twist or Lying Down Twist 5. Crocodile and/or 6. Lying Down Rest Form (Savasana) with Pause Button Mudra	1. Leg Stretch 1 with yoga band and Circles with yoga band 2. Clamshell Twist or Lying Down Twist 3. Baby Cobra 4. Knees to Chest 5. Lying Down Rest Form (Savasana) with Pause Button Mudra
Table	1. Table 2. Cat Flow 3. Rabbit Hop 4. Twisting Cat 5. Child or 6. Extended Child with Adhi Mudra	1. Table 2. Cat Flow 3. Tiger Flow (rest in Child) 4. Twisting Cat 5. Extended Child with Hakini Mudra
Seated	1. Seated Mountain 2. Seated Robin's Breath 3. Seated Half Moon (alternate arms) 4. Owl (Seated Twist) 5. Setting Sun 6. Seated Forward Fold (Optional: with Adhi Mudra hands on floor) 7. Seated Mountain with Pala or Bhu Mudra	1. Seated Mountain 2. Seated Rainbow Breath 3. Seated Robin's Breath 4. Owl (Seated Twist) 5. Seated Warrior 1 or 6. Seated Warrior 2 to Seated Windmill 7. Seated Mountain with Ushas or Hakini Mudra

Seated	1. Seated Mountain 2. Seated Extended Mountain with Band 3. Seated Side Bend with Band 4. Seated Twist with Band 5. Seated Forward Fold 6. Seated Mountain with Pala or Dvimukham Mudra	1. Seated Mountain 2. Seated Cat Flow or Seated Cat to Cobra 3. Seated Tiger Flow 4. Seated Twisting Cat 5. Seated Leg Stretches 6. Seated Tree 7. Seated Mountain with Ushas or Hakini Mudra
Standing	1. Mountain 2. Standing Half Moon (alternate arms or use both arms with yoga band) 3. Standing Twist (yoga band recommended) 4. Waterfall (with or without yoga band) 5. Standing Forward Fold 6. Mountain with Full Heart Mudra	1. Mountain 2. Airplane 3. Shining Star (with or without yoga band) 4. Standing Twist (with or without yoga band) 5. Warrior 1 6. Standing Forward Fold 7. Mountain with Ushas or Hakini Mudra
Standing	1. Mountain 2. Extended Mountain (with yoga band) 3. Standing Half Moon (with yoga band) 4. Standing Twist (with yoga band) 5. Standing Forward Fold (with yoga band) 6. Mountain with Ushas Mudra	1. Mountain 2. Waterfall 3. Shining Star (with or without yoga band) 4. Standing Twist (with or without yoga band) 5. Warrior 2 to Windmill (Optional for advanced) 6. Standing Forward Fold 7. Mountain with Ushas or Hakini Mudra

CHAPTER 14

Yoga Forms on a Mat

On the following pages, we present the **directions**, **modifications**, **precautions**, **benefits**, and **suggested sequencing** of the yoga forms that we include in the SMYLE™ program. Each set of directions includes information on what guidelines are addressed through the cues. When first teaching students the yoga forms, we suggest starting out with just three or four forms at a time, and emphasizing the "**Set-Up**" cues, that is, the cues relating to the set-up and execution of the form unrelated to the guidelines, as well as the cues for **Guideline #1**, relating to promoting a sense of ***safety*** through grounding, and **Guideline #2**, relating to promoting a sense of ***calm*** through control of the breath (see Table 14.1).

Table 14.1: Cuing yoga forms through the guidelines

Guideline #1	SAFE: Grounding to promote a sense of safety.
Guideline #2	CALM: Connecting movement with the breath.
Guideline #3	CLEAR: Bring mind to present moment through body sensing.
Guideline #4	UPLIFTED: Emotionally connect to the yoga forms to promote positive beliefs and attitudes.
Guideline #5	EMPOWERED: Empowering life lessons for "off the mat" (inferred, but might not be articulated).

Once the students become more familiar with the yoga forms, and have mastered coordinating movement with the breath, they will have more mental space available to take in more language. At that point, you can add more cues for **Guideline #3** (relating to body sensing, to promote ***clarity*** and presence of mind) and **Guideline #4** (positive suggestions to help students emotionally connect with the yoga forms to ***uplift*** their spirits). Certainly, some Guideline #3 cues can be added from the beginning during times that would otherwise be silent and when less mental effort is expected of them. Just be sure to not keep them in the yoga form too long by adding too much language. Remember—they are beginners! Also, please note that the *bold and/or italic* writing in each yoga description is not meant to be spoken to the students but is for the instructor's information. The **Guideline #5** statements, in bold, inform the instructor of the intended messages to be drawn into the body-mind when performing the yoga forms. They can also serve as lesson themes for on or off the mat as well.

At the end of each yoga form description you will find a key depicting the important sensory and breath benefits of the yoga form or movement. Table 14.2 provides the translation for these key codes. This code is not meant to imply that other forms do not offer the same types of sensory input, but rather that these particular yoga forms emphasize it to a greater degree.

Table 14.2: Key for sensory and breath benefits

BREATH	TAC	PROP	VEST	BAL
Breath awareness or coordinating movement with breath	Deep touch pressure	Enhanced proprioception	Slow, rhythmic movement	Balancing challenge

Also, please be aware that you could be encountering students who have experienced sexual abuse. This can be expected just based on the statistics: one in four girls and one in six boys will be sexually abused before they reach 18 years old (Townsend and Rheingold 2013). Unless you are working in a program geared for that population group, you will likely not know who they are. It is therefore important that you observe the precautions taught in Part 1 and avoid the Table forms unless mats are carefully positioned. For those working in specialized programs for students who have experienced sexual trauma, we recommend avoiding the Table forms altogether.

Some students will also need visual cues if they cannot discriminate between the right and left sides of their body. We suggest using a red bracelet (made from any material) on their right wrist, as both "red" and "right" start with the letter "R," and thus may be helpful in remembering. Also, we suggest *not* color-cuing the left side of the body. A 1976 study (old, but the most relevant study we could find) found that in contrast to previous studies using multiple colors, using a single color eliminates the possibility of discriminating *only* on the basis of color—that is, it forces the person to attend to the primary stimuli. In our case, the child needs to perceptually learn to associate the left/other side of their body based on position-in-space of the limb alone. In the study, vanishing the color cue gradually over time increased the effectiveness of the strategy (Allington 1976, p.190).

Finally, it is important to adapt these instructions for your population. These instructions were created to enhance receptive language processing in children and adolescents as well as older individuals who have special needs. For students who need even more concrete language, please adapt what we have written to best meet their needs. For example, compare these two sentences: "If you would like, lie down on your mat in a comfortable position with your legs straight and arms by your sides on the floor" vs. "Please lie down with straight legs and resting arms." You will notice that including invitational language, which is important in trauma-informed instruction, does add more language, and may be more difficult to implement for some populations. Remember—you know your student population best. Use our language as a template and adapt accordingly. Please feel free to contact us with any questions, comments, or suggestions. We are always looking to improve our program!

Whole Body Stretch

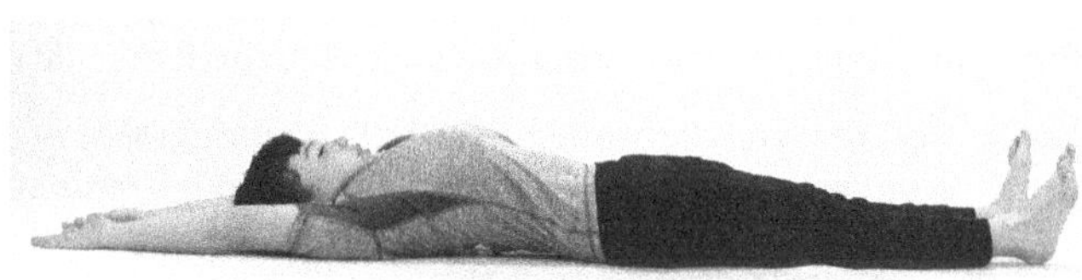

<table>
<tr><td colspan="5">1. When you're ready, lie down on your mat in a comfortable position, with your legs straight and your arms by your sides, on the floor.</td></tr>
<tr><td>Guideline #1:
SAFE</td><td colspan="4">2. Feel the firm support of the earth/ground below your body.</td></tr>
<tr><td colspan="5">3. Reach your arms above your head to the floor behind you.
4. Stretch your hands and feet away from each other, to make your body very long.</td></tr>
<tr><td>Guideline #3:
CLEAR</td><td colspan="4">5. Feel the stretch in your feet...legs...sides of your body...arms...and hands...</td></tr>
<tr><td>Guideline #2:
CALM</td><td colspan="4">6. Take three nice, slow, deep breaths, in...and out...
[State Guideline #4 during the three breaths.]</td></tr>
<tr><td>Guideline #4:
UPLIFTED</td><td colspan="4">7. Can you sense the whole length of your entire body? How does it feel to take up that much space?</td></tr>
<tr><td>Finishing step</td><td colspan="4">8. As you are ready, lower your arms back down to your sides to rest.
[Or proceed to Reclined Half Moon.]</td></tr>
<tr><td>Guideline #5:
EMPOWERED</td><td colspan="4">Some people don't like to take up space with their body, especially if they are feeling shy, sad, or bad about themselves. But when you stretch your body and let it take up more space, it can help you feel better about yourself, and more confident when talking with others.</td></tr>
<tr><td>BREATH</td><td></td><td>PROP</td><td></td><td></td></tr>
</table>

Reclined Half Moon

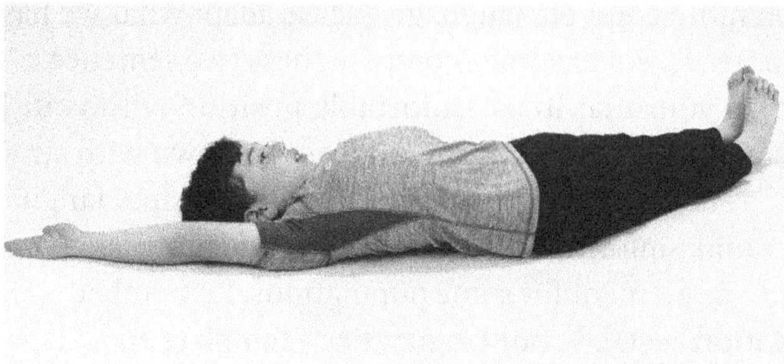

[From Whole Body Stretch]

1. Now, when you're ready, move your feet *way* over to the left, maybe even off your mat, to curve your body, like the sliver of the moon in the sky.
2. Now slide your arms and head to the left, keeping your arms and legs stretched long.

   Or: Bring your left arm down to your side while still stretching your [red] right arm overhead. Press your right foot away from you to stretch the right side of your body.

Guideline #3: CLEAR	3. Feel the stretch through the whole [red] right side of your body, from your foot and leg all the way up through your arm, hands, and fingers.			
Guideline #2: CALM	4. Breathe into the part of the body being stretched. *Or, for older students:* You might try sending your breath to the muscles of your ribcage, helping them to stretch and relax. *[Only keep them there for two breaths after this cue.]* *[Repeat steps 1–4 on the other side.]*			
Guideline #4: UPLIFTED	5. *[2nd side only]* Breathing into the stretch can help to relax the muscles, which helps to relax the mind.			
Finishing step	6. As you are ready, walk your feet back to the center of your mat and bring your arms back down to your sides. Feel the effects of that stretch in your body. *[Only pause for 3 seconds.]*			
Guideline #5: EMPOWERED	**When we breathe into a stretch, we release tightness and tension that we are holding inside our bodies, which helps to relax us.**			
BREATH		**PROP**		

Knees to Chest

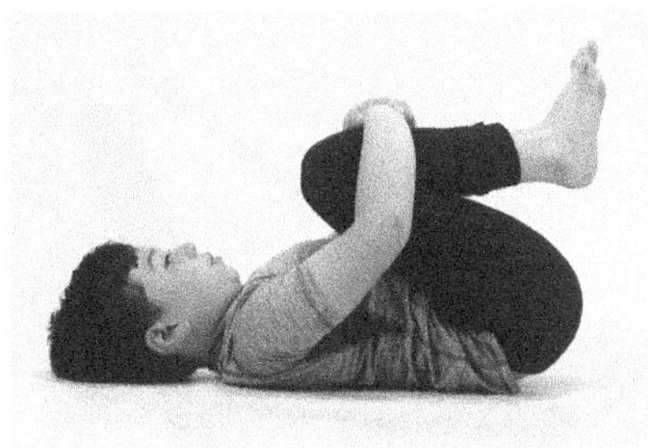

<table>
<tr><td colspan="5">1. If you would like, lie down on your mat in a comfortable position with your legs straight and arms by your sides on the floor. [Or from Reclined Half Moon.]</td></tr>
<tr><td>Guideline #1:
SAFE</td><td colspan="4">2. Feel the firm support of the earth/ground below your body.</td></tr>
<tr><td colspan="5">3. Take a slow breath in through your nose. As you breathe out, bring your knees into your body to fold yourself into a ball. Let your head rest on the floor.</td></tr>
<tr><td>Guideline #4:
UPLIFTED</td><td colspan="4">4. As you hug your knees close to you, imagine you are hugging a friend... Can you be your own friend during this yoga practice by listening to your body's messages? Remember to get out of a yoga form or breathing practice at any time if it does not feel right for you.</td></tr>
<tr><td>Guideline #2:
CALM
Guideline #3:
CLEAR</td><td colspan="4">5. Now, if you like, try breathing with me for three breaths: breathe in, belly blows up like a balloon, pushing against your leg. Breathe out, air flows out of the balloon and your stomach sinks back down.
6. Breathe in, belly rises...breathe out, belly sinks back down... Now breathe on your own as you feel how your breath moves your body.
[Stay for three breaths.]</td></tr>
<tr><td colspan="5">7. Now you may want to slowly rock your knees from side to side or move them in circles to help release any tightness in your lower back...</td></tr>
<tr><td>Finishing step</td><td colspan="4">8. As you are ready, straighten your legs back down on the floor and rest your body. Or: Place your feet on the floor, keeping knees bent, to prepare for... (Leg Stretches, Lying Down Twist, or Clamshell Twist).</td></tr>
<tr><td>Guideline #5:
EMPOWERED</td><td colspan="4">We need to be a friend to ourselves if we want to heal our hurt feelings. If we can care for ourselves just as we are, then we understand that we are worthy of love.</td></tr>
<tr><td>BREATH</td><td>TAC</td><td></td><td></td><td></td></tr>
</table>

Leg Stretch 1 with Band

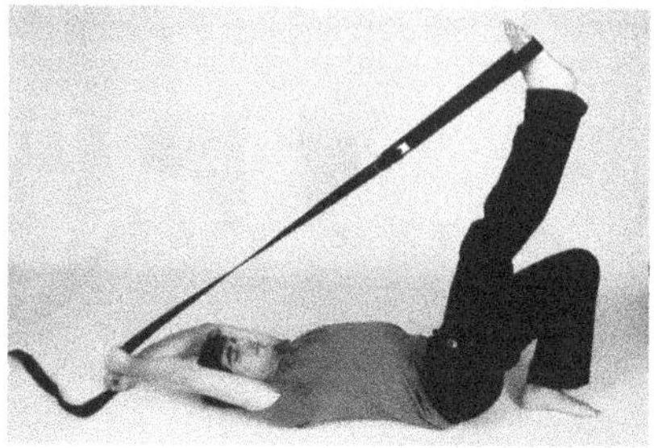

1. Lie down on your mat, with both knees bent and your feet on the floor.
2. Bend your [red] right leg close to your body and place the loop of the yoga band around your foot.
3. Slowly lift your leg up; try to keep your knee straight.
4. Slide both hands down the band so your arms are stretched over and behind your head.
5. Raise your leg only to the spot where you begin to feel a stretch.

Guideline #2: CALM	6. Breathe in and out through your nose. 7. Each time you breathe out, pretend you are sending your breath into your leg to soften the muscles and release any tightness or tension.			
Guideline #3: CLEAR Guideline #4: UPLIFTED	8. When you reach a tight spot, pause and breathe...soon it will open and you can move a little further, even if just a tiny bit... Just like in life...when you get stuck, pause and breathe...try again... Your breath can help you break through those tough times.			
Finishing step	*Proceed to Leg Stretches 2 and 3 on this side before switching to the other leg.* Take off the yoga band and rest your foot on the ground. *[Then repeat with the other leg.]*			
Guideline #5: EMPOWERED	**In life, you will face challenges. When things get hard, focus your attention on your breath. The power of your breath will help you handle difficult moments and give you strength to power through so you can reach your goals.**			
	TAC	**PROP**		

Leg Stretch 2 with Band

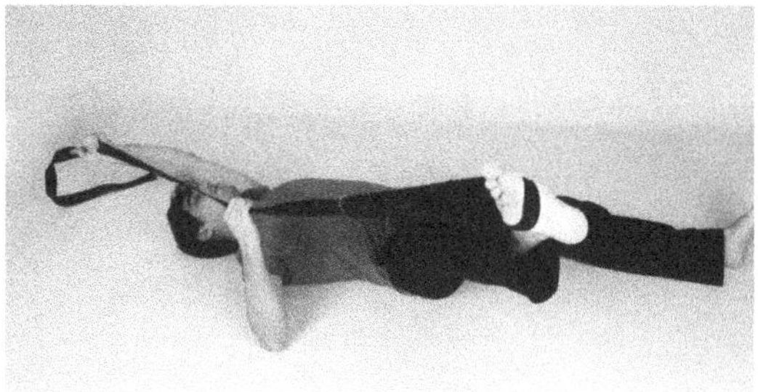

[From Leg Stretch 1]

1. Now straighten your other leg on the floor to get ready for the next stretch.
2. Bring your [red] right hand up on the yoga band toward your foot.
3. Lower your leg to the [red] right side, until your elbow rests on the floor.

Guideline #2: CALM	4. Slowly breathe in and out, through your nose, if you can.
Guideline #4: UPLIFTED	5. Each time you breathe out, pretend you are sending your breath into your leg to help let go of any tightness in your muscles.
Guideline #3: CLEAR	6. How does your leg feel in this stretch?
7. Then raise your leg back up to center.	
Finishing step	*Proceed to Leg Stretch 3.* *Or:* As you are ready, take the band off and rest your foot on the ground. *[Then repeat with the other leg.]*
Guideline #5: EMPOWERED	**In life, you will face challenges. When things get hard, focus on your breath. The power of your breath will help you handle difficult moments and give you strength to power through so you can reach your goals.**

	TAC	**PROP**		

Leg Stretch 3 with Band

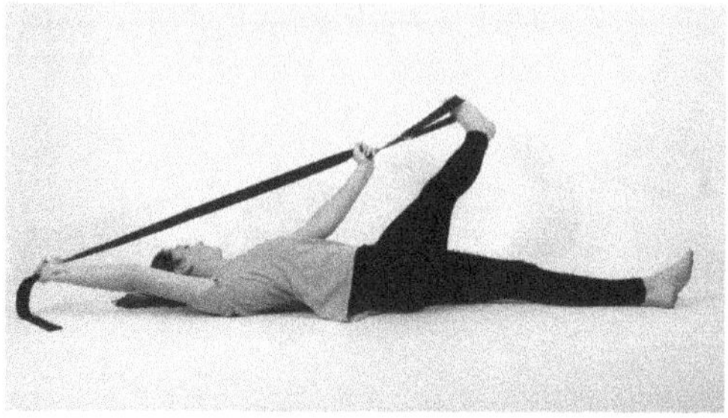

[From Leg Stretch 2]

1. Now switch your hands, so your left hand is holding the yoga band closer to your foot and your [red] right hand is holding the yoga band over your head, toward the floor behind you.

2. Now bring your leg over to the other side of your body, but keep your bottom on the floor.

Guideline #2: CALM	3. Slowly breathe in and out, through your nose if you can. *[Keep students here for about three breaths after this cue.]*			
Guideline #3: CLEAR	4. How does the stretch feel on this side of your body?			
Finishing steps	5. Then lift your leg back up to center. 6. Bend your knee close to your body and take the band off your foot. 7. Straighten your leg on the floor, and rest your body. *[Repeat Leg Stretches 1, 2, and 3 with the other leg, remembering to switch the left-right directional cues.]*			
Guideline #5: EMPOWERED	**In life, you will face challenges. When things get hard, focus your attention on your breath. The power of your breath will help you handle difficult moments and give you strength to power through so you can reach your goals.**			
	TAC	**PROP**		

Lying Down Twist

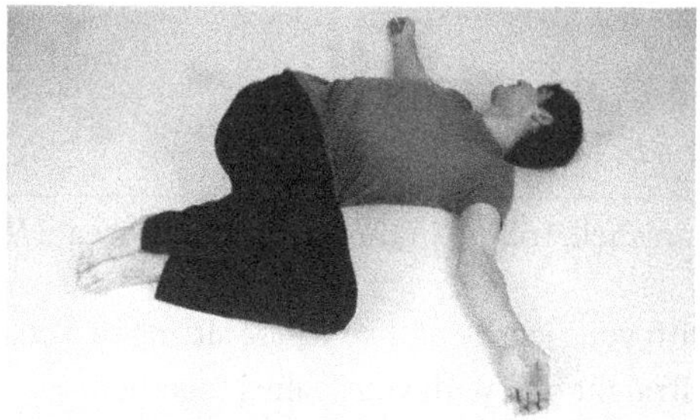

[From supine]

1. Bring your knees into your body.
2. Let go of your legs and lay your arms on the floor in a "T" position, with your palms facing up.
3. Keep your hips and knees bent.

Guideline #2: CALM	4. Take a breath in, and as you breathe out, lower your legs partway to the floor on one side. 5. Breathe in as you lift your legs back to center. 6. Breathe out as you lower your legs partway to the floor on the other side. 7. Continue moving like this... Breathe in as you lift your legs up... Breathe out as you lower them to the other side.
Guideline #3: CLEAR	8. How does it feel to slowly move your legs with your breath?
Guideline #4: UPLIFTED	9. Picture yourself squeezing out all the tightness and worries in your body, just like squeezing the water from a wet towel. *[Say all of the above within six repetitions, before resting on one side.]*

10. As you are ready, lower your legs to rest on the floor on one side.
11. If you would like, turn your head to look away from your legs.

Guideline #1: SAFE	12. Rest your shoulders down on the floor. 13. Sense your whole body sinking down into the support of the earth/ground.
Guideline #2: CALM	14. Breathe slowly in and out through your nose...
Finishing step	15. As you're ready, raise your legs back up and over to rest on the other side.
Guideline #5: EMPOWERED	**When we squeeze out our worries and doubts, we make room for more positive attitudes and experiences.**

BREATH	**TAC**	**PROP**		

Clamshell Twist[1]

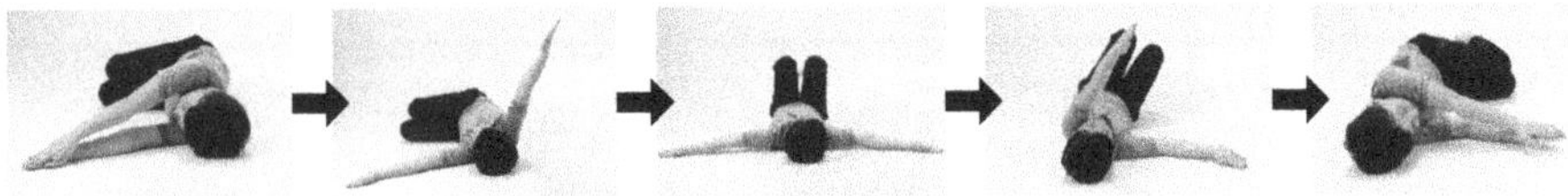

<table>
<tr><td colspan="2">1. Let's move like a clamshell, rolling in the waves of the ocean! Watch how I do it first [demonstrate].
2. Lie on your side, with your legs bent, like you're sitting in a chair.
3. Stretch your arms straight out, with your palms together.</td></tr>
<tr><td>Guideline #1:
SAFE</td><td>4. Can you feel the parts of your body that touch the floor? Maybe you feel your body getting heavy, like a clamshell sinking into the sand?</td></tr>
<tr><td colspan="2">5. As you breathe in, slowly open your clamshell. Raise your top arm up and over your body until it lands back on the floor behind you. Let your legs follow.
6. Slowly breathe out as you bring your other arm up and over to close your clamshell.
7. Again, on this side. [Repeat 5 and 6.]</td></tr>
<tr><td>Guideline #2:
CALM</td><td>8. Keep moving like a clamshell, gently side to side... Breathing in as you open your clamshell, breathing out as you close your clamshell.
9. If you want, you can make a "whoosh" sound whenever you close your clamshell, like the sound of the ocean waves.</td></tr>
<tr><td>Guideline #3:
CLEAR</td><td>10. How does it feel to be a clamshell rolling in the waves?</td></tr>
<tr><td>Guideline #4:
UPLIFTED</td><td>11. Rolling on the floor teaches us to let go, have fun, and trust in the present moment, just like we can learn to let go of worries and find joy in each moment.</td></tr>
<tr><td>Finishing step</td><td>12. The next time you close your clamshell, you can rest here or open your arms and look to the other side. Stay here for a few breaths. Then rest like this on the other side.</td></tr>
<tr><td>Guideline #5:
EMPOWERED</td><td>We can learn to let go of worries and embrace the spirit of playfulness, finding happiness and freedom in each moment.</td></tr>
</table>

BREATH	**TAC**		**VEST**	

1 Clamshell simulates one of the three exercises included in a study by Sai Sailesh Kumar Goothy *et al.* (2019), which found decreased depression, anxiety, and stress levels in elderly women with Type 2 diabetes.

Table

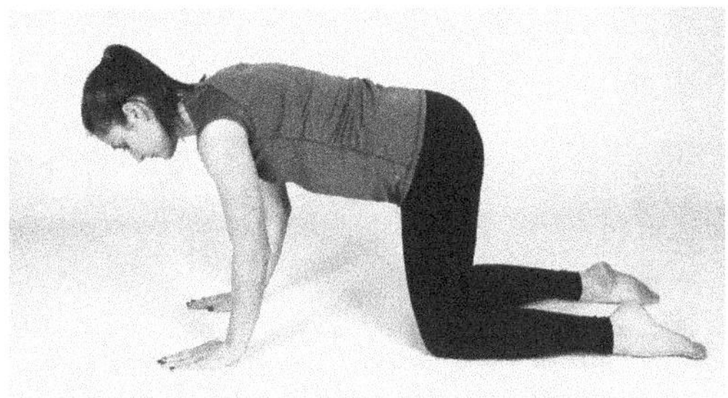

For younger children, it is helpful to place rubber "footprints" and "handprints" on the mat to facilitate proper positioning in Table form.

1. As you're ready...
    - Come on to your hands and knees.
    - Be sure your hands are under your shoulders.
    - Be sure your knees are under your hips.
2. Keep your belly and back strong and straight, like a table you could balance a glass of water on.
3. Look down at your hands.

Guideline #1: SAFE	4. Now, move your fingers apart and press your whole hand down to feel your solid contact with the ground. Notice how solid, firm, and stable it is. The ground is strong. It is not going anywhere. It will stay and support you wherever you go and whatever you do.			
Guideline #3: CLEAR	5. How does your body feel when you connect with the firm and steady ground?			
Finishing step	*From here, continue into Cat Flow or to another yoga form from Table.*			
Guideline #5: EMPOWERED	**Connecting your body to the solid earth/ground below can help you feel more safe and secure.**			
	TAC	**PROP**		

Cat Flow (Happy Cat/Angry Cat)

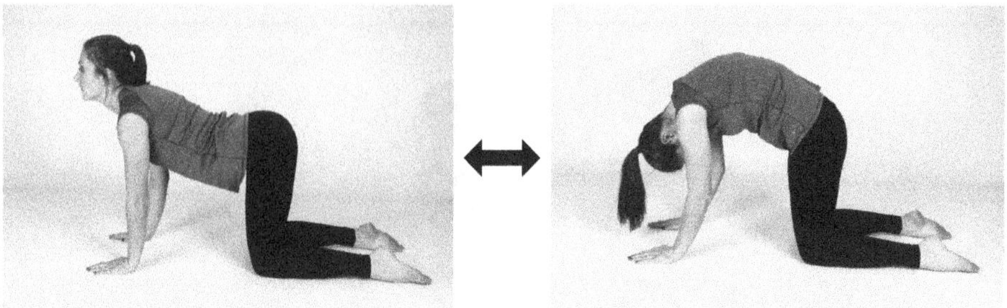

<table>
<tr><td>Guideline #1:
SAFE</td><td colspan="4">(From Table)
1. Move your fingers apart and press your palms and fingers down into the floor.</td></tr>
<tr><td colspan="5">2. Now, imagine you are a cat. You have a long tail.
3. Lift your tail to the sky, and look up. If you want, you can smile like a Happy Cat.
4. Now let's turn into an Angry Cat. The next time you breathe out, make a "hisss" sound as you tuck your tail between your legs, round your back, and drop your head to see your hidden tail.
[Practice a few times before introducing the breath flow.]</td></tr>
<tr><td>Guideline #3:
CLEAR</td><td colspan="4">5. How does it feel to be a Happy Cat?
6. How does it feel to be an Angry Cat?
[You can say this when teaching each form separately, before the flow.]</td></tr>
<tr><td>Guideline #2:
CALM</td><td colspan="4">7. Let's move back and forth from Happy Cat to Angry Cat with our breath.
8. As you breathe in...lift your tail...look up and smile—Happy Cat!
9. Breathe out with a "hisss"...as you tuck your tail and round your back—Angry Cat! [Repeat steps 8 and 9, two to five times.]
10. If appropriate: Now practice three times on your own.</td></tr>
<tr><td>Guideline #4:
UPLIFTED</td><td colspan="4">11. How does it feel to flow from a Happy Cat to an Angry Cat and back to a Happy Cat?</td></tr>
<tr><td>Finishing step</td><td colspan="4">12. As you are ready, rest in Child form.</td></tr>
<tr><td>Guideline #5:
EMPOWERED</td><td colspan="4">When you feel the support of the ground and move your body with your breath, you can more easily control how you feel.</td></tr>
<tr><td>BREATH</td><td>TAC</td><td></td><td>VEST</td><td></td></tr>
</table>

Cat Flow (classic, for older students)

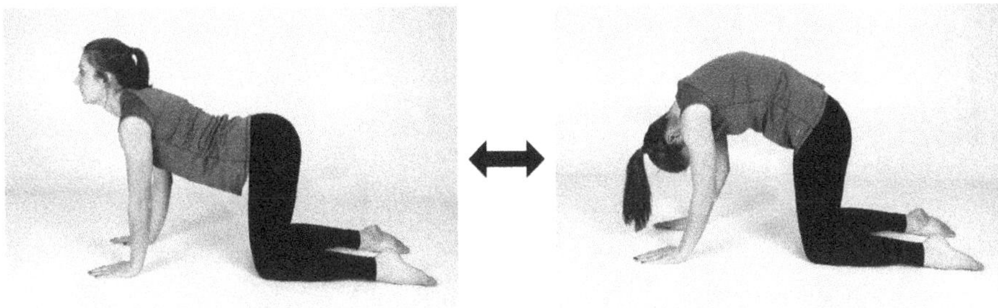

Guideline #1: SAFE	*(From Table)* 1. Move your fingers apart and press your palms and fingers down into the floor.
2. Now, imagine you are a cat. You have a long tail.	
Guideline #2: CALM	3. As you breathe in...lift your tail, drop your belly, and look up. 4. As you breathe out...tuck your tail under, round your back, and let your head drop between your arms. 5. Breathe in, lift your tail...look up. 6. Breathe out, tuck your tail under, round your back, and let your head hang down. 7. Continue this movement on your own with your breath.
Guideline #4: UPLIFTED	8. Let your strong connection with the ground provide the stability you need to smoothly ride the wave of your breath. *Or:* Let go of the effort and just let yourself ride the wave of your breath.
Finishing step	9. As you are ready, rest in Child form.
Guideline #5: EMPOWERED	**When you feel the support of the ground and move your body with your breath, you can more easily control how you feel.**

BREATH	**TAC**		**VEST**	

Tiger Flow

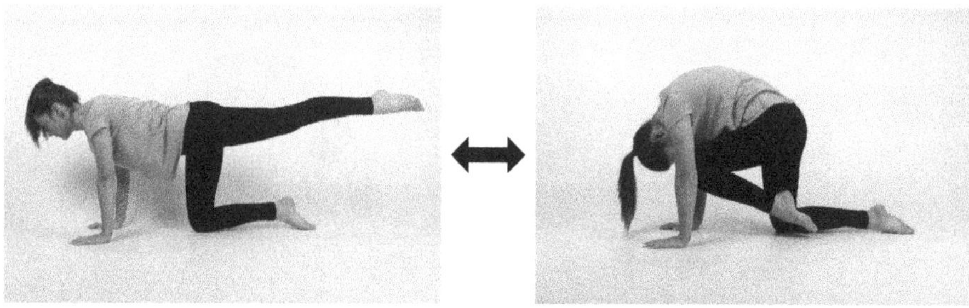

<table>
<tr><td>Guideline #1:
SAFE</td><td colspan="4">(From Table)
1. Move your fingers apart and press your palms and fingers down into the floor.</td></tr>
<tr><td>Guideline #2:
CALM</td><td colspan="4">2. As you breathe in, lift one leg off the floor, straight out behind you.
Or, from Cat Flow: The next time you breathe in, lift one leg off the floor, straight behind you.
3. As you breathe out, bend your knee toward your forehead. [Cue steps 2 and 3 1–3 more times.]
4. If appropriate: Now move like this, with your own breath.</td></tr>
<tr><td>Guideline #3:
CLEAR</td><td colspan="4">5. Fully sink into the sensations of movement and breath...
Or: Keep your strong connection with the earth/ground through your hands as you ride the rhythm of the flow.</td></tr>
<tr><td colspan="5">6. The next time you straighten your leg, hold it there and look down at the floor... keep breathing.
7. You can stay here or try lifting the arm on your other side just a little off the floor, or straighten that arm out in front of you.</td></tr>
<tr><td>Guideline #4:
UPLIFTED</td><td colspan="4">8. Strong and steady breath—strong and steady body.
9. When ready, slowly lower your hand and knee to the floor, and repeat on the other side.</td></tr>
<tr><td>Finishing step</td><td colspan="4">10. Rest in Child form.</td></tr>
<tr><td>Guideline #5:
EMPOWERED</td><td colspan="4">Our sense of confidence is felt from the upper belly area (below the ribs and above the belly button). [Cue students to place a hand on this area to locate it.] We can build confidence by moving and breathing in this area of the body.</td></tr>
<tr><td>BREATH</td><td>TAC</td><td>PROP</td><td>VEST</td><td>BAL</td></tr>
</table>

Twisting Cat

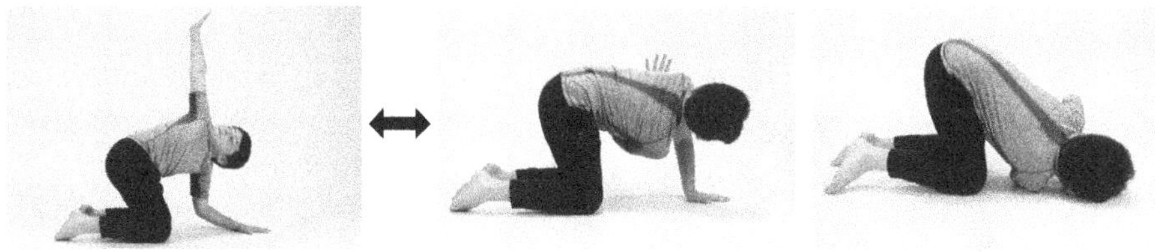

Guideline #1: SAFE	*(From Table)* 1. Move your fingers apart and press your palms and fingers down into the floor.			
Guideline #2: CALM	2. Take some nice slow breaths in and out... Then, as you breathe in, raise your [red] right arm out and up to the sky. 3. As you breathe out, reach that arm under your body to the other side, like this *[demonstrate: model a full twist with the shoulder close to touching the floor]*. 4. Then, as you breathe in, raise your [red] right arm back up to the sky. 5. As you breathe out, reach that arm under your body to the other side. 6. Continue moving with your breath, watching your hand as it moves.			
Guideline #3: CLEAR	7. How does it feel to move like this? 8. *[After four reps]* Next time you breathe out, reach your arm all the way under your body to the other side and rest down on your shoulder.			
Guideline #4: UPLIFTED	9. Notice how the room looks from this view. Do things look different upside down? How does that make you feel? 10. *[2nd side only]* You might notice things look a little different on this side, too. This helps us remember there's always another way to look at things!			
Finishing step	11. Slowly come back up to Table. Now let's repeat this on the other side.			
Guideline #5: EMPOWERED	**When we take the time to look at a problem in a different way, it can change our attitude about it and lead to better solutions.**			
BREATH	**TAC**	**PROP**	**VEST**	

Rabbit Hop

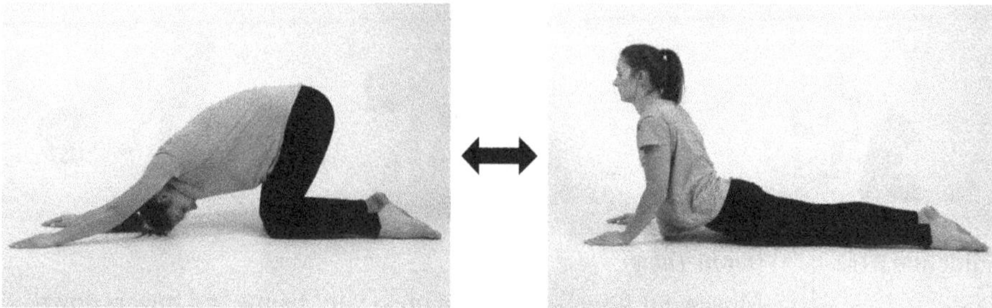

1. Meet me back in Table form. As you are ready, take a big "step" forward with your hands.
2. Lower the top of your head towards your mat, but don't touch it.
3. Keep your hips up and look back at your feet. This is rabbit ready to hop!

Guideline #1: SAFE	4. Move your fingers and press your whole hand into the ground. 5. The ground is strong and will support the rabbit wherever it goes on its journey.
Guideline #2: CALM	6. As you breathe in, push your hips forward to the floor and raise your chest up. Look straight ahead. This is one Rabbit Hop. 7. As you breathe out, come back into rabbit. 8. Breathe in, push your hips forward, and raise your chest. 9. Breathe out, hips come back, and head comes down. 10. Keep hopping like a rabbit, swinging your body slowly, back and forth. 11. Breathe in as you hop [swing your body] forward and breathe out as you fold back up.
Guideline #4: UPLIFTED	12. When you connect with the ground and move with your breath, it can help you feel ready for any new experiences that come your way. *[Perform 6–10 rounds and rest in Child form.]*
Finishing step	13. As you are ready, come back to Table. Sit back on your feet and rest your body over your legs, in Child form.
Guideline #5: EMPOWERED	**When we ground ourselves and move with our breath, it is easier to try new things.**

BREATH	TAC	PROP	VEST	

Down Dog

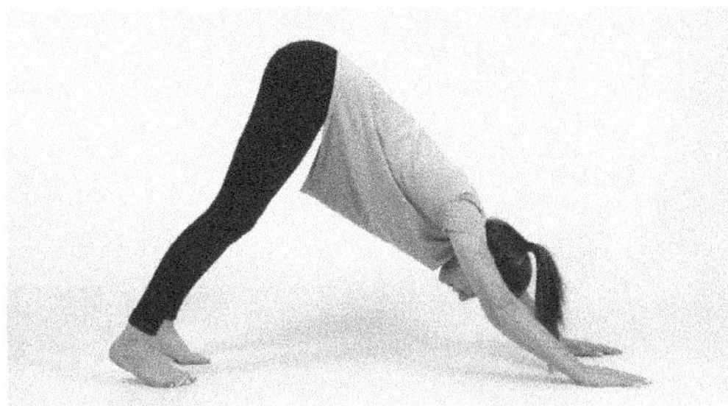

<table>
<tr><td colspan="5">1. If you would like, you can join me in doing a Down Dog stretch.
2. Meet me in a strong Table form.
3. Make sure your hands are under your shoulders and your knees are under your hips.
4. Now take one "step" forward with your hands.</td></tr>
<tr><td>Guideline #1:
SAFE</td><td colspan="4">5. Move your fingers and press down with your whole hand. Feel your solid contact with the ground.</td></tr>
<tr><td colspan="5">6. Curl your toes under, and then raise your hips high in the air, lifting your knees off the ground.
7. Keep your knees a little bent as you push the floor forward with your arms.
8. Lift your dog's tail as high as you can.</td></tr>
<tr><td>Guideline #2:
CALM</td><td colspan="4">9. Breathe in here, as you breathe out—try howling like a dog in the night! [This will encourage a longer exhale without needing to cue the breath.]</td></tr>
<tr><td>Guideline #3:
CLEAR</td><td colspan="4">10. If your arms or legs start to feel tired, notice it with curiosity ["witness" mentality]. But if you are too uncomfortable, come back down onto your hands and knees until you feel ready to try it again.</td></tr>
<tr><td>Guideline #4:
UPLIFTED</td><td colspan="4">[You can state this when students are resting in Child, after completing Down Dog, so they are not in Down Dog for too long.]
11. Learning to notice, as well as move away from, strong sensations in the body is an important skill so we don't get hurt. We call that "befriending" our body, which means to "be" a "friend" to our body and treat it with kindness.</td></tr>
<tr><td>Finishing step</td><td colspan="4">12. As you are ready, come back to Table. Sit back on your feet and rest your body over your legs, in Child form.</td></tr>
<tr><td>Guideline #5:
EMPOWERED</td><td colspan="4">We build fortitude when we learn how to mentally step back from situations and observe them from a place of equanimity.</td></tr>
<tr><td></td><td>TAC</td><td>PROP</td><td></td><td></td></tr>
</table>

Dolphin Flow

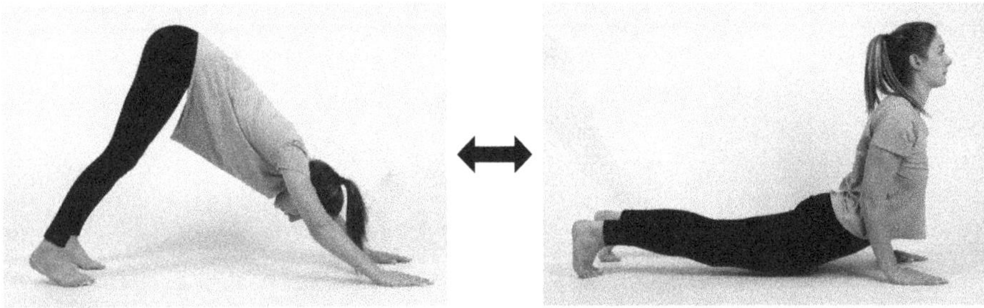

[For young students, begin with a video or visuals showing a dolphin diving in and out of the water.]

1. I invite you to join me in moving and breathing like a dolphin.
2. As you are ready, meet me in a strong Table form.
3. Make sure your hands are under your shoulders and your knees are under your hips.
4. Now take one "step" forward with your hands.
5. Then move your hands a little wider apart, if you can. *[This is to enable the chest to fit through the arms when coming up into Up Dog.]*

Guideline #1: SAFE	6. Move your fingers apart and press down with your whole hand to feel your solid contact with the ground.

7. Curl your toes under, and then lift your hips *high*, like you're a dolphin diving into the ocean *[demonstrate]*.
8. Now drop your hips down and raise your chest between your arms, like a dolphin coming up for air *[demonstrate]*.

Guideline #2: CALM	9. Breathe out as you dive down into the ocean. 10. Breathe in as you come up for air. 11. Continue this on your own.
Guideline #3: CLEAR	12. How does your body feel to move and breathe like a dolphin?
Guideline #4: UPLIFTED	13. What happens when you just let yourself "go with the flow?" *[Perform 6–10 rounds and rest in Child form.]*
Finishing step	14. As you are ready, come back to Table. Sit back on your feet and rest your body over your legs, in Child form.
Guideline #5: EMPOWERED	**When we ground ourselves and move with our breath, it is easier to "go with the flow."**

BREATH	TAC	PROP	VEST	

Child

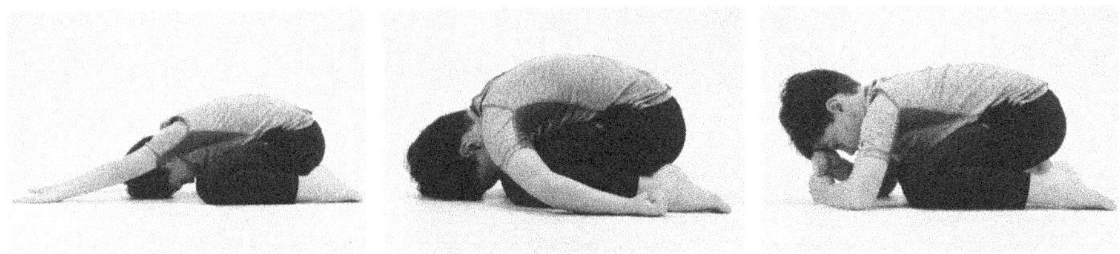

[From Table]

1. As you are ready, sit back on your feet and rest your body over your legs.
2. Let your forehead rest on the floor.
3. You may stretch your arms out in front of you on the floor (see left-hand photo above) or rest them next to your body (see center photo above). Or, if your forehead doesn't reach the floor, you can stack your fists on top of each other (see right-hand photo above).

<table>
<tr><td>Guideline #1:
SAFE</td><td colspan="4">4. Feel the weight of your body on your legs, inviting you to sink down into the safe support of the earth/ground.</td></tr>
<tr><td>Guideline #2:
CALM
Guideline #3:
CLEAR</td><td colspan="4">5. Follow your breath as it moves in and out, through your whole body.
6. Where do you feel your breath? Can you feel it in your back? In your belly? Pressing on your legs?
7. Each time you breathe out, sense/feel your body sinking down deeper and deeper onto the firm, solid, and stable earth/ground...</td></tr>
<tr><td>Guideline #4:
UPLIFTED</td><td colspan="4">8. Use this as a time of rest... There is no place to go...nothing to do... except be here now...
Or: How does it feel to be fully supported by the strength of the earth/ground?</td></tr>
<tr><td>Guideline #5:
EMPOWERED</td><td colspan="4">**Learning how to rise to a challenge, and completely release when it has passed, is crucial for developing resilience.**</td></tr>
<tr><td>**BREATH**</td><td>**TAC**</td><td></td><td></td><td></td></tr>
</table>

Mountain

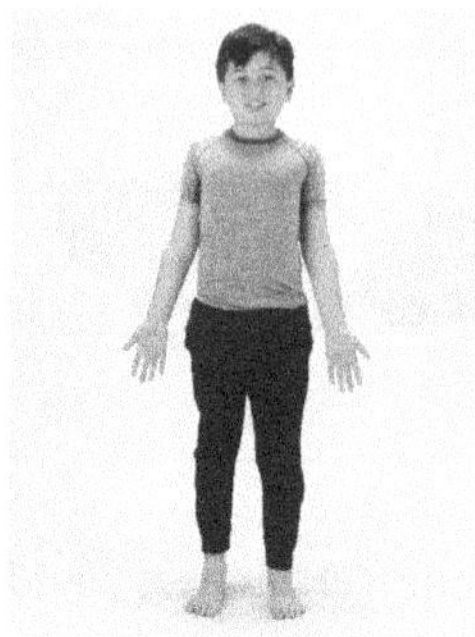

1. Stand up nice and tall, with your feet a little bit apart.
2. Point your toes to the front of your mat.

[Accommodations: You can put a block or pillow between the thighs or feet to help with proper alignment, or measure two fists' length between the feet.]

Guideline #1: SAFE Guideline #3: CLEAR	3. Without moving your feet, rock your body from side to side...and now from front to back, noticing how the floor feels under your feet. Now come back to center and press your feet down into the solid earth/ground. 4. Picture yourself as a strong, solid mountain: • Pull your belly in and stretch your head up nice and tall—this is the top of the mountain. • Lower your shoulders down away from your ears. • Stretch your hands down by your sides—these are the sides of the mountain.
Guideline #2: CALM	5. Breathe in through your nose. *Optional:* Smell flowers on the side of the mountain or fresh air. 6. Breathe out through your mouth like the wind blowing around the mountain *[demonstrate: purse your lips and make a wind sound]*. 7. How does it feel to breathe in and out as a mountain?
Guideline #4: UPLIFTED	8. You might imagine that a bunny is making a nest on the side of the mountain, right where your heart is. Can you stand strong like a mountain while keeping a nice soft spot for the bunny? • Strong mountain...soft bunny... • Strong body...soft heart...
Guideline #5: EMPOWERED	**People often harden their hearts to block out uncomfortable feelings, but when you do this, you also block out the good feelings, like joy and love. It takes emotional strength to let yourself feel what you feel, and when you do, it allows you to stay more present and engaged in life. In this Mountain form, feel the support of the earth/ground giving you the strength and courage to soften your heart and let the light in.**

BREATH		PROP		BAL

Extended Mountain with Band

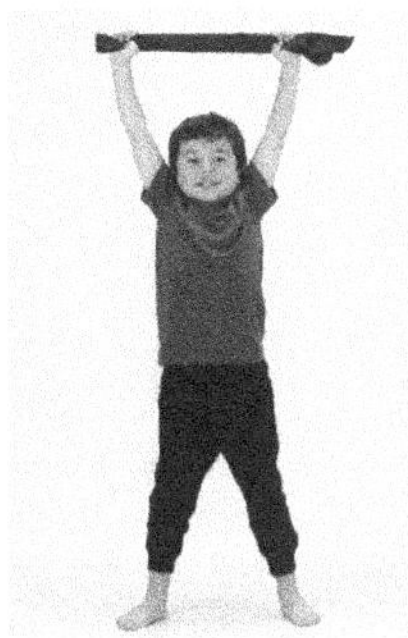
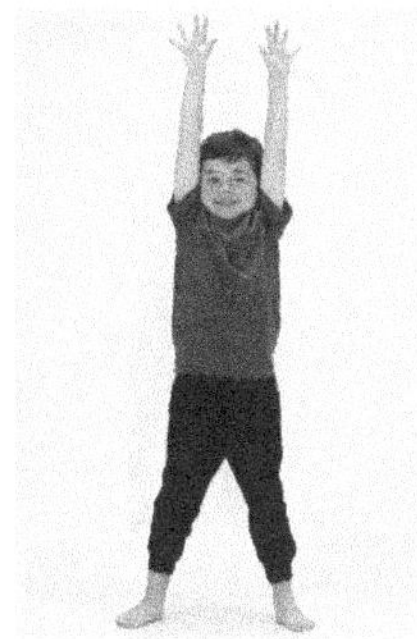

1. To prepare, fold the yoga band in half. *[Or do Extended Mountain without a yoga band (see right-hand photo above).]*
2. Hold the yoga band so your hands are a bit wider than your shoulders.

Or, from Mountain:

1. Step your feet a little apart.
2. Point your toes out a bit.

Guideline #1: SAFE	3. Press your feet into the floor to feel the support of the ground below you.

4. Stand tall and straight.
5. As you breathe in, raise your arms straight over your head.
6. Stretch the band tight by pulling your arms apart.
7. Lower your shoulders down away from your ears.

Guideline #3: CLEAR	8. Notice how that stretch feels in your arms...
Guideline #2: CALM	9. Take nice slow easy breaths...breathing in...breathing out...
Guideline #4: UPLIFTED	10. When our feet are grounded to the earth and our muscles are working, it can help us feel more solid, stable, and strong in both our body and mind... How does this make you feel in your *own* body?... In your *own* mind?
Finishing step	11. As you are ready, lower your arms to your sides and rest in Mountain.
Guideline #5: EMPOWERED	**As our bodies feel stronger, our minds feel stronger. We develop the confidence to try new things, and develop the mental strength to meet our goals.**

BREATH	**TAC**	**PROP**		**BAL**

Standing Half Moon with Band

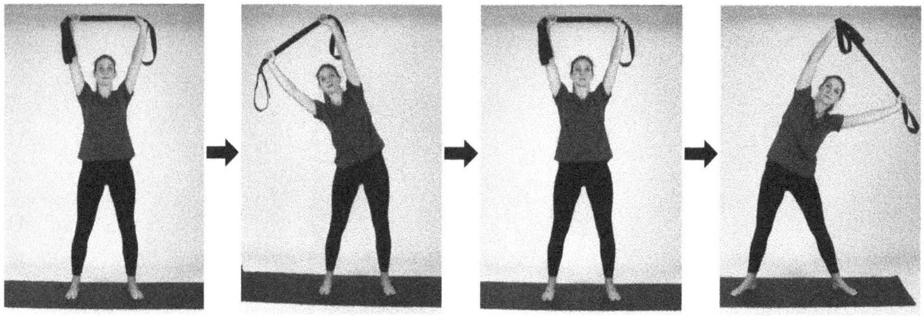

(From Extended Mountain with yoga band)

1. Now let's add some movement with our breath.

<table>
<tr><td>Guideline #2:
CALM</td><td colspan="4">2. Take a breath in through your nose.
3. Breathe out as you bend to your [red] right side.
4. Breathe in as you come back to center.
5. Breathe out as you bend to the left.
6. Breathe in as you come back to center.
7. Keep moving with your breath: breathe out to the side, breathe into the center.
[Do 3–5 sets, moving smoothly through the center; don't segment the movements.]</td></tr>
<tr><td>Guideline #3:
CLEAR</td><td colspan="4">8. How does it feel to stretch your body from side to side?
9. Notice if rooting your feet into the ground helps you feel more stable as you move from side to side...</td></tr>
<tr><td>Guideline #4:
UPLIFTED</td><td colspan="4">10. In the same way, when we ground ourselves, it can help us handle changes in our lives more easily.</td></tr>
<tr><td>Finishing step</td><td colspan="4">11. As you are ready, lower your arms to your sides and rest in Mountain.</td></tr>
<tr><td>Guideline #5:
EMPOWERED</td><td colspan="4">When you ground yourself, you are better able to bend and adapt to face whatever comes your way, with courage and resilience.</td></tr>
<tr><td>BREATH</td><td></td><td>PROP</td><td>VEST</td><td>BAL</td></tr>
</table>

Standing Twist with Band

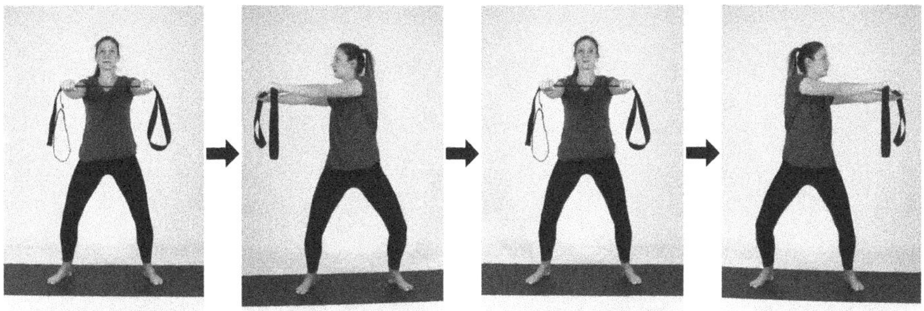

1. Fold your yoga band in half.
2. Step your feet a bit wider apart and point your toes out a bit.
3. Hold the band tight in front of your chest with your arms straight, a little wider than your shoulders.

Guideline #1: SAFE	4. Bend your knees and root your feet down into the ground. 5. Notice how solid your body feels when your muscles are actively working.			
Guideline #2: CALM	6. Breathe in here, and then breathe out as you twist to the [red] right side, watching your hands. 7. Breathe in, back to center. Breathe out, twist to the other side, watching your hands. *[This is one set.]* 8. Breathe in, back to center...breathe out, twist to the other side. 9. Continue to move like this with your breath. *[Do 3–4 sets total.]*			
Guideline #3: CLEAR	10. How does it feel to twist your body from side to side?			
Guideline #4: UPLIFTED	11. Picture yourself squeezing out all the tightness and worries in your body, just like squeezing the water from a wet towel.			
Finishing step	12. As you are ready, twist back to center, lower your arms to your sides, stand up tall, and rest in Mountain.			
Guideline #5: EMPOWERED	**When we squeeze out our worries and doubts, we make room for more positive attitudes and experiences.**			
BREATH		**PROP**	**VEST**	**BAL**

Star

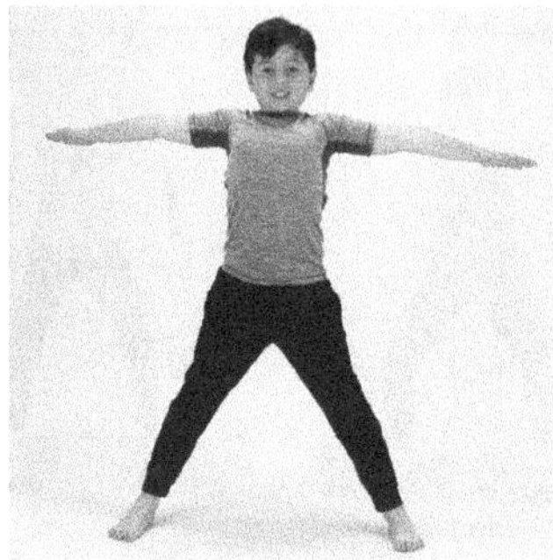

1. Now, I invite you to join me in Star. In Star, we use our head, legs, and arms to form the five points of a star.
2. As you are ready, turn to face the side of your yoga mat.
3. If you like, step your feet wider apart, to a comfortable spot. This can help you feel more stable.

   [Demonstrate a wide stance, but let the students stay within own comfort zone.]
4. Point your toes out a little bit.

<table>
<tr><td>Guideline #1:
SAFE</td><td colspan="4">5. Press your feet down and sense the strength of your legs firmly planting you on the ground.
6. Stand tall and straight.</td></tr>
<tr><td>Guideline #3:
CLEAR</td><td colspan="4">7. As you're ready, lift your arms straight out to each side.
8. Feel the stretch in your arms, all the way to your fingertips.
9. Pull in the muscles in your belly.
10. Stretch your head up nice and tall, to make your star even taller.
11. Notice the muscles in your face...are they soft or tight?
12. Invite the muscles to soften and rest.</td></tr>
<tr><td>Guideline #2:
CALM
Guideline #4:
UPLIFTED</td><td colspan="4">13. Notice your breath, in...and out...in...and out...
14. Imagine breathing in light and positive energy.
15. As you breathe out, shine that positivity and light to the world around you.</td></tr>
<tr><td>Finishing step</td><td colspan="4">16. As you are ready, lower your arms to your sides, step your feet together, and rest in Mountain.</td></tr>
<tr><td>Guideline #5:
EMPOWERED</td><td colspan="4">Shine your light and positive energy to the world around you.</td></tr>
<tr><td>BREATH</td><td></td><td>PROP</td><td></td><td>BAL</td></tr>
</table>

Shining Star with or without Band

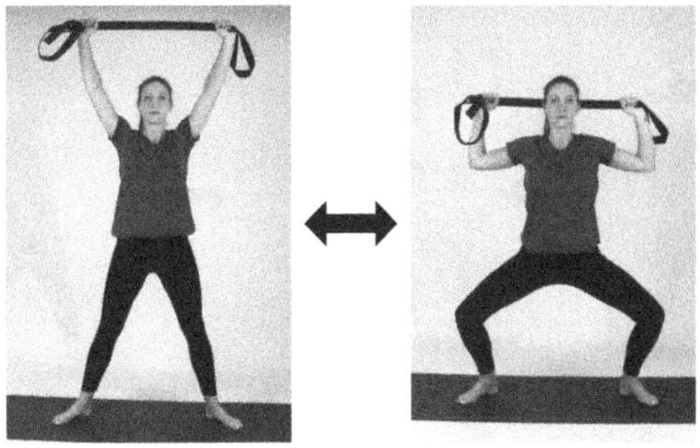

Guideline #2: CALM	*[From Star]* 1. Now, if you like, try adding some movement with your breath. 2. Watch me first, while you rest your arms for a moment. 3. You can do this with your feet apart or closer together. *[Demonstrate both options.]* • If you step your feet closer together, point your toes straight ahead. • If your feet are further apart, point the toes out more. 4. When ready, breathe in, stand tall, and stretch your arms stright. 5. If you are holding a yoga band, stretch the band tight overhead. If you are not holding a yoga band, keep your arms stretched out to the sides in Star. 6. As you breathe out, bend your knees and elbows like this *[demonstrate]*. 7. Breathe in, stand up tall, and stretch your arms straight. 8. Breathe out, and bend your knees and elbows *[demonstrate]*. 9. Continue to move this way with your breath.
Guideline #4: UPLIFTED	10. Imagine your Star getting brighter and brighter with each breath in and out, shining light and joy/positive energy to the world.
Guideline #3: CLEAR	11. How does it feel to move with your breath like this?
Finishing step	12. As you are ready, lower your arms to your sides and rest in Mountain.
Guideline #5: EMPOWERED	**Shine your light and positive energy to the world around you.**

BREATH	**TAC**	**PROP**	**VEST**	

Airplane

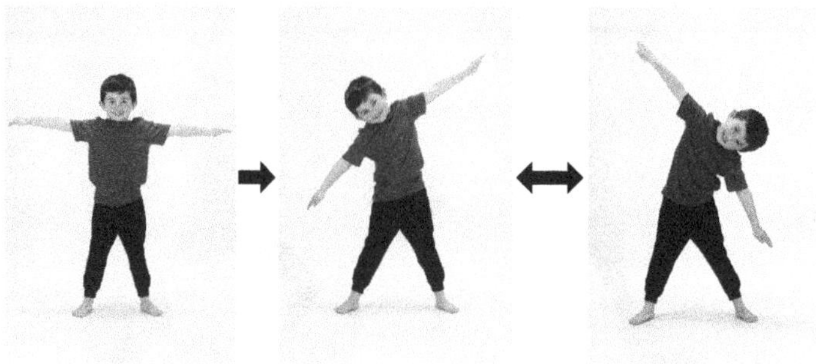

(From Star, with arms outstretched)

1. Now let's pretend to fly like an airplane.

Guideline #1: SAFE	2. Press your feet down to feel the support of the ground below you.
Guideline #2: CALM	3. As you breathe in, bend to one side to turn your airplane. 4. As you breathe out, bend to the other side to turn your airplane the other way. 5. Keep flying your airplane from side to side with your breath. 6. Breathe in as you turn your airplane one way. 7. Then breathe out as you turn it the other way. *[Repeat 3–4 times to each side.]*
Guideline #3: CLEAR	8. How does it feel to move like this? 9. Does it feel different flying one way or the other? *Or:* How does it feel to stretch your body from side to side? *Or:* Notice if rooting your feet into the ground helps you feel more stable as you change position from side to side...
Guideline #4: UPLIFTED	10. *If appropriate, you may add:* In the same way, when we ground ourselves, it can help us handle changes in our lives more easily.
Finishing step	11. When you are ready, come back to center, lower your arms to your sides, step your feet together, and rest in Mountain.
Guideline #5: EMPOWERED	**In life, things change, and it's important to learn how to be flexible and move with the changes. Just as your body moves more easily when it is grounded, your mind can more easily "go with the flow" when it is grounded and stable.**

BREATH		PROP	VEST	BAL

Warrior 1

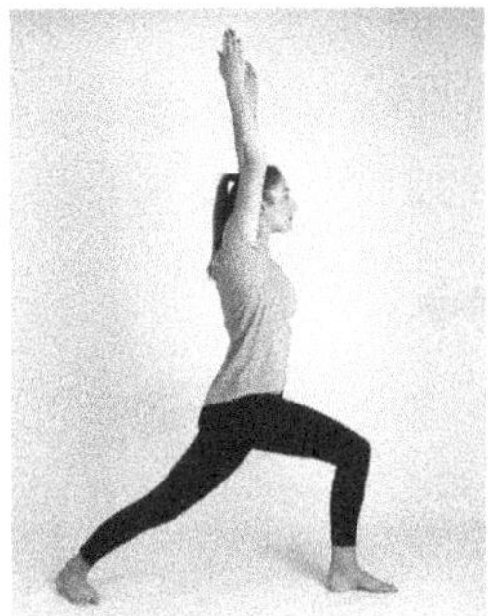

1. Stand at the back of your mat and take a big step forward with your [red] right leg.
2. Turn the toes of your back foot out just a little.
3. Place your hands on your hips and turn your hips to face your front leg.

Guideline #1: SAFE	4. Bend your front knee over your ankle. 5. Push your feet away from each other, like you are trying to stretch your mat longer. 6. Keep your front knee bent as you straighten and reach your arms up to the sky. 7. Turn your hands to face each other. 8. Feel the earth/ground through your strong legs.			
Guideline #2: CALM	9. As you breathe in, reach up higher to the sky. 10. As you breathe out, hold this reach, nice and strong.			
Guideline #3: CLEAR	11. How does it feel to press your feet into the earth/ground as you reach up to the sky with your arms?			
Guideline #4: UPLIFTED	12. *[1st side]* Standing like a Warrior brings out different feelings in different people...you may feel grounded...strong...balanced...or confident... How does standing like a Warrior make *you* feel? *[2nd side]* As you reach your arms to the sky, welcome good things to come your way... Open arms...open mind.			
Finishing step	13. When you are ready, step your back foot forward to come into Mountain. *[Repeat with the other leg (switch leg cues).]*			
Guideline #5: EMPOWERED	**We learn to be true to ourselves and more empowered when we listen to our body's messages, and nurture the positive messages.**			
	TAC	**PROP**		**BAL**

Dynamic Warrior 1

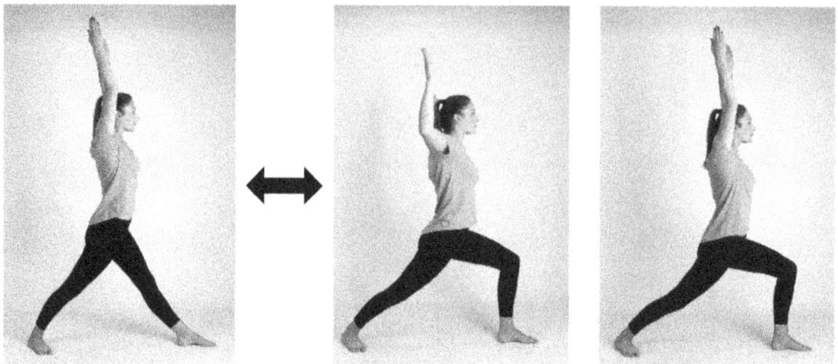

1. Stand at the back of your mat and take a big step forward with your [red] right leg.
2. Turn the toes of your back foot out just a little.
3. Place your hands on your hips and turn your hips to face the front of your mat.

Guideline #2: CALM	4. Breathe in as you straighten your arms overhead, with your hands facing each other (photo to left of arrow above). 5. Breathe out as you bend your front knee over (not past) your ankle and pull your elbows back (photo to right of arrow above). 6. Breathe in, straighten your knee and arms. 7. Breathe out, bend your knee and arms. 8. Continue to move like this with your breath.
Guideline #3: CLEAR	9. The next time you bend your knee, keep it there and stretch your arms overhead into Warrior 1 (photo furthest right above). 10. How does it feel to press your feet into the earth/ground as you reach up to the sky?
Guideline #4: UPLIFTED	11. *[1st side]* You may feel grounded...or strong...or balanced... confident. How does standing like a Warrior make *you* feel? *[2nd side only]* As you reach your arms to the sky, welcome good things to come your way... Open arms...open mind...
Finishing step	12. When you are ready, step your back foot forward to come into Mountain. See if you notice any different sensations in your body. *[Repeat steps with the other leg (switch leg cues).]*
Guideline #5: EMPOWERED	**We learn to be true to ourselves and more empowered when we listen to the messages arising from our own body, and nurture the positive messages.**

BREATH	TAC	PROP	VEST	BAL

Warrior 2

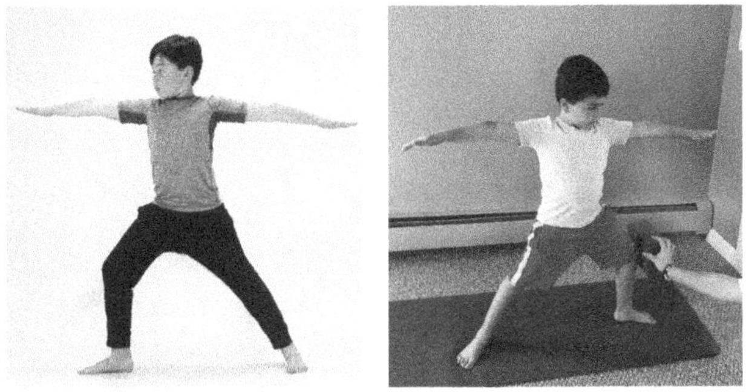

1. As you're ready, face your body to the side of your mat, and step your feet wide apart.
2. Turn your [red] right foot to the side and turn your left foot in just a little *[demonstrate].*
3. Place your hands on your hips and turn your hips more to the long side of the mat.
   [Due to body mechanics, the hips will be positioned diagonally.]

Guideline #1: SAFE	4. Bend your right knee so it is over your ankle (not past). *[Use a yoga block as a tactile cue if necessary (see right-hand photo above).]* 5. Push your feet away from each other as if you're trying to stretch the mat longer. Feel the earth/ground through your strong legs.
Guideline #2: CALM	6. Reach the top of your head, up to the sky. 7. As you breathe in, raise your arms out to the sides, as high as your shoulders *[demonstrate].* Turn your head to look over your front fingers.
Guideline #3: CLEAR	8. *[1st side]* Is there a place in your body where you feel strong in Warrior 2? Try sending your breath to that area. How does it make you feel? The more you notice your strength and power, the easier it is to move past challenges in our lives.
Guideline #4: UPLIFTED	9. *[2nd side] [For "witness" mentality]* If you start to feel strong muscle sensations, just notice them with a sense of curiosity. But if the feeling gets too uncomfortable, please come out of Warrior 2 to rest.
Finishing step	*[Repeat steps on the other side or move into Windmill.]* 10. When you are ready, straighten your legs and step your feet together to rest in Standing Mountain. See if you notice any feelings or sensations in your body.
Guideline #5: EMPOWERED	**We develop strength in our bodies when we learn to accept stronger muscle sensations. In the same way, we can learn to deal with challenges without getting caught up in our strong feelings about them. But if the sensation or situation is too intense, we need to move away from it so we don't get hurt.**

	TAC	**PROP**		**BAL**

Windmill (from Warrior 2)

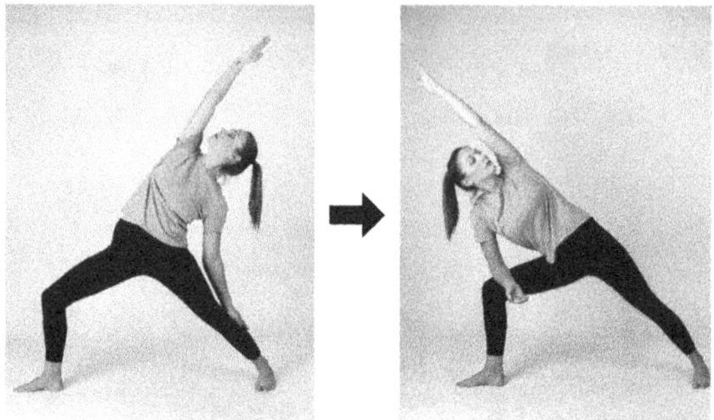

[Make sure Warrior 2 is mastered before attempting Windmill.]

[From Warrior 2, shorten Warrior 2 cues to preserve strength.]

1. Now let's try Windmill. Your arms will be the blades of the windmill. As you are ready, turn your [(red) right *or* front] palm up.

Guideline #2: CALM	2. As you breathe in, slide your left hand down your back leg as you lift your [red] right arm straight overhead (left-hand photo above). 3. As you breathe out with a "whoosh," bend your body to the other side, rest your arm on your bent leg, and raise your left arm up close to your ear (right-hand photo above). 4. Keep moving like a windmill. 5. Breathe in to the left, slide your arm down your leg, reach your other arm overhead. 6. Breathe out to the right, rest your arm on your bent leg, reach your other arm overhead. *[Complete three sets on each side of Warrior 2.]*
Guideline #4: UPLIFTED	7. Pressing your feet into the ground can help you to feel more stable as you change position... In the same way, when we ground ourselves, it can help us handle changes in our lives more easily.
Finishing steps	8. When you're ready, lower your arms to your sides and turn your feet to face the long side of the mat. Now let's do Warrior 2 on the other side. 9. When you are ready, straighten your legs and step your feet closer together to rest in Standing Mountain. See if you notice any different feelings or sensations in your body.
Guideline #5: EMPOWERED	**In life, things change and it's important to learn how to be flexible. Just as your body moves more easily and smoothly when it is well grounded, your mind can more easily "go with the flow" when it is grounded and stable.**

BREATH	TAC	PROP	VEST	BAL

Standing Forward Fold with or without Band

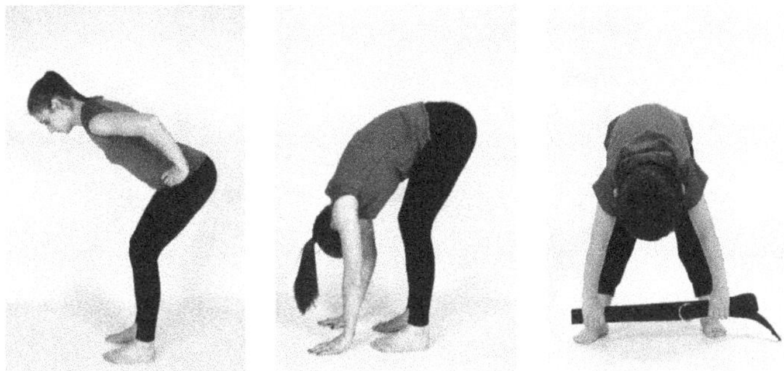

1. Fold your yoga band, if using one.
2. Step your feet a bit wider apart and point the toes of your feet out a bit.
3. Pull the band tight in front of your chest with your arms straight, a little wider than your shoulders.

   Or: You may place hands on your hips if not using a yoga band.

Guideline #1: SAFE	4. Root your feet down into the earth/ground.			
Guideline #2: CALM	5. Breathe in and raise your arms to the sky, pulling your band tight. *Or:* You may keep your hands on your hips if not using a band. 6. Breathe out, bend your knees, and bend forward at your hips with a long, flat back (left-hand photo above). You may rest your arms on your legs or let your arms hang as you continue to breathe in and out.			
Guideline #4: UPLIFTED	7. Imagine letting any stress, tightness/tension, or worries from the day simply roll off your back.			
Finishing step	8. As you are ready, bend your knees a bit more, place your hands on your thighs, and slowly come back up to standing.			
Guideline #5: EMPOWERED	**Learning how to rise to a challenge and completely release when it has passed is crucial for developing resilience.**			
		PROP		**BAL**

Waterfall with or without Band

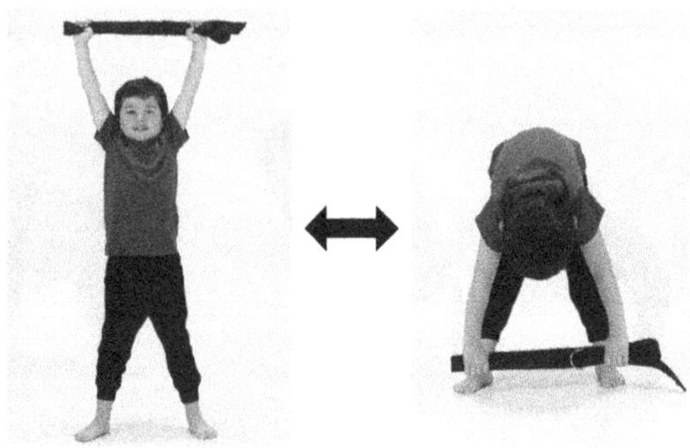

[From Mountain with or without yoga band]

1. Do you want to use a yoga band?
   - If yes, fold the yoga band in half and hold it with both hands a bit wider than your shoulders.
   - If no, just stand with your arms at your side, in Mountain.

<table>
<tr><td>Guideline #1:
SAFE
Guideline #3:
CLEAR</td><td colspan="4">[Guideline #1 cues are embedded in Mountain]
2. As you're ready, raise your arms straight overhead.
3. If you have a band, stretch it tight by pulling your arms apart (left-hand photo above).
4. Notice how that stretch feels in your arms...</td></tr>
<tr><td>Guideline #2:
CALM</td><td colspan="4">5. Now let's add some movement with the breath.
6. As you breathe in, reach your arms up even higher to the sky.
7. As you breathe out, bend your knees a little and flow your body like a waterfall, all the way to the ground, like this [demonstrate].
8. Breathe in, bend your knees, reach up to the sky (stretch the band tight).
9. Breathe out, flow like a waterfall to the ground...
10. Continue this movement with your breath...</td></tr>
<tr><td>Guideline #4:
UPLIFTED</td><td colspan="4">11. Breathe in happy thoughts as you reach up to the sky...
12. Then breathe out your worries as you flow like a waterfall to the ground.
[Start with a total of three (check for dizziness), and then work up to a total of four to six Waterfalls over time (if well tolerated).]
13. The next time your waterfall flows down to the ground, stay here and let your body rest. Let all your worries roll off your back, like they are flowing down the waterfall.</td></tr>
<tr><td>Finishing step</td><td colspan="4">14. As you're ready, push on your upper legs to help you stand back up.</td></tr>
<tr><td>Guideline #5:
EMPOWERED</td><td colspan="4">Bring in light and let go of worries or tightness in the bodymind.</td></tr>
<tr><td>BREATH</td><td></td><td>PROP</td><td>VEST</td><td>BAL</td></tr>
</table>

Tree

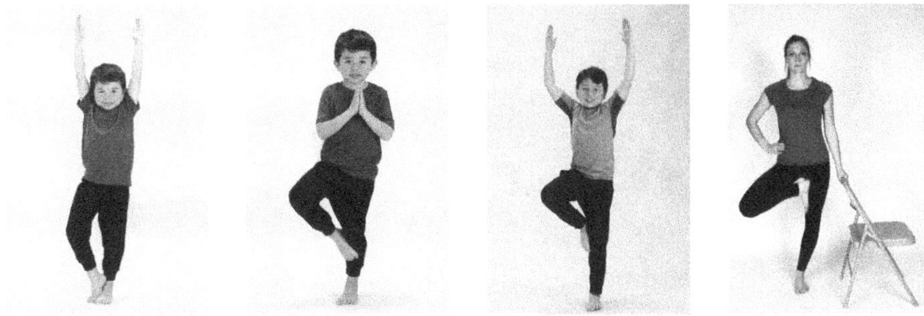

1. Meet me in a strong Mountain form.
2. For extra support, stand near a wall or a sturdy, slip-proof chair (photo furthest right above).
3. Press your hands together in front of your chest.
4. Look at something straight in front of you that is not moving.

Guideline #1: SAFE	5. Press your feet down to feel the support of the ground below you. 6. Tap your left leg; this will be our first balancing leg. 7. Bring your hands back to your chest as you lean your body weight into the left leg. 8. Turn your right foot out and put your right heel on the left ankle. (Photo furthest left above.)
Guideline #3: CLEAR	9. How do you feel here? Do you feel balanced and stable? 10. You can stay here or lift your right foot up to your lower (center-left photo above) or upper leg (center-right photo above). Make sure you do not rest your foot on your knee. 11. Keep facing forward, as your bent knee points to the side. 12. If you feel balanced here, you may slowly raise your arms up to the sky (hands facing each other), to grow the branches of your tree.
Guideline #2: CALM	13. As you breathe in, imagine breathing in fresh air to help the tree grow. 14. Then breathe out your worries in the wind.
Guideline #4: UPLIFTED	15. Feel your body sway side to side as it tries to find balance. Welcome this swaying...as this is how we learn to find balance. Just like in life...you need to first feel off-balance to learn what it means to be balanced.
Finishing step	16. Slowly lower the arms and place your right foot back on the floor. *[Repeat on the other side.]*
Guideline #5: EMPOWERED	**It is an important life lesson to be aware of when you are off-balance, in order to make changes to find balance in the body and mind.**

		PROP		**BAL**

Baby Cobra

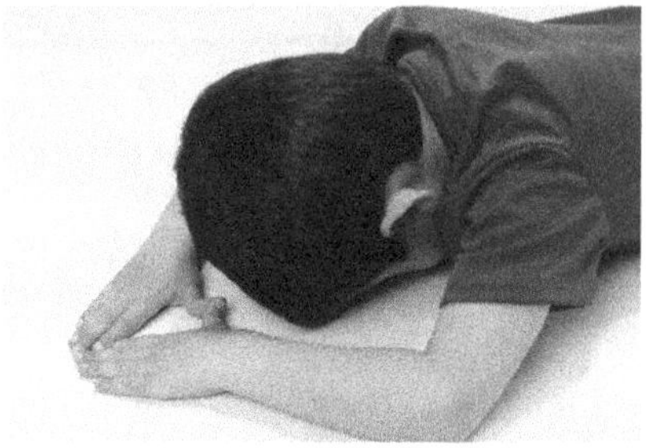

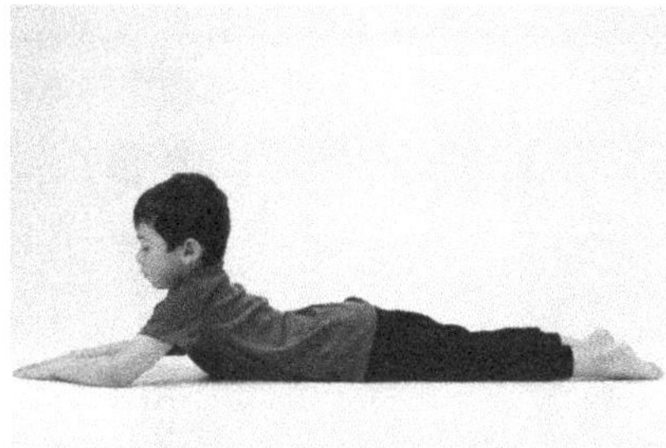

1. Lie on your belly/stomach, with your legs touching or a little apart.
2. Rest your forehead on the floor.
3. Place your hands on the mat just above your head and touch your thumbs and pointer fingers together to make a diamond shape *[demonstrate]* (left-hand photo above).

Guideline #1: SAFE	4. Push your hips and the tops of your feet into the ground. 5. Push your arms and hands down as you lift your head and chest up. 6. Keep your elbows on the mat (right-hand photo above). 7. Feel your body's connection to the ground.
Guideline #2: CALM	8. Let's pretend to be cobra snakes now. *[Make the breathwork fun.]* 9. Breathe in through your nose...breathe out with a "hissssssss." *[Do this three times.]*
Guideline #3: CLEAR	10. How does your body feel when you pretend to be a cobra? *Or:* Feel the ground under your belly as you breathe. This pressure can be calming for the body and mind. 11. Listen to your body...does it want to stay here longer or rest? 12. *If you need to rest:* Fold your arms on top of each other to make a pillow and rest your forehead on top of them in Crocodile.
Guideline #4: UPLIFTED	13. It's important to listen to our body as it lets us know what we are feeling and how to control our feelings.
Finishing steps	14. As you are ready, slowly lower your belly back to the ground. Then bend your knees so your feet are up in the air *[demonstrate]*. 15. Move your feet from side to side like "windshield wipers" on a car, to release any stress/tightness in your back. 16. As you are ready, move onto your back and bring your knees to your chest, to rest your back even more.
Guideline #5: EMPOWERED	**As we listen to our body, we can more easily control how we feel.**

BREATH	**TAC**	**PROP**		

Crocodile

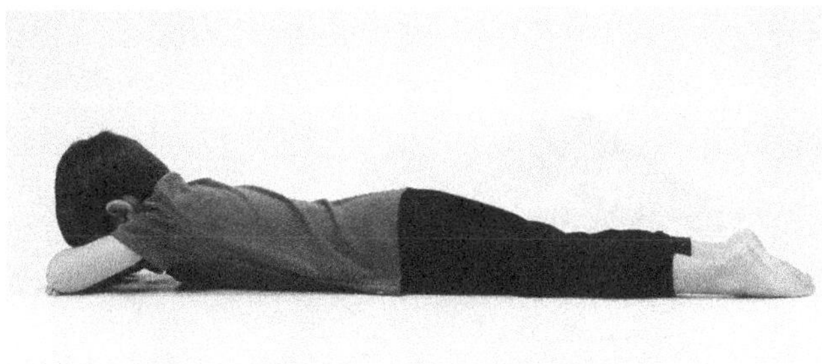

1. Lie on your belly/stomach, with your legs a little bit apart.
2. Now make a pillow with your arms, like this:
    - First, fold your arms on top of each other and hold near the elbows *[demonstrate]*.
    - Pull your elbows a bit closer to you, so your chest is lifted.
    - Then rest your forehead on your arms.

<table>
<tr><td>Guideline #1:
SAFE</td><td colspan="4">3. Rest here and notice where your legs, belly, and arms touch the floor.
4. Feel your body's connection to the ground.</td></tr>
<tr><td>Guideline #2:
CALM
Guideline #3:
CLEAR</td><td colspan="4">5. You may feel your belly press against the floor as you breathe in and out.
6. Feeling this pressure on your belly as you breathe can help to relax your body and mind.</td></tr>
<tr><td>Guideline #4:
UPLIFTED</td><td colspan="4">7. Notice any calming effects as you connect with the earth/ground and your own breath.</td></tr>
<tr><td>Finishing step</td><td colspan="4">8. As you are ready, move on to your back and bring your knees to your chest, to release any tightness in your lower back.</td></tr>
<tr><td>Guideline #5:
EMPOWERED</td><td colspan="4">As we learn to connect with the earth/ground and our breath, it helps us to feel more safe and calm.</td></tr>
<tr><td>BREATH</td><td>TAC</td><td>PROP</td><td></td><td></td></tr>
</table>

Lying Down Rest Form (Savasana)

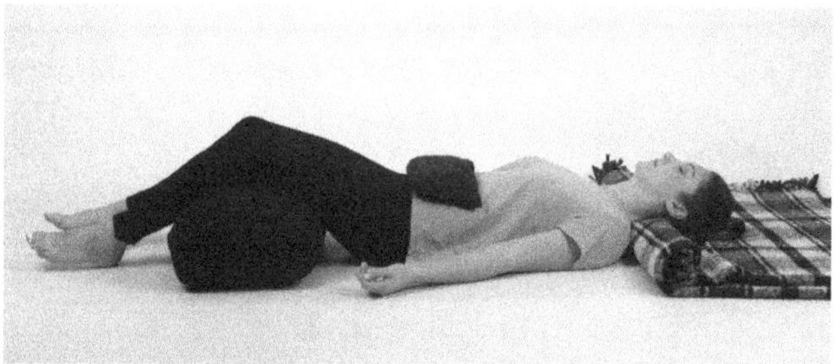

1. When you're ready, lie down on your mat in a comfortable position, with your legs straight and arms resting by your sides.
2. You may wish to place a bolster or rolled blanket under your knees and a folded blanket or small pillow under your head.
3. *Optional:* During breathwork, you may wish to place a weighted yoga bag or a "breathing buddy" on your belly.
4. Think about softening the muscles of your arms and legs to let them completely rest on the floor.

Guideline #1: SAFE Guideline #3: CLEAR	5. Feel the firm support of the ground below your body. 6. How does it feel to be fully supported by the earth/ground?			
Guideline #2: CALM	7. Breathe slowly in and out through your nose.			
Guideline #4: UPLIFTED	8. Invite waves of relaxation to flow up from your legs all the way into your heart and mind.			
Finishing step	9. Roll on to your side and slowly push yourself up to a seated position.			
Guideline #5: EMPOWERED	**We can use bodily sensations to spread a sense of healing and relaxation through the bodymind.**			
BREATH	**TAC**			

CHAPTER 15

Yoga Forms Using a Chair

Yoga classes frequently include one or more students who have some sort of mobility challenge. In an effort to "fit in" with the rest of the class (or because no other option was offered to them), some of these students may perform the yoga forms and movements on the mat when a chair version of the yoga form might actually be the safer route to go. This may be especially true for ambulatory students who have "invisible" mobility challenges, such as wrist conditions that make upper extremity weight bearing painful or even harmful. It is therefore strongly suggested that all students be provided with the option to use a mat and/or chair during the yoga session, and that every effort be made to eliminate any stigma attached to the use of a chair for yoga.

On the flipside, please be aware that students who may need a chair for most of the practice may be capable of and interested in performing the standing yoga forms. And although they may choose not to recline on the mat—or get on their hands and knees—for most of the practice, some may decide it is worth the effort to recline at the end for the final guided meditation. So it is always a good idea to remind students of their various options.

Chair yoga forms usually produce just as strong a muscle challenge for the torso and arms as their counterpart forms on the mat. However, a sense of grounding may be lessened due to reduced engagement of the leg muscles and reduced body weight through the legs, resulting in less pressure of the feet into the ground. An alternate source of grounding occurs from contact of the sitting bones on the surface of the chair, from which point the spine is lengthened upward. However, we also cue pressing the feet down into the ground even while seated in a chair, as this provides deep touch pressure through the soles of the feet as well as proprioceptive input through engagement of the leg muscles. This combination of tactile and proprioceptive input promotes a greater sense of grounding, which can enhance a sense of safety and security.

Also, do not feel intimidated if you find yourself in a position where you need to teach yoga to a class of students with mixed mobility levels. Remember that in most cases the cues for the spine, shoulders, arms, and Guidelines #2, #3, and

#4 will be identical. It is primarily the "set-up" and lower body instructions that will differ. Please refer back to Chapter 12 for more detailed information on how to work with groups of students who have mixed mobility levels. Also please read the introduction of Chapter 14, most of which applies to working with students who are using a chair, and not just those performing yoga on a mat.

Finally, as these are our last words in the book, we would like to take this opportunity to thank you for your interest and hours spent reading it. We hope you enjoyed the learning process and gained the knowledge you were looking for. We know it was a lot to digest, but each time you re-read this book you will absorb more of the information, some of which may inspire and energize your professional practice in ways you hadn't foreseen. Please feel free to contact us through the Sensory-Enhanced Yoga® Institute to share your successes and challenges as you incorporate this material into your work with children, adolescents, and/or individuals who have special challenges. We are always available to answer a question, hear your suggestions, or take any other feedback.

Also remember to keep up to date on your own internet research as there is an explosion of studies right now on the topics of trauma and yoga, and much still to be learned! Hopefully most future study findings will be consistent with the information presented in this book. There are still many questions left unanswered regarding most of the topics discussed. Perhaps some of you will be inspired to conduct your own research to help connect some of the remaining dots. So this is by no means the end of the story on working with individuals who are healing from trauma, toxic stress, or related conditions using yoga as a healing modality. We hope you will consider helping to expand this knowledge base, as there are so many people around the world who can benefit from this important work! We wish you well on your journey forward, and don't forget to SMYLE™!

Seated Mountain

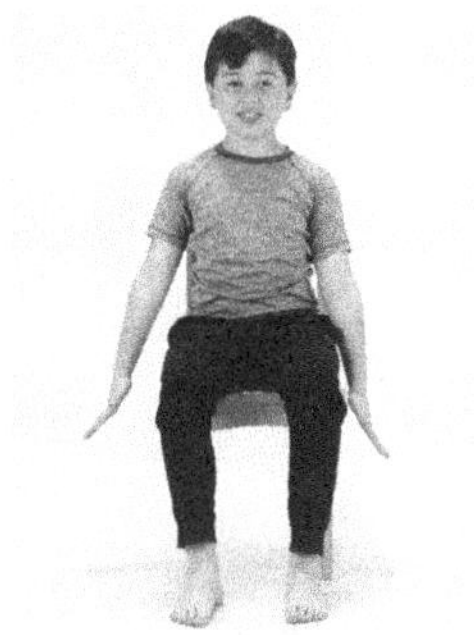

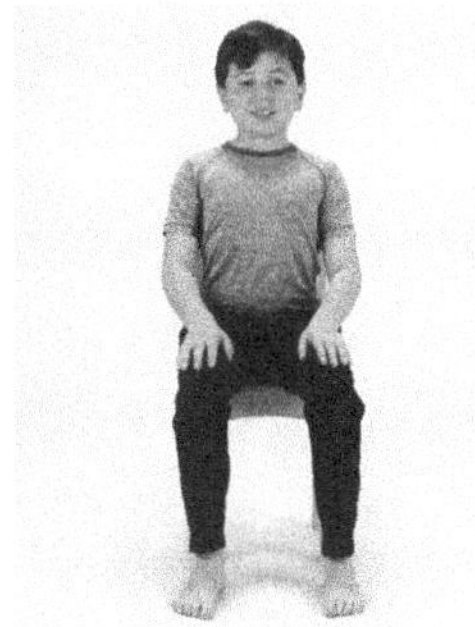

<table>
<tr><td>Guideline #1:
SAFE</td><td colspan="4">1. Sit forward so your back isn't touching the chair.
2. Point your toes forward.
3. Press your feet down and feel the ground below you.
4. Press your bottom into the seat of the chair.</td></tr>
<tr><td colspan="5">5. Stretch your head up nice and tall—this is the top of the Mountain.
6. Stretch your hands down by your sides to form the sides of the Mountain (left-hand photo above).
Or: You can rest your hands on your lap (right-hand photo above). Do what feels right for you.
7. Drop/relax your shoulders down away from the ears.
8. You are as strong and solid as a Mountain.
9. You may close your eyes or look down.</td></tr>
<tr><td>Guideline #2:
CALM</td><td colspan="4">10. Breathe in through your nose. Optional: Smell flowers on the side of the mountain or fresh air.
11. Breathe out through your mouth like the wind blowing around the mountain [demonstrate: purse your lips and make a wind sound].
12. How does it feel to breathe in and out as a mountain?</td></tr>
<tr><td>Guideline #4:
UPLIFTED</td><td colspan="4">13. You might imagine that a bunny is making a nest on the side of the mountain, right where your heart is.
14. Can you sit strong like a mountain and keep a soft spot for the bunny?
• Strong mountain...soft bunny...
• Strong body...soft heart...</td></tr>
<tr><td>Guideline #5:
EMPOWERED</td><td colspan="4">People often harden their hearts to block out uncomfortable feelings, but when you do this you also block out good feelings, like joy and love. It takes emotional strength to let yourself feel your emotions. When you do, it helps you stay more present and engaged in life. In Mountain form, feel the support of the earth/ground giving you the strength and courage to soften your heart and let the light in.</td></tr>
<tr><td>BREATH</td><td></td><td>PROP</td><td></td><td></td></tr>
</table>

Seated Whole Body Stretch

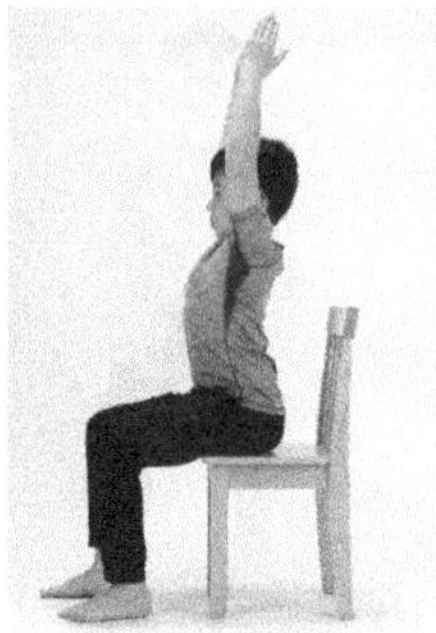

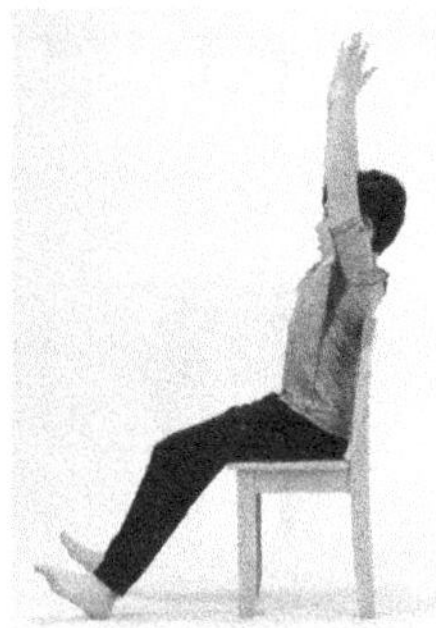

Guideline #1: SAFE	1. Meet me in a strong Seated Mountain. Sit forward from the back of your chair. Keep your feet under your knees (left-hand photo above). *Or:* Straighten your legs in front of you and press your heels down into the ground (right-hand photo above). 2. Raise your arms overhead. 3. If you want, you can make a pencil point with your hands, like this *[demonstrate]*. 4. Reach your arms up high to make your body really long.
Guideline #3: CLEAR	5. Where do you feel the stretch in your body...maybe your legs... sides...arms...hands?
Guideline #2: CALM	6. Take three slow, deep breaths, in and out.
Guideline #4: UPLIFTED	7. Can you feel how long your whole body is? 8. How does it feel to take up that much space?
Finishing step	9. When you're ready, slowly lower your arms down to your sides and rest in Seated Mountain. See if you notice any sensations or feelings in your body. *Or:* Move into Seated Rainbow Breaths *or* Seated Half Moon.
Guideline #5: EMPOWERED	**Some people don't like taking up space with their body, especially if they're feeling shy, sad, or bad about themselves. But actually, when you stretch your body and let it take up more space, it can help you feel better and more confident when talking with others.**

BREATH		**PROP**		

Seated Rainbow Breaths

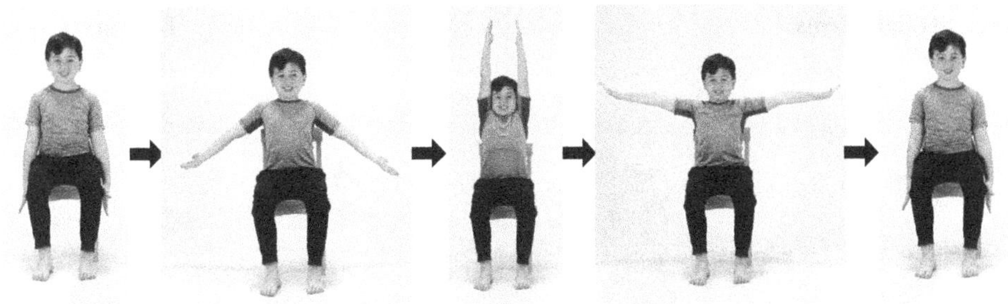

<table>
<tr><td>Guideline #1:
SAFE</td><td colspan="4">[From Seated Mountain, with arms down by the sides of the body]
1. From here, let's do a few Rainbow Breaths.
2. Press your feet down and feel the ground below you.
3. Press your bottom down into your chair.</td></tr>
<tr><td>Guideline #2:
CALM</td><td colspan="4">4. As you breathe in, lift your arms up toward the sky, like you are painting a rainbow with your hands.
5. As you breathe out, blow your arms back down to your sides.</td></tr>
<tr><td>Guideline #4:
UPLIFTED</td><td colspan="4">6. Keep painting the rainbow with your breath...breathing in...and blowing out your worries with each breath out.</td></tr>
<tr><td>Guideline #3:
CLEAR</td><td colspan="4">7. How does this feel in your body?
[Perform 3–6 reps total.]</td></tr>
<tr><td>Finishing step</td><td colspan="4">8. When you're ready, slowly lower your arms back down and rest in Seated Mountain. See if you notice any sensations or feelings in your body.</td></tr>
<tr><td>Guideline #5:
EMPOWERED</td><td colspan="4">Connecting your movement with your breath can help to clear the worries from your mind.</td></tr>
<tr><td>BREATH</td><td></td><td>PROP</td><td></td><td></td></tr>
</table>

Seated Half Moon

Arm variation 1: Straight arms	**Arm variation 2: Bent arms**

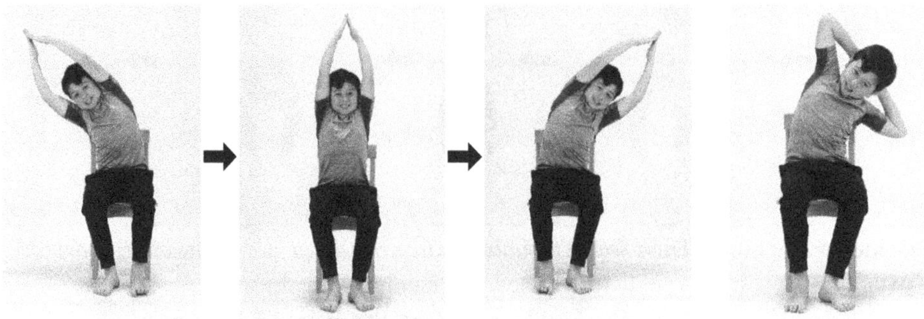

[From Seated Whole Body Stretch, with bent legs, feet on floor]

1. From here, let's try Seated Half Moon Stretch.

Guideline #2: CALM	2. Decide if you want to do bent arms or straight arms *[demonstrate both]*. 3. As you breathe in through your nose, reach up with your arms. 4. Breathe out as you bend to your [red] right side. 5. Breathe in, and come back to center. 6. Breathe out as you bend to the left. 7. Breathe in, and come back to center. 8. Continue to move like this with your breath. 9. Try not to stop and just flow from side to side, like a swing.		
Guideline #3: CLEAR	10. How does it feel to stretch your body from side to side? 11. Notice if pressing your feet into the ground and your bottom into the chair helps you feel more stable as you bend from side to side...		
Guideline #4: UPLIFTED	12. In the same way, when you ground yourself, it can help you handle changes in your life more easily.		
Finishing step	13. As you're ready, slowly lower your arms and rest in Seated Mountain. See if you notice any different feelings or sensations in your body.		
Guideline #5: EMPOWERED	**When we ground ourselves, we are better able to bend and adapt to face whatever comes our way, with courage and resilience.**		
BREATH		**PROP**	**VEST**	**BAL**

Seated Knee to Chest

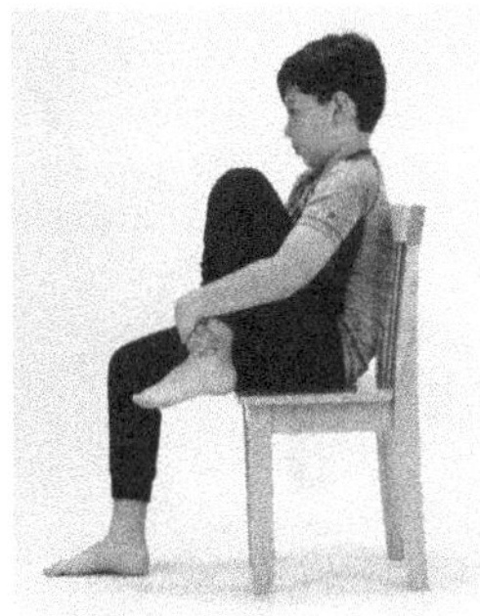

[From Seated Mountain]

1. As you're ready...bring one knee up to your chest.
2. Imagine you are folding yourself into a ball.

Guideline #4: UPLIFTED	3. As you hug your knee, imagine you are hugging a friend... 4. *[1st side]* Can you be your own friend during this yoga practice by listening to your body's messages? 5. Remember to get out of a yoga form or breathing practice at any time if it does not feel right for you.
Guideline #2: CALM	6. Now, if you like, try breathing with me for three breaths: • Breathe in, belly blows up like a balloon, pushing against your leg... • Breathe out, air flows out of the balloon, stomach sinks down. • Breathe in, belly rises...breathe out, belly sinks back down. *[Repeat one more time.]* 7. Continue to breathe on your own now as you feel how your breath moves your body.
Finishing step	8. As you're ready, lower your leg back to the floor and rest your body. See if you notice any different sensations or feelings in your body. *[Repeat the steps on the other side.]*
Guideline #5: EMPOWERED	**We need to be a friend to ourselves if we want our emotional wounds to heal. It's only when we feel self-love that we fully understand we deserve love and are loved by others.**

BREATH	**TAC**	**PROP**		

Seated Leg Stretches

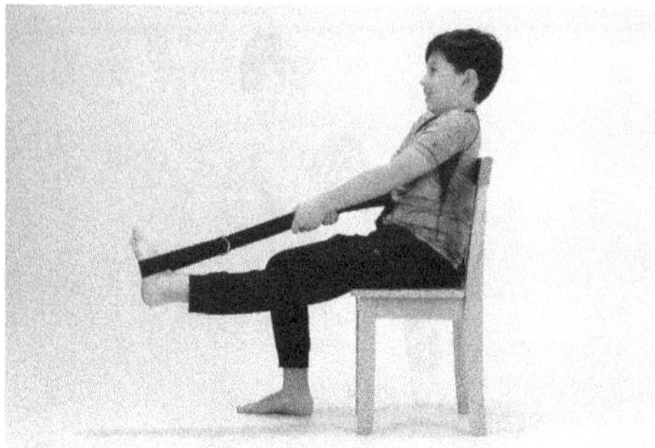

[From Seated Mountain]

1. I invite you to join me for some Leg Stretches.
2. When you are ready, decide if you want to use a yoga band or not.
   - *With a yoga band:* please make a small loop at the end.
   - *Without a yoga band:* try holding your thigh to support your leg.
3. Sit forward in your seat so your back is not touching the chair.

Guideline #1: SAFE	4. Place the loop of the yoga band over [the ball of] your right foot. 5. Straighten your leg and sit up tall. 6. Hold the band close to your foot so you can feel a good stretch all the way through your leg. 7. Feel how strong your leg muscles are when you push your foot into the band.
Guideline #2: CALM	8. Breathe in and out through your nose. 9. Each time you breathe out, imagine blowing the air into your leg to help soften the muscles [release any tightness].
Guideline #3: CLEAR Guideline #4: UPLIFTED	10. Notice when you connect your breath to harder body movements, your breath gives you power to work through it. Your breath can help you do hard things. 11. Now, if you'd like, move your leg in a circle to loosen up the muscles in your hip. Draw a circle in one direction and then go the other way. 12. Which way feels better for you?
Finishing step	13. As you are ready, take the band off your foot and rest your foot on the ground. *[Repeat the steps on the left side.]*
Guideline #5: EMPOWERED	**In life, you will face challenges. When things get hard, focus on your breath. The power of your breath will help you get through difficult times, and give you strength to reach your goals.**

BREATH	TAC	PROP		

Owl (Seated Twist)

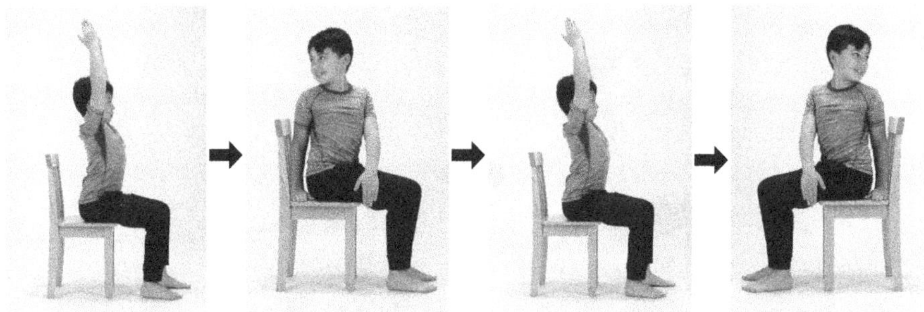

<table>
<tr><td>Guideline #1:
SAFE</td><td colspan="4">[Grounding cues are incorporated into Seated Mountain.]</td></tr>
<tr><td>Guideline #2:
CALM</td><td colspan="4">[From Seated Mountain]
1. Breathe in, as you sit up tall, and raise your arms up overhead.
2. Breathe out, twist your body, and drop your arms to the [red] right side.
3. If you want, you can turn your head to look behind you.
Optional: You look just like an owl!
4. As you breathe in, bring your arms back up overhead.
5. As you breathe out, twist your body to the other [left] side, drop your arms, and turn your head to look behind you.
Optional: If you want you can "hoooottt" like an owl when you breathe out.
6. Keep twisting from side to side, moving with your breath.</td></tr>
<tr><td>Guideline #4:
UPLIFTED</td><td colspan="4">7. Picture yourself squeezing out all the tightness and worries in your body, just like you squeeze out water from a wet towel.
8. By twisting out the stress it can help you feel lighter and more energized.
Optional: Now let's try to hold it on each side for a few breaths. [Stay for 2–3 breaths on each side.]</td></tr>
<tr><td>Finishing step</td><td colspan="4">9. As you're ready, twist your body back to center, lower your arms by your sides, and rest in Seated Mountain. See if you notice any different feelings or sensations in your body.</td></tr>
<tr><td>Guideline #5:
EMPOWERED</td><td colspan="4">Stress builds up over time in everyone. It is important to slow down and squeeze out the stress, so you can make room for new, positive experiences.</td></tr>
<tr><td>BREATH</td><td></td><td>PROP</td><td>VEST</td><td></td></tr>
</table>

Seated Cat Flow (Happy Cat/Angry Cat)

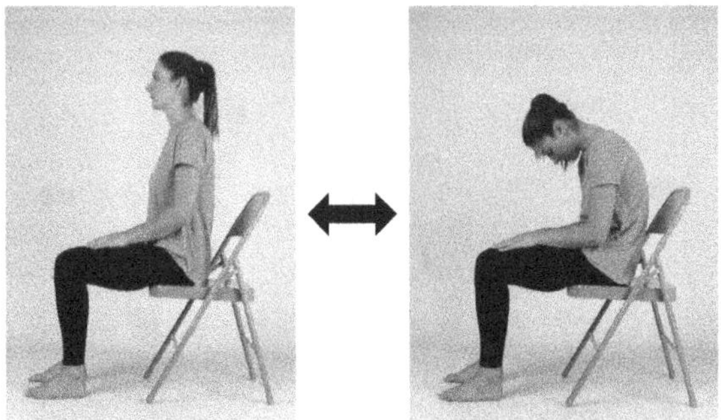

<table>
<tr><td>Guideline #1:
SAFE</td><td colspan="4">[From Seated Mountain]
1. Imagine you are a cat. You have a long tail.
2. Lift your tail to the sky, and look up (left-hand photo above).
3. If you want you can smile like a Happy Cat.
4. Now let's turn into an Angry Cat...tuck your tail between your legs, round your back, and drop your head to see your hidden tail (right-hand photo above).</td></tr>
<tr><td>Guideline #3:
CLEAR</td><td colspan="4">5. How does it feel to be a Happy Cat?
6. How does it feel to be an Angry Cat?
7. Which feels better to you right now...in this moment?
[Practice a couple of times before introducing the breath flow.]</td></tr>
<tr><td>Guideline #2:
CALM</td><td colspan="4">8. Let's switch back and forth from Happy Cat to Angry Cat using our breath.
9. As you breathe in...lift your tail...look up and smile—Happy Cat!
10. Breathe out with a "hisss" as you tuck your tail and round your back—Angry Cat!
[Repeat steps 9 and 10, three to five times.]
If appropriate: Now practice three times on your own.</td></tr>
<tr><td>Guideline #4:
UPLIFTED</td><td colspan="4">11. How does it feel to flow from a Happy Cat to an Angry Cat...and back to a Happy Cat?</td></tr>
<tr><td>Guideline #5:
EMPOWERED</td><td colspan="4">When you feel the support of the ground and move your body with your breath, you more easily can control how you feel.</td></tr>
<tr><td>BREATH</td><td>TAC</td><td></td><td>VEST</td><td></td></tr>
</table>

Seated Tiger Flow

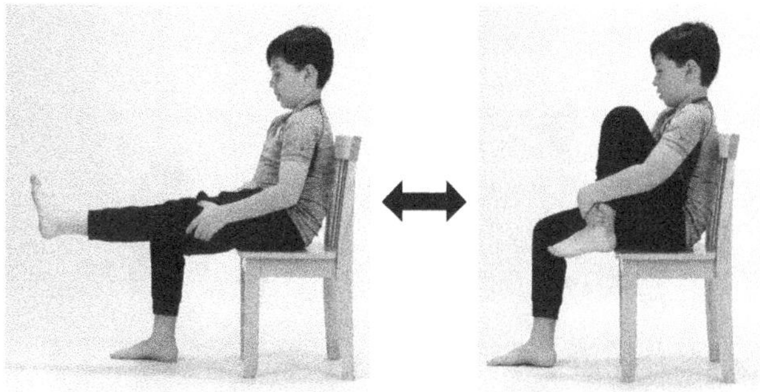

<table>
<tr><td>Guideline #1:
SAFE</td><td>[Grounding cues are incorporated into Seated Mountain.]</td></tr>
<tr><td>Guideline #2:
CALM</td><td>[If necessary, demonstrate and practice without the breath first.]
[From Seated Mountain]
1. As you breathe in, lift one leg off the floor, straight out in front of you (left-hand photo above).
Or from Cat Flow: The next time you breathe in, lift one leg off the floor, straight out in front of you.
2. As you breathe out, bring one knee up to your chest. You may also round your back to bring your forehead to your knee*, or keep your head up and your back straight (right-hand photo above).
[Cue one to three more times.]
If appropriate: Now move like this with your own breath.</td></tr>
<tr><td>Guideline #3:
CLEAR</td><td>3. Keep your strong connection with the ground through your resting foot as you sense the rhythm of the flow...</td></tr>
<tr><td colspan="2">4. Next time you breathe in, straighten your leg, hold it, and look straight ahead... Keep breathing...
5. You can stay here or try lifting the arm on your other side...keep breathing...</td></tr>
<tr><td>Guideline #4:
UPLIFTED</td><td>6. Strong and steady breath—strong and steady body.
7. When ready, slowly lower your arm to your side and foot to the floor.
[Repeat on the other side.]</td></tr>
<tr><td>Guideline #5:
EMPOWERED</td><td>Our sense of confidence is felt from the upper belly area (below the ribs and above the belly button). [Cue students to place a hand on this area to locate it.] We can build confidence by moving and breathing in this area of the body.</td></tr>
</table>

BREATH	TAC	PROP	*VEST	BAL

Seated Twisting Cat

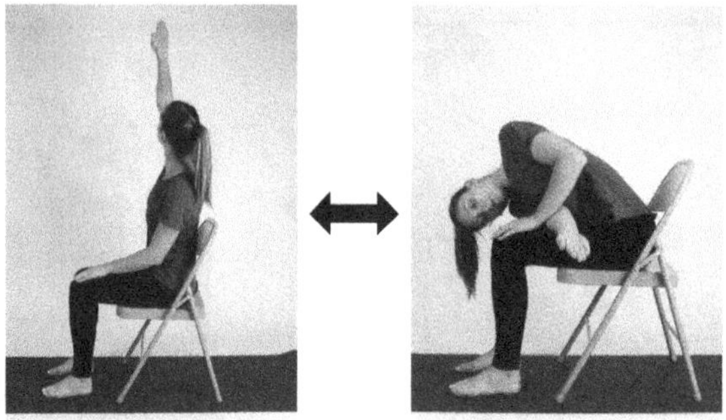

Guideline #1: SAFE	*[From Seated Mountain]* 1. As you're ready...meet me in a strong Seated Mountain, with your hands resting on your legs. *[Cue Seated Mountain.]*
Guideline #2: CALM	*[If necessary, demonstrate and practice without the breath first.]* 2. As you breathe in, raise your [red] right arm out and up to the sky, and look at your hand (left-hand photo above). 3. As you breathe out, reach that arm under your other arm, like this *[demonstrate]*, watching your hand as it moves (right-hand photo above). *[Model full twist with forearm/elbow close to touching upper leg/thigh.]* 4. Breathe in, raise your right arm up to the sky. 5. Breathe out, reach under your other arm. 6. Continue moving like this, watching your hand as it moves.
Guideline #3: CLEAR	7. How does it feel to move like this? 8. *[After four reps]* The next time you breathe out, reach your arm all the way under your body and rest down on your arm.
Guideline #4: UPLIFTED	9. Notice how the room looks from this view. 10. Do things look different upside down? How does that make you feel? 11. *[2nd side]* You might notice how things look a little different on this side, too. This helps us remember there is always another way to look at things!
Finishing steps	12. Slowly come back up to Seated Mountain. 13. Now let's repeat this on the other side.
Guideline #5: EMPOWERED	**When we take the time to look at a problem in a different way, it can change our attitude about it, and lead to better solutions.**

BREATH	TAC	PROP	VEST	

Setting Sun

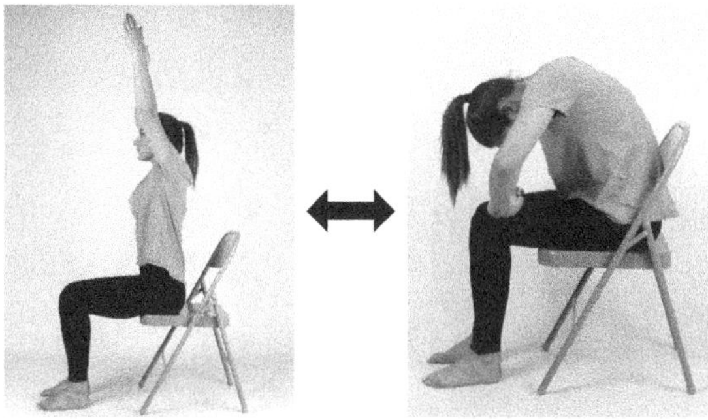

Guideline #1: SAFE	*[Grounding cues are incorporated into Seated Mountain.]*
Guideline #2: CALM	*[From Seated Mountain]* 1. As you breathe in, raise your arms out and up to the sky (left-hand photo above). 2. As you breathe out, bend forward with "Airplane arms," and let your hands land on your legs, like this *[demonstrate]* (right-hand photo above). 3. Breathe in, and push your body up as you raise your arms out and up to the sky. 4. Breathe out, bend forward with "Airplane arms," and bring your hands to your legs. 5. Breathe in, push yourself up, and raise your arms to the sky. 6. Continue to move like this with your breath, back and forth, like you are swinging on a swing.
Guideline #4: UPLIFTED	7. What happens when you just let yourself "go with the flow?" *[Perform 6–10 rounds.]*
Finishing step	8. As you are ready, come back and rest in Seated Mountain. See if you notice any different feelings or sensations in your body.
Guideline #5: EMPOWERED	**When we ground ourselves and move with our breath, it is easier to move past challenges.**

BREATH	TAC	PROP	VEST	

Seated Forward Fold

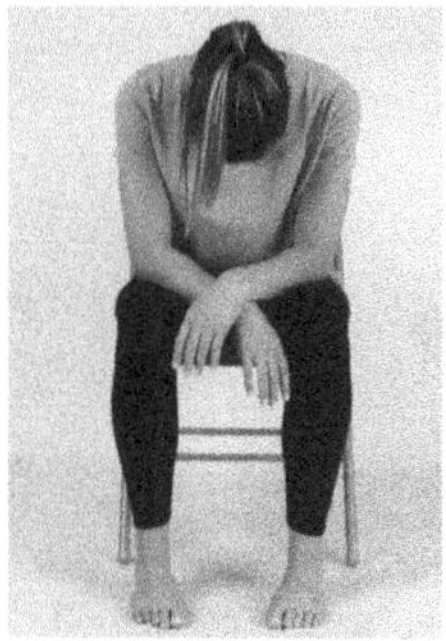 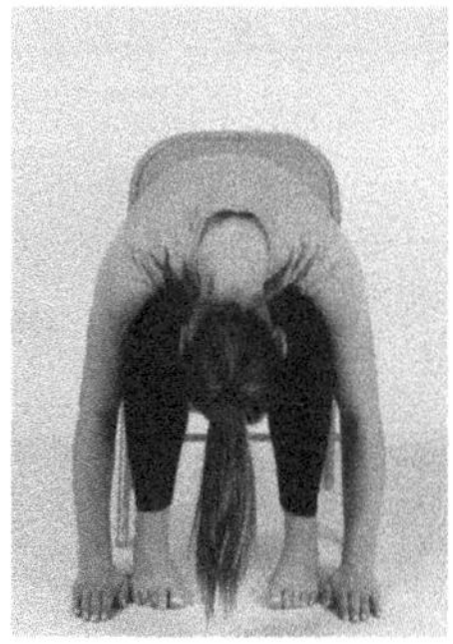

<table>
<tr><td>Guideline #1:
SAFE</td><td colspan="4">[From Seated Mountain]
1. Step your feet just a bit wider apart.
2. Point the toes of your feet in a tiny bit.
3. Bend forward at your hips [with a long, flat back].
4. Rest your arms/forearms on your legs.
5. Let your head hang down.
6. Let's stay here for a few breaths (left-hand photo above).
7. [After a few breaths] You can stay here, or if you want, you can let your arms hang down to the floor (right-hand photo above).</td></tr>
<tr><td>Guideline #2:
CALM</td><td colspan="4">8. Follow your breath as it moves in and out of your body.
9. Where do you feel your breath? Can you feel it in your back? In your belly? Pressing on your legs?
10. Each time you breathe out, sense/feel your body sinking down deeper and deeper on to the firm, solid, and stable earth/ground.</td></tr>
<tr><td>Guideline #4:
UPLIFTED</td><td colspan="4">11. Imagine letting any stress, tightness/tension, or worries from the day simply roll off your back.</td></tr>
<tr><td>Finishing steps</td><td colspan="4">12. As you are ready, bring your elbows to your legs if they are not here already, and rest here for a few breaths.
13. Then place your hands on your legs, and come back up to Seated Mountain. See if you notice any different feelings or sensations in your body.</td></tr>
<tr><td>Guideline #5:
EMPOWERED</td><td colspan="4">Learning how to rise to a challenge and completely release when it has passed is crucial for developing resilience.</td></tr>
<tr><td>BREATH</td><td>TAC</td><td>PROP</td><td></td><td></td></tr>
</table>

Seated Extended Mountain

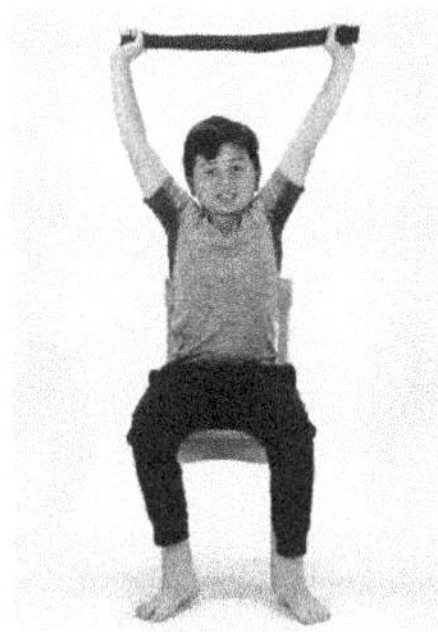

<table>
<tr><td>Guideline #1:
SAFE</td><td colspan="4">[From Seated Mountain]
1. Decide if you want to use a yoga band or not.
• With a yoga band: fold the yoga band in half and hold it with both hands a bit wider than your shoulders.
• Without yoga band: keep your hands shoulder-width apart.
2. Point your toes to the front of your mat.
3. As you breathe in, raise your arms straight overhead.
4. Stretch the band tight by pulling your arms apart.
5. Lower your shoulders down away from your ears.</td></tr>
<tr><td>Guideline #3:
CLEAR</td><td colspan="4">6. Notice how that stretch feels in your arms...</td></tr>
<tr><td>Guideline #2:
CALM</td><td colspan="4">7. Take nice slow easy breaths...breathing in...breathing out...</td></tr>
<tr><td>Guideline #4:
UPLIFTED</td><td colspan="4">8. When our feet are grounded to the earth/ground and we squeeze our muscles, it can help us to feel more solid, stable, and strong in both our body and mind... How does this make you feel in your own body?... In your own mind?</td></tr>
<tr><td>Finishing step</td><td colspan="4">9. As you're ready, slowly lower your arms to your sides and rest in Seated Mountain. See if you notice any different feelings or sensations in your body.</td></tr>
<tr><td>Guideline #5:
EMPOWERED</td><td colspan="4">As our bodies feel stronger, our minds feel stronger. We develop the confidence to try new things and meet our goals.</td></tr>
<tr><td>BREATH</td><td>TAC</td><td>PROP</td><td></td><td></td></tr>
</table>

Seated Half Moon with Band

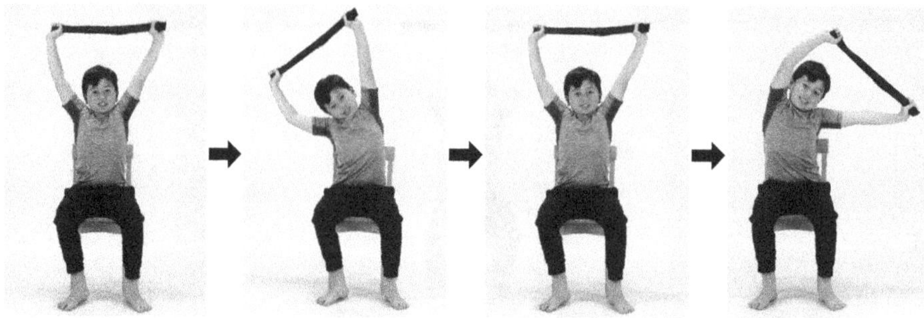

Guideline #1: SAFE	*[Grounding cues are incorporated into Seated Mountain.]*
Guideline #2: CALM	*[From Seated Mountain]* 1. Let's add some movement with our breath. 2. As you're ready...take a breath in through your nose (photo furthest left above). 3. Breathe out as you bend to your [red] right side (center-left photo above). 4. Breathe in as you come back to center (center-right photo above). 5. Breathe out as you bend to the left (photo furthest right above). 6. Breathe in as you come back to center. 7. Keep moving with your own breath...breathe out to the side... breathe into the center. *[Do 3–5 total sets. Keep moving through the center; don't segment the movements.]*
Guideline #3: CLEAR	8. How does it feel to stretch your body from side to side? 9. Notice if pressing your feet into the ground and your bottom into your chair helps you feel more stable as you bend from side to side...
Guideline #4: UPLIFTED	10. In the same way, when you ground yourself, it can help you handle changes in your life more easily.
Finishing step	11. As you're ready, slowly lower your arms and rest in Seated Mountain. See if you notice any different feelings or sensations in your body.
Guideline #5: EMPOWERED	**When we ground ourselves, we are better able to bend and adapt to face whatever comes our way, with courage and resilience.**

BREATH	TAC	PROP		BAL

Seated Twist with Band

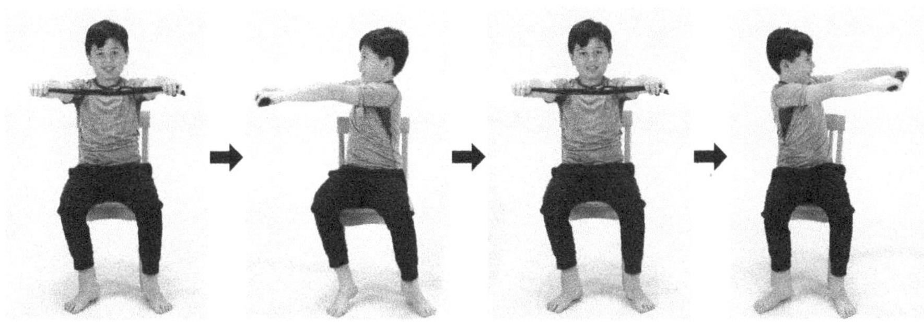

<table>
<tr><td>Guideline #1:
SAFE</td><td colspan="4">[Grounding cues are incorporated into Seated Mountain.]</td></tr>
<tr><td colspan="5">[From Seated Mountain]
1. Hold the band in front of your chest with your arms straight, a little wider than your shoulders.
2. Pull the band tight (photo furthest left above).</td></tr>
<tr><td>Guideline #2:
CALM</td><td colspan="4">3. Breathe in here, and then breathe out as you twist to the [red] right side, watching your hands (center-left photo above).
4. Breathe in, and twist back to center (center-right photo above). Breathe out, and twist to the other side, watching your hands [one set] (photo furthest right above).
5. Breathe in, come back to center...breathe out, twist to the other side. [Complete a total of three sets with step-by-step cues.]</td></tr>
<tr><td>Guideline #3:
CLEAR</td><td colspan="4">6. How does it feel to twist your body from side to side?</td></tr>
<tr><td>Guideline #4:
UPLIFTED</td><td colspan="4">7. Picture yourself squeezing out all the tightness and worries in your body, just like when you squeeze water from a wet towel.</td></tr>
<tr><td>Finishing step</td><td colspan="4">8. As you're ready, come back to center, lower your arms, and rest in Seated Mountain. See if you notice any different feelings or sensations in your body.</td></tr>
<tr><td>Guideline #5:
EMPOWERED</td><td colspan="4">When we squeeze out our worries and doubts, we make room for more positive attitudes and experiences.</td></tr>
<tr><td>BREATH</td><td>TAC</td><td>PROP</td><td>VEST</td><td>BAL</td></tr>
</table>

Seated Star

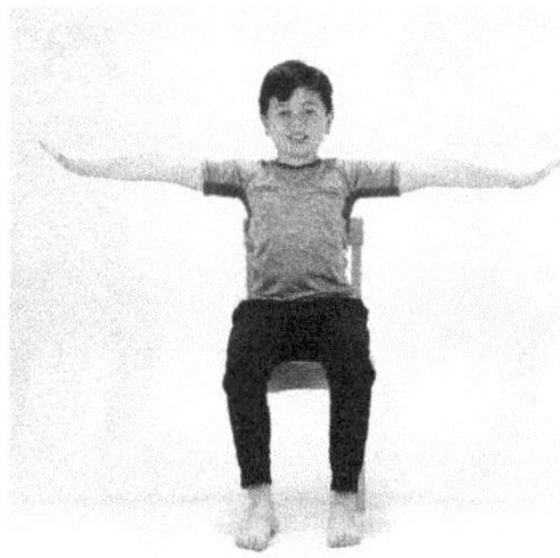

Guideline #1: SAFE	*[Grounding cues are incorporated into Seated Mountain.]*
Guideline #3: CLEAR	*[From Seated Mountain]* 1. As you're ready, lift your arms out straight to each side *[demonstrate]*. 2. Feel the stretch in your arms all the way to your fingertips. 3. Pull in the muscles in your belly. 4. Stretch your head up nice and tall. 5. Notice the muscles in your face...are they soft or tight? 6. Invite the muscles to soften and rest.
Guideline #2: CALM Guideline #4: UPLIFTED	7. Notice your breath, in...and out...in...and out... 8. As you breathe in, imagine bringing light and positive energy into your body. 9. As you breathe out, shine that positivity and light to the world.
Finishing step	10. As you're ready, lower your arms and rest in Seated Mountain. See if you notice any different feelings or sensations in your body.
Guideline #5: EMPOWERED	**Shine your light and positive energy to the world around you.**

BREATH		**PROP**		

Seated Shining Star

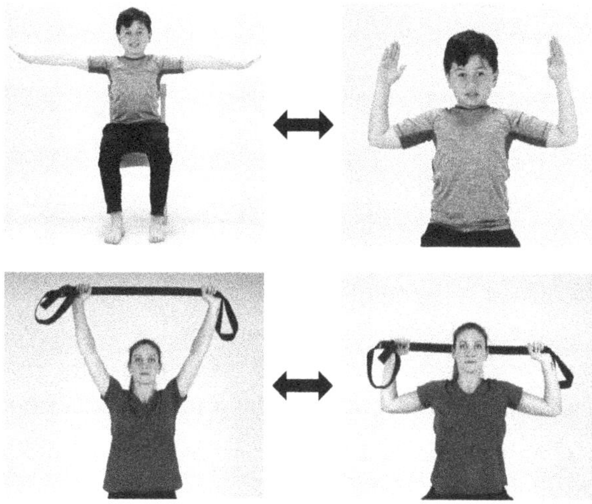

<table>
<tr><td colspan="1">Guideline #1:
SAFE</td><td colspan="4">[Grounding cues are incorporated into Seated Mountain.]</td></tr>
<tr><td>Guideline #2:
CALM</td><td colspan="4">[From Seated Mountain]
1. Let's add some movement with our breath.
2. If you are not holding a yoga band, lift your arms out straight to each side [demonstrate] (top-left photo above).
If you are holding a yoga band, pull the band tight overhead (bottom-left photo above).
3. As you breathe out, bend your elbows like this [demonstrate "goal post" arms) (top-right photo above).
If you are using a yoga band, pull it down behind your head (bottom-right photo above).
4. Breathe in, sit up tall, and stretch your arms.
5. Breathe out, and bend your elbows.
6. Continue to move like this with your breath.
[Repeat 3–5 times.]</td></tr>
<tr><td>Guideline #4:
UPLIFTED</td><td colspan="4">7. Imagine your Star getting brighter and brighter with each breath in and out, shining light and joy/positive energy to the world.</td></tr>
<tr><td>Guideline #3:
CLEAR</td><td colspan="4">8. How does it feel to move with your breath like this?</td></tr>
<tr><td>Finishing step</td><td colspan="4">9. As you're ready, lower your arms and rest in Seated Mountain. See if you notice any different feelings or sensations in your body.</td></tr>
<tr><td>Guideline #5:
EMPOWERED</td><td colspan="4">Shine your light and positive energy to the world around you.</td></tr>
<tr><td>BREATH</td><td>TAC</td><td>PROP</td><td></td><td></td></tr>
</table>

Seated Airplane

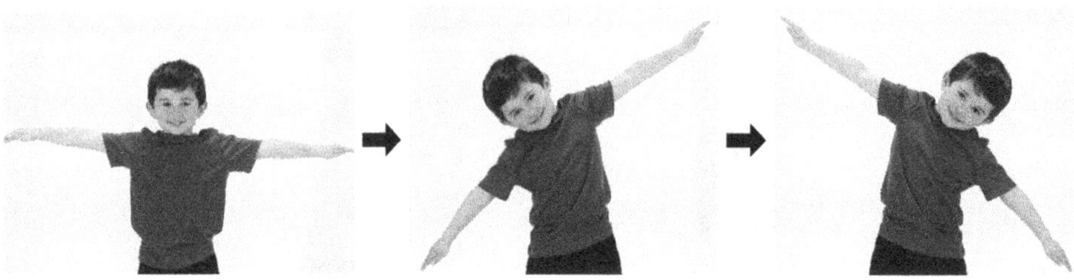

Guideline #1: SAFE	*[From Seated Star]* 1. Let's pretend to fly like an airplane. 2. Press your feet down to feel the support of the ground below you. 3. Lift your arms straight out to your sides (left-hand photo above).
Guideline #2: CALM	4. As you breathe in, bend to one side to turn your Airplane (center photo above). 5. As you breathe out, bend your body to the other side to turn your Airplane the other way (right-hand photo above). 6. Keep flying your Airplane from side to side with your breath. 7. Breathe in as you turn your Airplane one way. 8. Then breathe out as you turn it the other way. *[Repeat 3–4 times to each side.]*
Guideline #3: CLEAR	9. How does it feel to move like an airplane?... Does it feel different flying one way or the other? *Or:* How does it feel to stretch your body from side to side? *Or:* Notice if rooting your feet into the ground helps you feel more stable as you change position from side to side...
Guideline #4: UPLIFTED	10. In the same way, when we ground ourselves, it can help us handle changes in our lives more easily.
Finishing step	11. As you're ready, lower your arms and rest in Seated Mountain. See if you notice any different feelings or sensations in your body.
Guideline #5: EMPOWERED	**In life, things change, and it's important to learn how to be flexible and move with the changes. Just as your body moves more easily when it is well grounded, your mind can more easily "go with the flow" when it is grounded and stable.**

BREATH		PROP	VEST	BAL

Seated Warrior 1

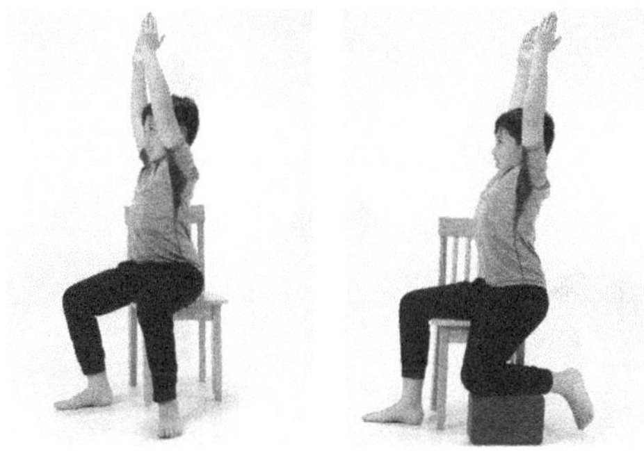

[Make sure the student is sitting on a well-fitted chair.]

1. Sit on the corner of your chair, with your [red] right leg facing the right side of your chair and your left leg facing the front of your chair (left-hand photo above).
2. Place your feet flat on the floor.

   [Check that hips and knees are at 90-degree angles.]
3. Separate your legs only to what is comfortable for you [the angle can be less than 90 degrees].

   Or: If you like, sit facing the [red] right side of your chair and rest your left shin on a yoga block placed on the floor at a height that is comfortable to you (right-hand photo above).

   [Demonstrate both positions.]

Guideline #1: SAFE	4. Press your feet [and/or leg] down, and feel the ground below you. 5. Press your sitting bones/bottom into the seat of the chair.			
Guideline #3: CLEAR	6. Put your hands on your hips and turn them to face toward the [red] right side of the chair. *Do not over-twist.* 7. As you breathe in, reach your arms to the sky. 8. As you breathe out, hold this reach, nice and strong. 9. Feel the strength from the earth/ground moving through your whole body, from your feet and legs all the way to your fingertips. *[If you want, go to Dynamic Warrior 1 from here.]*			
Guideline #4: UPLIFTED	10. *[If staying in Seated Warrior 1]* Warrior 1 brings out different feelings in different people...you may feel grounded...or strong...or balanced...confident... How does Warrior 1 make *you* feel? *Or:* As you reach your arms to the sky, welcome good things to come your way... Open arms...open mind... *[Repeat the steps on the other side.]*			
Finishing step	11. As you are ready, lower your arms and come back to Seated Mountain.			
Guideline #5: EMPOWERED	**We learn to be true to ourselves and more empowered when we listen to our body's messages, and nurture the positive messages.**			
		PROP		**BAL**

Dynamic Seated Warrior 1

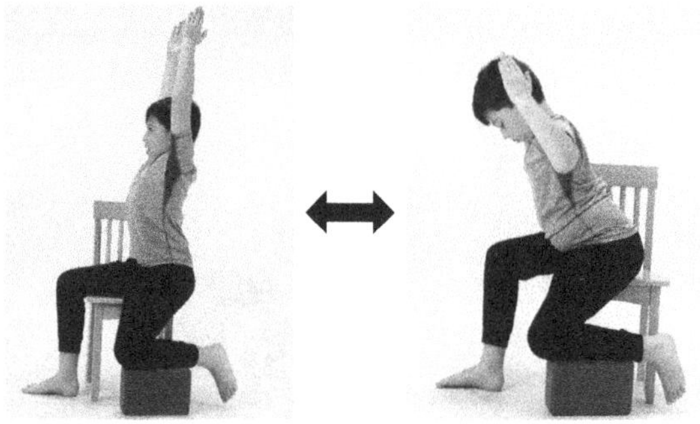

[Caution: Only do the dynamic version IF the lower leg is positioned on a yoga block placed on the floor OR substitute with Setting Sun.]

Guideline #1: SAFE	*[Grounding cues are incorporated into Seated Mountain.]*
Guideline #2: CALM	*[From Seated Warrior 1]* 1. Breathe in, sit straight up, and reach your arms to the sky (left-hand photo above). 2. Breathe out, and bend forward with bent elbows, pulling your arms back (right-hand photo above). 3. Continue to move like this with your breath.
Guideline #3: CLEAR	4. How does it feel to move with your breath like this?
Transitioning to hold	5. The next time you straighten and reach your arms up to the sky, stay here and continue to breathe in and out.
Guideline #4: UPLIFTED	6. Warrior 1 brings out different feelings in different people...you may feel grounded...or strong...or balanced...confident... How does Warrior 1 make *you* feel? *Or:* As you reach your arms to the sky, welcome good things to come your way... Open arms...open mind... *[Repeat the steps on the other side.]*
Finishing step	7. As you are ready, lower your arms and come back to Seated Mountain.
Guideline #5: EMPOWERED	**We learn to be true to ourselves and more empowered when we listen to the messages coming from our own body, and nurture the positive messages.**

BREATH	TAC	PROP	VEST	BAL

Seated Warrior 2

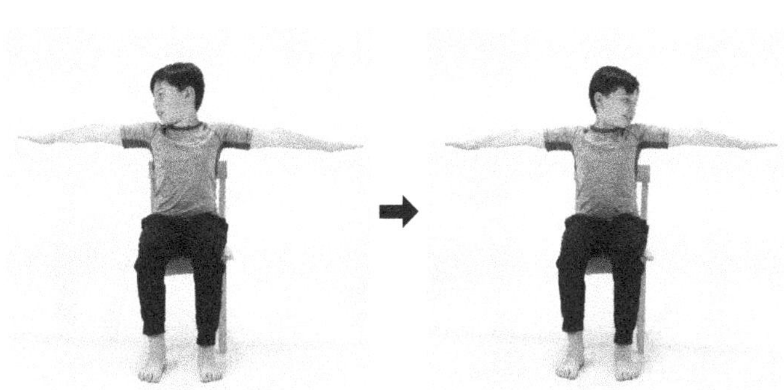

Guideline #1: SAFE	*[From Seated Mountain]* 1. If you like, step your feet wider apart, to a comfortable spot. 2. Push your feet down to root them into the ground. 3. Feel the earth/ground through your strong legs supporting you as a Warrior.			
Guideline #2: CALM	4. Reach the top of your head up to the sky. 5. The next time you breathe in, raise your arms out to the sides, as high as your shoulders *[demonstrate]*. 6. Turn your head to look over the fingers of your [red] right hand (left-hand photo above).			
Guideline #3: CLEAR	7. Warrior 2 can increase power and strength. Is there a place in your body where you feel strong in Warrior 2? Even if only in one spot, try to send your breath to that area. Do you notice any changes in how you feel?			
Guideline #4: UPLIFTED	8. The more we can sense our own strength and power, the easier it is to move past challenges in our lives. 9. *[For "witness" mentality]* If you start to feel strong muscle sensations, just notice them with a sense of curiosity. But if the feeling gets too uncomfortable, please come out of Warrior 2 to rest. *[Repeat steps on the other side (right-hand photo above).]*			
Finishing step	10. As you are ready, lower your arms and come back to Seated Mountain.			
Guideline #5: EMPOWERED	**We develop strength in our bodies when we learn to accept stronger muscle sensations. In the same way, we can learn to accept harder situations without letting our minds get caught up in our strong feelings about them.**			
	TAC	**PROP**		**BAL**

Seated Windmill (from Warrior 2)

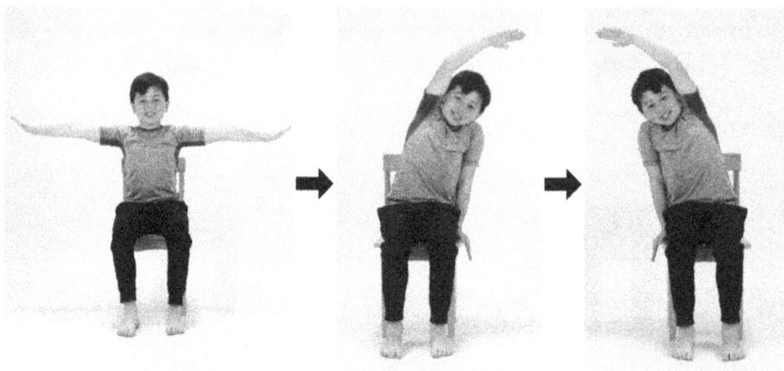

Guideline #1: SAFE	*(From Star)* 1. Now if you like, you can try Windmill with me. Your arms will be the blades of the windmill (left-hand photo above). 2. As you are ready, root your feet into the ground.
Guideline #2: CALM	3. As you breathe in, bend your body to the left, holding the chair with your left hand as you lift your [red] right arm up and over close to your ear (center photo above). 4. As you breathe out with a "whoosh," bend to the right, hold your chair with your [red] right hand as you lift your left arm up and over close to your ear (right-hand photo above). 5. Keep moving like a windmill. 6. Breathe in to the left, hold the chair, and reach your [red] right arm overhead. 7. Breathe out to the right, hold the chair, and reach your other arm overhead. *[Complete three sets to each side.]*
Guideline #4: UPLIFTED	8. Notice if pressing your feet into the ground helps you feel more stable when moving from side to side. In the same way, when we ground ourselves, it can help us feel more stable and able to handle changes in our lives.
Finishing step	9. As you are ready, lower your arms and come back to Seated Mountain.
Guideline #5: EMPOWERED	**In life, things change and it's important to learn how to be flexible and move with the changes. Just as your body moves more easily when it is well grounded, your mind can more easily "go with the flow" when it is grounded and stable.**

BREATH	TAC	PROP	VEST	BAL

Seated Waterfall

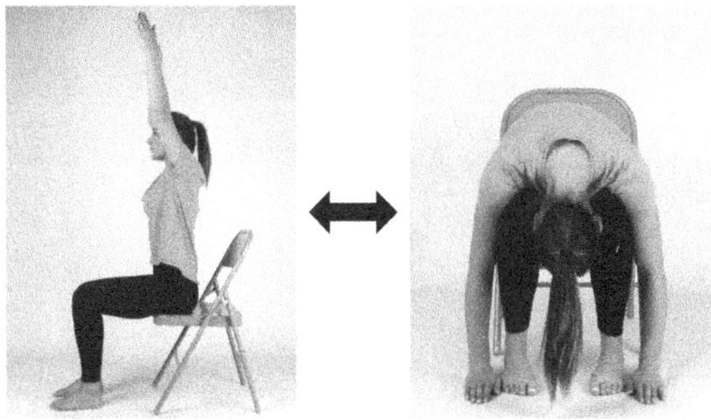

[From Seated Mountain with or without a yoga band]

1. Please decide if you want to use a yoga band or not.
   - *With yoga band:* fold the band in half and hold with both hands a bit wider than your shoulders.
   - *Without yoga band:* sit with your arms at your sides in Seated Mountain.

Guideline #1: SAFE	*[Grounding cues are incorporated into Seated Mountain.]*
Guideline #3: CLEAR	2. If you have a band, stretch it tight by pulling your arms apart.
Guideline #2: CALM	3. As you breathe in, reach your arms up high to the sky (left-hand photo above). 4. As you breathe out, flow your arms and body down like a Waterfall toward the ground, like this *[demonstrate]*. 5. Bend as far as is comfortable for you (right-hand photo above). 6. Breathe in, push off your legs, and reach your arms to the sky. *[Pushing off the legs helps to protect the back.]* 7. Stretch the band tight. 8. Breathe out, and flow like a Waterfall to the ground.
Guideline #4: UPLIFTED	9. Breathe in happy thoughts as you reach up to the sky... 10. Then breathe out your worries as you flow like a Waterfall to the ground. *[Repeat 3–5 times based on the student's comfort level.]*
Finishing steps	11. The next time your Waterfall flows down to the ground, stay here and let your body rest. Let all your worries roll off your back, like they are flowing down the Waterfall. 12. As you're ready, put your hands on your upper legs and slowly push yourself back up to Seated Mountain.
Guideline #5: EMPOWERED	**Bring in light and let go of worries.**

BREATH		**PROP**	**VEST**	**BAL**

Seated Tree

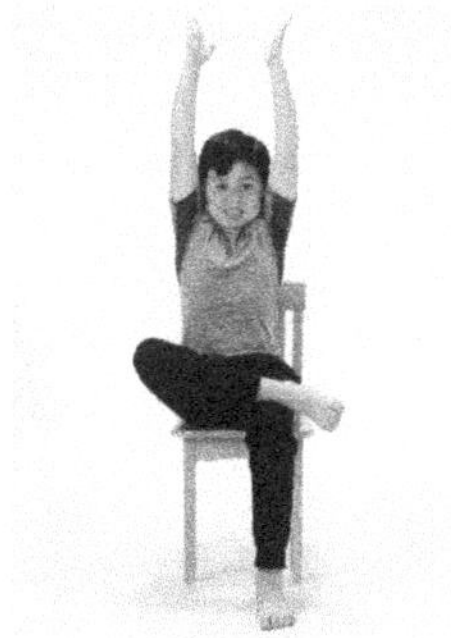

1. If you would like/as you're ready, meet me in Seated Mountain with your hands resting on your legs. *[Cue Seated Mountain.]*
2. Rest your [red] right ankle on your left leg/lower thigh *or* cross your [red] right thigh over your left thigh.
3. Press your hands together in front of your chest.

Guideline #1: SAFE	4. Press your left foot down to root your tree into the ground. 5. Press your sitting bones/bottom into the seat of the chair. 6. Reach your head up to the sky to grow your tree tall.		
Guideline #3: CLEAR	7. How do you feel here? Do you feel balanced and stable? 8. You can stay here or slowly raise your arms up to the sky [hands facing each other], to grow the branches of your tree.		
Guideline #2: CALM	9. As you breathe in, imagine breathing in fresh air to help your tree grow. 10. Then breathe out your worries in the wind.		
Guideline #4: UPLIFTED	11. If you want, you can sway your body from one side to the other side, to let your tree blow in the wind. 12. How does it feel when your tree sways off-balance, and then comes back to center to find balance? 13. Just like in life...you need to first feel off-balance to learn what it means to be balanced.		
Finishing steps	14. Slowly lower your arms and place your right foot back on the floor. 15. Repeat on the other side.		
Guideline #5: EMPOWERED	**It is an important life lesson to be aware of when you are off-balance, in order to make changes to find balance in the body and mind.**		

		PROP		**BAL**

Seated Cat to Cobra)

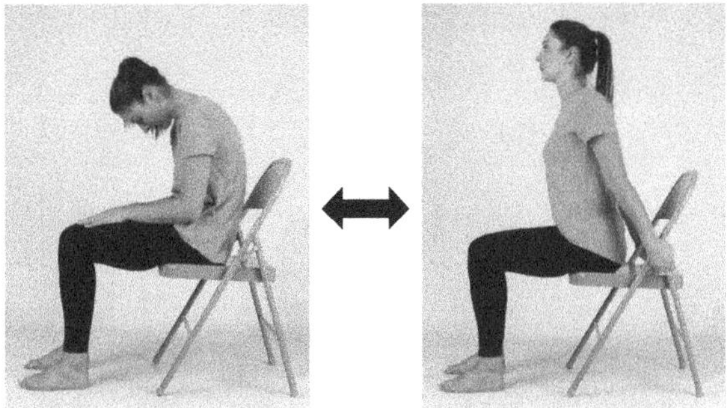

Guideline #1: SAFE	1. As/when you're ready...meet me in Seated Mountain with your hands resting on your legs. *[Cue Seated Mountain.]*
Guideline #2: CALM	2. Let's pretend to be Cobra snakes. 3. Breathe in here...then breathe out with a "hisssssss" as you round your back and drop your head (left-hand photo above). 4. As you breathe in, lift your chest and head, and reach back to hold the chair *[demonstrate holding the back of the chair]* (right-hand photo above). 5. Breathe out with a "hisssssss," round your back, and drop your head. 6. Breathe in, lift your chest and head, and hold the chair. *[Repeat the last two steps two more times.]* 7. Try moving this way with your own breath.
Guideline #3: CLEAR	8. How does it feel to move your body with your breath? *Or:* How does it feel to move and breathe like a cobra?
Guideline #4: UPLIFTED	9. Listen to your body...do you want to keep moving or stop? 10. If you want to stop, rest your elbows on legs and let your head hang down. 11. It's important to listen to your body as it lets you know *what* you are feeling and how to *control* your feelings.
Finishing step	12. As you're ready, put your hands on your upper legs and slowly push yourself back up to Seated Mountain.
Guideline #5: EMPOWERED	**By listening to our body, we can more easily control how we feel.**

BREATH	**TAC**	**PROP**	**VEST**	

Seated Crocodile

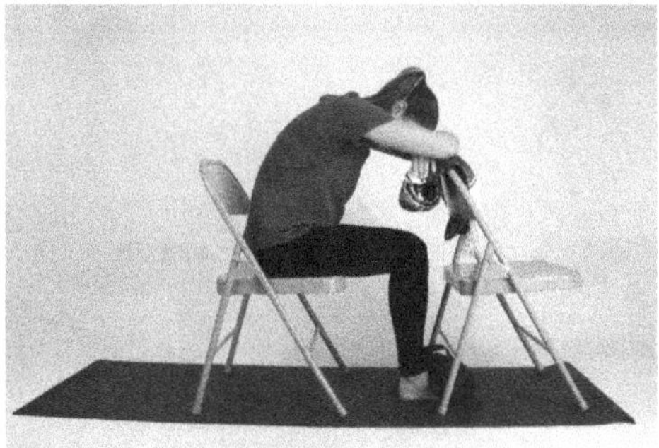

Guideline #1: SAFE	1. Sit at a table/desk *or* place a second chair in front of you. 2. Rest your arms on the table/desk or on the back of a chair. 3. Make a pillow with your arms like this: • First, fold your arms on top of each other and hold near the elbows, like this *[demonstrate]*. • Place your arms on the back of the chair, on top of the blanket. • Then rest your forehead on your arms. 4. As you rest here, notice where your legs, feet, and arms touch the floor or a chair. 5. Feel your body's connection to the ground.
Guideline #2: CALM	6. Take nice slow easy breaths in...and out...in...and out...
Guideline #4: UPLIFTED	7. Notice any calming feelings as you connect with the earth/ground and your own breath.
Finishing step	8. As you're ready, slowly push yourself back up to Seated Mountain. See if you notice any different feelings or sensations in your body.
Guideline #5: EMPOWERED	**As we learn to connect with the earth/ground and our breath, it helps us to feel more safe and calm.**

BREATH	**TAC**	**PROP**		

References for Part 3

CHAPTER 12

Brain Balance (2021) "Normal Attention Spans By Age." www.brainbalancecenters.com/blog/normal-attention-span-expectations-by-age

Levine, P.A. (1997) *Waking the Tiger: Healing Trauma*. Berkeley, CA: North Atlantic Books.

Paul, J.A., Baker, H.M., and Cochran, J.D. (2012) "Effect of online social networking on student academic performance." *Computers in Human Behavior 28*, 6, 2117–2127. www.sciencedirect.com/science/article/pii/S0747563212001665

Figure attributions

Figures 12.2, 12.3, and 12.4, breathing in: by Government of Aragón, Creative Commons BY NC SA 4.0, https://globalsymbols.com/symbolsets/arasaac/symbols/23055?locale=en

Figures 12.2, 12.3, and 12.4, breathing out: by Mada, Creative Commons BY SA 4.0, https://globalsymbols.com/symbolsets/tawasol/symbols/8100?locale=en

CHAPTER 13

Rothschild, B. (2009) "Safe trauma recovery [Video]. www.youtube.com/watch?v=LhuzpUlaX_k [Also available at www.somatictraumatherapy.com/videos]

Figure attributions

Figure 13.1, breathing in: by Government of Aragón, Creative Commons BY NC SA 4.0, https://globalsymbols.com/symbolsets/arasaac/symbols/23055?locale=en

Figure 13.1, breathing out: by Mada, Creative Commons BY SA 4.0, https://globalsymbols.com/symbolsets/tawasol/symbols/8100?locale=en

CHAPTER 14

Allington, R. (1976) "Color as an Attentional Cue in Discrimination Learning." State University of New York at Albany. Doctoral Thesis.

Goothy, S.S.K., Padmanabha, B.V., Goothy, S., and Mukkadan, J.K. (2019) "Effect of selected vestibular exercises on depression, anxiety and stress in elderly women with type 2 diabetes." *International Journal of Biochemistry and Physiology 4*, 4, 000169.

Townsend, C. and Rheingold, A.A. (2013) *Estimating a Child Sexual Abuse Prevalence Rate for Practitioners: A Review of Child Abuse Prevalence Studies*. Charleston, SC: Darkness to Light. www.d2l.org/wp-content/uploads/2017/02/PREVALENCE-RATE-WHITE-PAPER-D2L.pdf

Subject Index

Author Index